SMITH AUDIO RELAXATION INSTRUCTION SERIES (SARIS)

A seven-CD series containing recorded instructions of all the major exercises in this book.

SMITH RELAXATION INVENTORY SERIES

Includes reproducable user templates for the entire Smith Relaxation Inventory Series

DISC 1: Yogaform Stretching
Full Yogaform Stretching (29 minutes)
Brief Yogaform Stretching (20 minutes)

DISC 2: Progressive Muscle Relaxation
Full Progressive Muscle Relaxation (26 minutes)
Brief Progressive Muscle Relaxation (19 minutes)
Letting Go (11 minutes)

DISC 3: Autogenic Training
Verbal Suggestions (16 minutes)
Visual Suggestions (16 minutes)

DISC 4: Breathing Exercises
Breathing Stretches (12 minutes)
Diaphragmatic Breathing (5 minutes)
Passive Breathing (10 minutes)

DISC 5: Imagery
Sense Imagery (30 minutes)
Insight Imagery (23 minutes)

DISC 6: Meditation and Mindfulness
Eight Meditations (28 minutes)
Graduated Mindfulness (24 minutes)
Mindful Walking (15 minutes)

DISC 7: Relaxation Sampler (30 minutes)

Presenter: Jonathan C. Smith, PhD

For purchasing information, contact: stressinstitute@aol.com

A self-help book on relaxation and stress management, *The Stress Management Companion*, is available at www.lulu.com/stress

---

We invite you to explore the Roosevelt University Stress Institute Web site: www.roosevelt.edu/stress

This site contains useful information about the Stress Institute's Certificates in Relaxation and Stress Management. The Web site also contains a free demonstration of relaxation training from DISC 7: Relaxation Sampler: www.roosevelt.edu/stress/sampler.htm

Jonathan C. Smith, PhD, is a Licensed Clinical Psychologist, a Professor of Psychology at Chicago's Roosevelt University, and is founding Director of the Roosevelt University Stress Institute. He has taught stress management and multiple relaxation and meditative techniques to thousands of individuals for over 30 years. Dr. Smith is author of 14 books and over 3 dozen articles.

Relaxation, Meditation, &Mindfulness

Jonathan C. Smith, PhD

 Springer Publishing Company

Springer Publishing Company, Inc.
11 W. 42nd Street, 15th Floor
New York, NY 10036-8002

Acquisitions Editor: Sheri W. Sussman
Production Editor: Pamela Lankas
Cover design by Joanne Honigman

05 06 07 08 09 / 5 4 3 2 1

Smith, Jonathan C.
   Relaxation, meditation, and mindfulness : a mental health practitioner's guide to new and traditional approaches / Jonathan C. Smith
       p. cm.
   Includes bibliographical references and index.
   ISBN 0-8261-2745-2
   1. Relaxation. 2. Meditation. 3. Attention. I. Title.
BF637.R45S62 2005
613.7'92—dc22   2005001030

Printed in the United States of America by Maple-Vail Book Manufacturing Group.

To: Clyde

Contents

List of Tables and Figures   *ix*

PART I: Basic Concepts

1   Introduction   3
2   Six Families of Techniques: An Historical Overview   7
3   The Relaxation Engine   19
4   The Six Access Skills of Relaxation   29
5   The Paths and Landscapes of Relaxation   45
6   The Destinations of Relaxation: 59
    Ten Great Goals
7   Summary of ABC_2 Relaxation Theory: Psychological   71
    Relaxation Theory

PART II: The Relaxation Instruction Manual

8   General Instructions for All Approaches to Relaxation   77
9   Yogaform Stretching   79
10   Progressive Muscle Relaxation   93
11   Breathing Exercises   113
12   Autogenic Training   131
13   Imagery and Relaxing Self-Talk   147
14   Meditation and Mindfulness   161

PART III: Training Issues

15   Overview of Relaxation Training Formats   179
16   Orientation   187
17   Assessment Tools   201
18   Troubleshooting and Enhancing Relaxation   219

PART IV: Combination Training Formats

19   Scripting   235
20   Abbreviated Programs   271
21   Workshops and Group Relaxation   283

PART V: Special Applications

22   Relaxation for Children   293
23   Relaxation and Pain Management   315
24   Spirituality, Religion, and Relaxation   331

Appendix   *347*
References   *357*
Index   *361*

List of Tables and Figures

TABLES

4.1	Self-Stressing, Relaxation Access Skills, and Relaxation Families	44
9.1	Yogaform Stretching Instruction Scripts	85
10.1	List of "Let-Go" Phrases	102
10.2	Progressive Muscle Relaxation Scripts	105
11.1	Breathing Exercise Scripts	120
12.1	Autogenic Training Scripts	137
13.1	Menu of Sense Imagery Themes	151
13.2	Imagery Scripts	154
14.1	Meditation and Mindfulness Scripts	170
16.1	Relaxation Precautions Fact Sheet	189
16.2	Brief Introduction to Stress and Relaxation	190
16.3	Self-Stressing and the Six Families of Relaxation	191
17.1	Target Symptom Fact Sheet	202
17.2	Behavioral Signs of Relaxation Rating Scale	203
17.3	Smith Relaxation Preferences Inventory (SRPI)	206
17.4	Smith Relaxation Goals Inventory (SRGI)	207
17.5	Smith Relaxation States Inventory Revised (SRSIr)	208
17.6	Smith Relaxation States Inventory Revised (SRSIr) Scoring Key	209
17.7	Smith Relaxation States Inventory Brief Version (SRSIbv)	210
17.8	Smith Relaxation States Inventory Brief Version (SRSIbv): Summary Sheet	211
17.9	Smith Relaxation States Inventory—Alternative Brief Version (SRSIabv)	214
17.10	Smith Relaxation States Inventory Alternative Brief Version (SRSIabv) Summary Sheet	215
19.1	Scripting Schedule	238

19.2	Scripting Schedule for Clients	239
19.3	Suggestions for Combining and Sequencing Exercises	252
19.4	Scripting Workbook	260

FIGURES

3.1	The nervous system.	21
5.1	R-State pyramid.	48
6.1	The 10 great goals of relaxation.	60
17.1	Simplified R-State Pyramid map.	218
21.1	Example of blackboard summary of group-generated imagery themes and sense details.	288

NOTE

Part I

Basic Concepts

1

Introduction

Everyone is a relaxation expert. Some may take walks, others listen to songs on the radio, still others sip tea, and so on. But there are times when such casual relaxation is not enough.

For example, take Gil, who has suffered from a weight problem for over a decade. Every time he goes on a diet, he fails. The pattern is the same. When Gil faces a serious problem, such as an unpaid bill or a dispute with the family, he walks the dog. Then he starts eating to "soothe my nerves." For Gil, walking the dog is not enough to reduce stress and calm the craving.

Or consider Ernie, a student of vocal music at a Midwestern university. He is paralyzed by performance anxiety. Whenever Ernie has to sing, he "freezes" and forgets his lines. Ernie needs more than Mozart; he needs the skill of deep relaxation.

And then there's Lois, a young waitress at a famous vegetarian restaurant. Lois works very long hours and runs out of energy by 5 p.m. But she has to work until midnight. Lois needs more energy and a cup of tea won't do it.

Fortunately, over a half century of solid scientific research, with studies numbering in the thousands, informs us of a set of tools that go beyond casual, everyday relaxation. These are the techniques and strategies of *professional deep relaxation*. When practiced well, professional deep relaxation can be journeying vehicle, with a remarkable engine of body and brain processes that can move us through wonderful psychological paths and landscapes to some very important life destinations—including reducing stress, enhancing resistance to disease, speeding recovery from illness, increasing energy and stamina, and even cultivating insight, creativity, and spirituality.

THE SIX FAMILIES OF PROFESSIONAL
DEEP RELAXATION

There are many techniques and strategies to try. Some, like yoga and deep breathing, may sound familiar; others may have exotic or imposing scientific names. How does one cope with so many options? Traditionally, there have been two approaches. One is to focus on a single technique and consider it in great detail. It is quite possible to devote decades to the study of several thousand yoga exercises and just scratch the surface. The other approach is to present very superficial samples of all techniques. In this volume I will present the major families of relaxation, and for each I will devote just enough detail for the serious instructor and practitioner. We will not, however, consider exercises that have dubious validity, pose some risk (advanced yoga), or require substantial professional supervision (hypnosis, biofeedback).Our first step is to organize these techniques into six families of professional deep relaxation, which will form the core of this book.

The first three families are primarily physical:

- **Yoga stretching** involves slowly, smoothly, and gently stretching out tension in the muscles and joints.
- **Progressive muscle relaxation** involves reducing tension by tensing up (or squeezing) a muscle, and then going limp.
- **Breathing exercises** involve learning to inhale and breathe out tension in a deeply relaxing way.

The last three families are primarily mental:

- **Autogenic suggestion** involves thinking powerfully suggestive relaxing phrases, such as "Imagine you are sitting in a warm and wonderfully relaxing pool. You feel warm and heavy."
- **Imagery and relaxing self-talk** incorporate a type of daydream or fantasy of a relaxing setting or activity, or the repetition of relaxing words and affirmations.
- **Meditation** involves easily sustaining focus on a very simple stimulus. For **concentrative meditation** the simple stimulus is just one thing, such as a waterfall or candle, whereas **mindfulness** involves quietly observing the flow of all simple stimuli, without thought or worry, much as one might watch clouds float by on a lazy day.

What are the effects of these approaches? How do they go beyond casual, everyday activities? For over a decade, a number of us at the Roosevelt University Stress Institute in Chicago have been studying the promise of relaxation (Smith, 1999a, 1999b, 2001). We cast a wide net and looked at the six families just described as well as dozens of other activities such as massage, hot tubs, pleasure reading, going to church, walking the dog, listening to Mozart, and even sipping tea. Our project involved thousands of relaxers and produced nearly fifty articles. Put simply, we found that not only can relaxation go beyond stress management, but that different families of relaxation have different effects. The fruits of this research form the basis of this book.

This volume takes us on a journey into the worlds of relaxation. We begin in Part I with an historical overview of six families of relaxation most used by health professionals and continue with the question of how relaxation works. I offer a comprehensive psychological theory of relaxation that explains why there are six families of techniques, and what their different psychological effects may be. Part II offers concrete and practical instructions for all families of techniques and Parts III and IV continue with advanced training issues. We conclude in Part V with three applications: relaxation with children; relaxation and pain management; and relaxation, spirituality, and religion.

Let me emphasize that this book does not review relaxation research; beginning scholars might consider Lichtstein (1988), Smith (1990, 1999a, 2001), or any of the excellent volumes of Lehrer, Woolfolk, and their colleagues (e.g., Lehrer & Woolfolk, 1993).

Finally, all relaxation instructional texts are based on personal opinion, theoretical insight, clinical experience, and a modest dose of relaxation research. *Relaxation, Meditation, and Mindfulness* continues in this tradition. Except where indicated, my training suggestions are hypotheses founded primarily on personal experience.

2

Six Families of Techniques: An Historical Overview

This book considers six families of relaxation techniques. We begin with a brief historical overview of the approaches used most by health professionals.

PROGRESSIVE MUSCLE RELAXATION

Progressive muscle relaxation (PMR) is perhaps the most widely used professional approach to relaxation in America. For years it has dominated textbooks and relaxation research and, even now, we see the term "progressive relaxation" used interchangeably (and incorrectly) with "relaxation."

Physiologist and physician Edmund Jacobson began work on relaxation as a doctoral student at Harvard in 1907, prompted in part by his desire to cure his own insomnia (Jacobson, 1938). After graduating, Jacobson developed a private practice, often making use of relaxation procedures. At first he used reductions in the knee-jerk reflex as a sign of relaxation and a tool for refining relaxation techniques. Later he enlisted the aid of scientists at Bell Telephone Laboratories and invented the integrated neurovoltmeter, essentially a biofeedback device capable of measuring tension-related action potentials from muscle groups and nerves. Such a tool fit well Jacobson's hypothesis that all stressful worry had neuromuscular manifestations, and that reducing these manifestations would in turn reduce stressful worry.

Jacobson's Minimal PMR

Jacobson's (1929) approach (which I term "minimal PMR") involved training subjects to detect and recognize increasingly subtle levels of muscle tension and remain relaxed throughout the day. In each session a client would focus on a body part, for example, the hand, generate the smallest amount of tension, and let go. Jacobson felt it was very important to avoid suggestive patter, fearing it might introduce what he felt were the confounding effects of hypnotic suggestion (ironically, some hypnosis scholars consider Jacobson's approach to be a form of hypnosis; Edmonston, 1986). Clients would be taught to relax two or three muscle groups per 60-minute session, eventually covering 50 groups for the entire body. Training required 50 or more sessions that could last from 3 to 6 months to a year.

Illustration of Minimal Progressive Muscle Relaxation

Quietly attend to your right hand. When your mind wanders, simply return. Gently begin to tense up the muscles in your right hand, very, very slowly. The moment you notice the slightest increase in tension, let go. Relax.

Overt PMR

Jacobson's minimal method was cumbersome and not widely used. In 1958 Joseph Wolpe introduced the first abbreviated version of progressive relaxation. Earlier Wolpe had found that a conditioned fear reaction in cats could be eliminated by evoking a response incompatible with fear concurrently with a feared stimulus. Progressive relaxation could work as such a "reciprocal inhibitor" and became a part of Wolpe's well-known desensitization treatments.

The abbreviated approach of Wolpe and others involves overtly creating a considerable level of relaxation starting in the first session. One consciously "tenses up" for about 5–10 seconds and then "lets go," attending to the release of tension for 30 seconds or so. Often up to 16 muscle groups, rather than one to three, are separately targeted in each session. As training progresses, muscle groups are combined until eventually one can simply detect and relax tension without first overtly creating tension.

The version of PMR taught in this text is similar to overt PMR. Eleven muscle groups are targeted. One vigorously tenses and then releases tension. However, unlike traditional overt PMR, the version in this text attempts to present relatively "pure" exercises that involve only tensing up and letting go. Occasional stretching, breathing, and imagery components have been eliminated so that practitioners can readily identify the effects of tensing and letting go, independently of other relaxation strategies.

Covert PMR

Covert PMR involves letting go of muscle tension without first tensing up. Often it is presented as an advanced lesson, after weeks of training in overt PMR. Occasionally, covert PMR is introduced alone, without prior practice in overt PMR, and is often combined with autogenic training. One focuses on letting go.

In the most abbreviated format, termed "conditioned relaxation" (Paul, 1966) and "cue-controlled relaxation" (Russell & Matthews, 1975), one simply thinks a relaxing cue word, such as "relaxed" or "calm," immediately after practicing progressive relaxation. In time, thinking the cue itself is sufficient to evoke relaxation.

Illustration of Overt Progressive Muscle Relaxation

Quietly attend to your right hand. Tense up the muscles in your right hand now. Keep the rest of your body relaxed. Notice the tension grow in your right hand. Then let go. Let the tension flow away. Notice the sensations of relaxation. Can you tell the difference between how your hand feels now and how it felt when you were tensing it?

Illustration of Covert Progressive Muscle Relaxation

Quietly attend to your right hand. Let go of any feelings of tension you may feel. There is nothing you have to do but let the tension flow and dissolve away.

AUTOGENIC TRAINING

Autogenic training is a popular European approach to relaxation, one that has had modest impact in North America (Schultz & Luthe, 1969). Its roots can be traced to authoritarian hypnosis of nearly a century ago. At the beginning of the 20th century, Berlin neurophysiologist Oskar Vogt developed a nonauthoritarian and directive approach to hypnosis that involved gently hinting at what he wanted a patient to do or perceive. His wish was not to disturb the patient's freedom of will. In addition, Vogt introduced a step-by-step approach, the "fraction method," in which a patient would be hypnotized for a few minutes, and then wakened. The effects of each brief hypnosis would be ascertained and used to adjust subsequent suggestions. Finally, Vogt made the important observation that patients could induce their own hypnotic-like states (Schultz & Luthe, 1969) and that these states, when evoked a few times a day, appeared to have relaxing, therapeutic value.

Around the same time dermatologist Johannes Schultz shifted to neurology and psychiatry and began practicing hypnosis. Schultz made use of the notion that thinking of physical sensations related to relaxation can often evoke relaxation. Importantly, he was convinced that hypnosis was not something imposed upon a patient by a domineering hypnotist, but an inner ability that patients permitted to unfold.

In the 1920s and 1930s, Schultz (1932) introduced autogenic training, a relaxation therapy based on a somewhat overstated notion of "self-generated" (autogenic) healing. Central to this idea is that the brain has powerful self-healing potential, which can be activated in part through what Benson (1975) later termed "the relaxation response" (see chapter 3). During the course of his career, Schultz published more than 400 articles and several books. His system became widely known in Europe and was introduced in the Western hemisphere by Wolfgang Luthe (1965).

Standard and Organ-Specific Exercises

Traditional autogenic training is a highly structured sequential program (Linden, 1990; Luthe, 1969–1973). It begins with six "standard exercises" that involve mentally repeating verbal formulae or suggestive phrases targeted to the following somatic sensations:

- Heaviness
- Warmth

- Cardiac regulation (slowly, evenly beating heart)
- Respiration (relaxed breathing)
- Abdominal warmth
- Cooling of the forehead

This book focuses on warmth, heaviness, cardiac regulation, and abdominal warming because of their similar physiological effect; respiration and forehead cooling are not presented because they overlap with separately presented breathing and meditation exercises.

Autogenic training places considerable emphasis on "passive volition," that is, repeating formulae passively, while maintaining complete indifference about the result. A beginning client might be instructed to let the phrase "hands are warm . . . hands are warm" to repeat in his or her mind, quietly attending to the repeating words much as one might attend to the slow repetition of an echo. After mastering beginning warmth and heaviness exercises, a client progresses to phrases targeted to the heart ("heartbeat strong and even"), respiration ("it breathes me"), abdominal warmth ("warmth radiates from my stomach"), and forehead ("forehead cool and calm").

Many traditional relaxation techniques have elements that resemble autogenic suggestion. One type of Zen meditation involves focusing on abdominal warmth. Kundalini yoga involves meditating on chakras or presumed "energy centers," which loosely correspond to autogenic standard exercises. Some forms of Christian prayer involve attending to feelings of loving warmth radiating from the heart.

Illustration of Autogenic Standard Exercise

Gently let these words float through your mind: "Hand and arms, warm and heavy. Hand and arms, warm and heavy." There is no need to deliberately try to conjure up these feelings. Just let the words float through your mind.

Once the standard exercises are mastered, a variety of special exercises may be introduced. "Organ-specific formulas" tailor the standard exercises to the particular needs of the patient. For example, a backache patient may use the phrase "My back is warm," a headache patient, "My forehead is cool," and so on. "Intentional formulas" are phrases targeted to behavioral change objectives ("I will study more, drink less.").

Autogenic "Meditation"

Traditional autogenic training teaches a series of seven "meditative" (or more accurately, "imagery") exercises after the standard exercises have been mastered. One begins with an imagery preparation exercise that involves attending to vague retinal sensations that spontaneously occur with eyes closed in relaxation. Such sensations might include faint and formless clouds of light, spots, and so on. Once a trainee can sustain attention on such phenomena, he or she graduates to increasingly challenging images, including colors, then simple shapes (square, circle) and concrete objects (chairs, vases) until they can be produced and modulated on demand. The most advanced images include abstract constructs (truth, justice, friendship), emotional states, and other people. Eventually, exercises are directed toward seeking "answers from the unconscious," i.e., asking questions ("What is the source of my frustration") and passively waiting for a spontaneous answer to emerge in the form of a change in image (an answer spontaneously appearing on an imagined blackboard, TV screen).

Today, autogenic training more or less in full form is popular in Europe and Canada, whereas highly abbreviated forms (usually targeting "warmth and heaviness") prevail in the United States. In addition, abbreviated and somewhat controversial variations have emerged with highly specific suggestions targeted, for example, to individual cancer tumors, the immune system, and so on (Simonton, Matthews-Simonton, & Creighton, 1978).

BREATHING AND YOGA STRETCHING

The histories of breathing and yoga stretching (as well as meditation) are intertwined. We begin with two oriental religions, Hinduism and Buddhism. Hinduism, one of the ancient religions of India, has incorporated a diverse assortment of yoga stretching, breathing, and meditation exercises for thousands of years. In the second century B.C., such exercises were codified in the yoga aphorisms of Patanjali (Eliade, 1969; Prabhavananda, 1963). Patanjali emphasized an eight-step path for cultivating of a meditative state of mind conducive to spiritual insight. The steps included various initial ascetic practices, yoga postures and stretches, breathing relaxation exercises, and finally meditation. The easiest of meditative practices, often called concentrative meditation, involved withdrawing the senses from troubling and distracting influence of external stimuli, memories, and so on, and concentrating on a single point.

Through the centuries, numerous variations of Hindu thinking appeared, some emphasizing devotion to a theistic God and others an impersonal nontheistic absolute (the "flow of energy everywhere," "consciousness and being"). This latter position, associated with the eighth century Indian philosopher, Shankara, was eventually to form the basis of most Western forms of Hinduism, yoga, and meditation, including transcendental meditation.

Many Yogas

Yoga is primarily associated with exercises involving stretching and maintaining various postures. However, there is no single yoga tradition. Over the past 5,000 years, thousands of exercises and hundreds of systems have evolved. Indeed, someone who claims to "practice yoga" has said very little about what she actually does; she might as well claim to "practice fitness," "do holistic health," or "believe in moral living." Some of the specific systems include hatha yoga, prana yoga, kundlini yoga, bhakti yoga, raja yoga, kriya yoga, and tantra yoga. Virtually every year, a new yoga system emerges.

Some preliminary distinctions can be made. Hatha yoga focuses on stretching and maintaining specific postures (such as the famous "lotus" cross-legged sitting position) and to some extent developing muscles; breathing exercises are traditionally included (Coulter, 2001). Prana yoga focuses on breathing; kundalini yoga emphasizes chakra energy centers in the body, bhakti yoga emphasizes prayer and worship, raja yoga focuses more on philosophical inquiry, kriya yoga tends to consider sources of energy, and tantra yoga is often associated with sexual energies.

It should be noted that in the West simple stretching exercises can be traced back to Olympic athletes in ancient Greece. Such exercises, although sometimes similar to hatha yoga, have primarily been used to prepare for and recover from athletic activity. Other contemporary fitness routines, ranging from the Alexander technique to Pilates, incorporate some form of stretching.

This book focuses on simple stretches and postures somewhat similar to those found in hatha yoga.

Illustration of a Yoga Stretching Exercise

Let both arms hang to each side. Slowly swing your right hand and arm up tracing a circle in the air to your side. Do this very slowly, smoothly, and gently, as if you were balancing a feather on your fingertips. Let your hand and arm easily move higher until

> it is pointing straight up into the sky. Continue attending to your hand and arm as you slowly, smoothly, and gently return it to your side.

Many Breathing Exercises

As we have noted, prana yoga focuses primarily on breathing exercises. It is an approach, over 5,000 years old, that has generated thousands of specific breathing exercises. Breathing exercises are almost always deployed as part of another technique. One popular Western approach is Lamaze, a natural childbirth method. Breathing exercises vary considerably, and include active yoga stretches, active diaphragmatic breathing, and some passive approaches. Generally, the goal of breathing exercises is to foster diaphragmatic breathing and a pace that is slow and even. One initially learns to breathe deeply, then breathing becomes effortless and shallow.

This book presents three types of breathing exercise, each increasingly passive: breathing and stretching, active diaphragmatic breathing, and passive breathing.

> **Illustration of a Breathing Exercise**
>
> Gently take a deep breath. Pause. Then slowly exhale, letting the air flow through your lips, as if you were blowing on a candle flame. Attend to the flow of breath. Notice how it quietly moves in through your nostrils, and down into your lungs. Follow the flow of breath in and out.

IMAGERY AND RELAXING SELF-TALK

Imagery involves creating in one's mind a passive, relaxing setting or activity, often accompanied by the repetition of relaxing words or self-statements. Alternatively, one might simply engage in relaxing self-talk and passively repeat relaxing phrases and affirmations.

Imagery (and to some extent relaxing self-talk) have scientific roots in both hypnosis and autogenic training, as well as antecedents in 19th century religious and self-help cults and in many Eastern and Western religious traditions. Images and phrases often form an important part of hypnotic induction and the production of hallucination is a frequently suggested hypnotic response. Advanced autogenic exercises incorporate a graduated series of simple and complex images. It should be noted that yoga and meditation traditions have their own imagery exercises, although these are rarely employed in the West. Here, focal stimuli can be as complex as circular patterned mandala artwork or as simple as a candle flame. Kundalini meditation, a form of yoga, involves attending to sensations and images associated with various internal "chakras," or somatic energy centers such as the heart ("attend to the feelings of warmth in your heart"), throat, spine, and center of the forehead.

Many forms of imagery do not have relaxation as a goal. Active and discursive imagery is often used in psychotherapeutic traditions as diverse as psychoanalysis and behavior therapy. For example, a psychodynamic therapist might instruct a client to engage in "free association." Here, a word or topic ("Your dream about a domineering old bear") is selected that is salient to a therapy session. Then the client, with eyes closed, lets thoughts and images spontaneously emerge without any censorship, modification, or selection. During this activity, he or she shares with the therapist whatever thoughts arise.

Behavior therapists might use a different type of "coping imagery." Here imagery is a mental rehearsal of confronting and coping with a stressor, including possible setbacks. A client suffering from fear of public speaking might visualize approaching a podium, taking a few deep breaths, opening lecture notes, repeating the supporting phrase "one step at a time, I can do it," beginning the speech, perhaps forgetting a point, coping by successfully checking his or her notes, resuming, and successfully completing the speech. It should be emphasized that coping imagery does not involve visualizing just the successful outcome. Although self-help books and programs often offer a strategy of visualizing success ("Imagine yourself rich . . . successful . . . in love . . . powerful . . . etc."), such imagery simply does not work.

Relaxation imagery involves creating a cognitive or mental representation of a real or hypothetical relaxing setting or activity, perhaps supplemented by relaxing self-statements. Unlike therapeutic imagery, it involves a minimum of thought, activity and effort, greater sustained focus, and some indirect intention to evoke positive states of mind. Most forms of relaxation imagery can be divided into three categories: sense, narrative, and insight imagery. This text emphasizes sense and insight imagery.

Sense imagery involves passively attending to sense stimulation without engaging in an activity. One might imagine a beach and attend to the waves, sky, sound of birds, and so on. Again, all senses are involved. Narrative imagery involves attending to a simple and somewhat plotless relaxing story, for example, walking through the woods, floating through the air, riding a horse, and so on. One attends to simple relaxing sensations (sights, sounds, feelings, smells) that arise while completing a relaxing activity. Insight imagery has as its objective evoking deeper understanding or appreciation of a topic or question.

Illustration of an Imagery Exercise (Sense Imagery)

Enjoy a fantasy about a pleasing vacation spot on the beach. Involve all of your senses. What do you see? The blue sky above? The green trees? The clear blue water? What do you hear? Perhaps the gentle rustle of trees, or the splashing of waves. What do you feel touching your skin? Perhaps the warm sun or cool breeze. And what relaxing fragrances are there? The clean scent of water? Flowers?

MEDITATION AND MINDFULNESS

Health professionals who use meditation teach either concentrative meditation (such as transcendental meditation), which involves restricting attention to a simple stimulus, or mindfulness meditation, which involves nonjudgmental attention to all stimuli.

Concentrative Meditation

Concentrative meditation is most often traced to ancient Hinduism and Tibetan Buddhism. This book presents a summary of seven types of concentrative meditation based on a schema that summarizes approaches that have emerged over the millenia (Smith, 1999a). Three involve attending to relaxing body sensations, two on mental activities, and two on external sensations:

Meditations of the Body

Body sense meditation involves focusing on the relaxing physical sensations one may have after practicing a relaxation, such as feeling "warmth," "heaviness," or a warm "abdominal glow."

Rocking meditation involves attending to the gentle movement of rocking back and forth.

Breathing meditation involves attending to the flow of breath.

Meditations of the Mind

Mantra meditation involves attending to the passive mental repetition of a syllable, word, or meaningless sound, often termed a "mantra." Transcendental meditation is one form of mantra meditation.

Visual image meditation involves selecting an utterly simple image, such as a visualized spot of light or star, and focusing attention on it.

Meditation of the Senses

Sound meditation involves selecting and attending to a simple, relatively unchanging sound (a meditation gong, a waterfall, the blowing wind, or even the gentle hum of an air conditioner).

External image meditation involves attending to a very simple and unchanging external visual stimulus, such as a candle flame.

Mindfulness Meditation

Mindfulness meditation (also called Zazen, just sitting, or Vipassana) traces its roots to Buddhism. Buddhism gave birth to Zen, one of the most popular approaches to meditation in Japan, and to some extent in the West. Around 500 B.C. Buddhism emerged as a reform offshoot of Hinduism (Conze, 1959; Layman, 1976). Buddha taught that existence is permeated with suffering caused by self-centered thought. Selfish thought can be reduced by following an "eightfold path" of right motivation and conduct eventually culminating in a passive focusing exercise, meditation.

In the sixth century Buddhism was carried to China and appeared 600 years later in Japan as Zen. Unlike concentrative meditation, Zen meditation involves calmly attending to the flow of all stimuli, not a continuous single stimulus. One does so without thought, judgment, or analysis. This is typically called mindfulness meditation. Today health professionals outside of the Buddhist tradition teach simple mindfulness awareness techniques, often in combination with stretching, breathing, and other concentrative meditation techniques (Kabat-Zinn, 1990). Although some teach mindfulness in isolation, Kabat-Zinn's preference is to deploy mindful meditation in a variety of contexts (being mindful of taste, movement, thoughts, etc.) in order to enhance the transfer of training to life at large.

Illustration of a Meditation Exercise

Let the word "one" easily float through your mind, over and over. There is no need to force it to repeat at any speed or volume. Just let the word gently repeat again and again. All you need to do is attend to the word "one." Whenever your mind wanders, gently return to attending to the word "one" as it repeats over and over.

3

The Relaxation Engine

Relaxation is a remarkable vehicle that can take us to many wonderful places. In fact, the vehicle metaphor is useful for summarizing much of what happens in relaxation training and practice. The "engine" consists of core physiological processes that "get things moving" by reducing stress. These processes are "under the hood," generally out of sight and outside of voluntary control. To continue, in the driver's cabin we find control devices to drive the vehicle, for example, the accelerator, brakes, and various switches and knobs. These are processes we explore in the following chapter. The landscape and paths through which our vehicle travels represents the psychological effects of relaxation, ranging from feeling physically limp, feeling energized and joyful, and feeling spiritual. Our destination consists of the overall goals of relaxation, that is why we have chosen to practice. Together, the metaphor of the vehicle, complete with engine, control panel, landscape and paths, and destination, summarize what we consider in the chapters the constitute Part I of this book. In this chapter we begin with the relaxation engine, which in simple terms is the counterpart of what can be called the stress engine.

THE STRESS ENGINE

We are built for a brute and primitive world. Without deliberation, our brains and bodies energize to attack, defend, or run—to fight the enemy, chase away the bear, to flee. Once mobilized with stress energy, we make rapid choices for emergency action. This is the engine of stress, one that serves us well in times of violence and threat. Its opposite is the relaxation engine, the processes whereby stress is relieved and the brain and body are readied for deeper relaxation.

Briefly, the stress engine consists of activating and energizing processes that are more or less outside of direct conscious control. First, we need to define some terms.

The Nervous System

To review the basics, the nervous system is divided into the peripheral nervous system (PNS) and the central nervous system (CNS). The PNS is, in turn, divided into the somatic and autonomic nervous systems, and the CNS includes the brain and spinal cord.

The Somatic (Musculoskeletal) Nervous System

The somatic nervous system is primarily involved in sensory input (sight, hearing, touch) and voluntary skeletal muscular activity (walking, gesturing, deliberate facial expressions).

The Autonomic Nervous System

In contrast, the autonomic nervous system regulates physical functions over which people have relatively little control, including heart rate, breathing, digestion, and regulation of blood flow. The autonomic nervous system is divided into sympathetic and parasympathetic branches as well as the enteric nervous system situated in the abdomen.

Both the sympathetic and parasympathetic nervous systems leave the spine and extend to basic internal organs, including the heart, lungs, intestines, and so on. As we shall see later, the sympathetic nervous system "revs us up" for stress. In contrast, the parasympathetic nervous system dampens the effects of the sympathetic nervous system and is responsible for vegetative life-support functions (e.g., heart rate) and conserving energy. The enteric nervous system is a bit different in that it surrounds the intestines in the gut and regulates digestion and gut movement; however, it is also involved with a variety of positive and stress-related "gut feelings" (the positive "warm inner glow" of satisfaction; "butterflies" in the stomach, etc.). See Figure 3.1 for a summary.

ADVANCED MATERIAL: All nervous system activity, including stress and relaxation processes, is modulated by neurotransmitter substances including acetylcholine,

NERVOUS SYSTEM			
CENTRAL NERVOUS SYSTEM		**PERIPHERAL NERVOUS SYSTEM**	
BRAIN	SPINAL CORD	SOMATIC NERVOUS SYSTEM	AUTONOMIC NERVOUS SYSTEM
		1. Nerves to muscles	1. Sympathetic Nervous System
		2. Nerves from sense organs	2. Parasympathetic Nervous System
			3. Enteric Nervous System

FIGURE 3.1   The nervous system.

norepinephrine, serotonin, dopamine, GABA or gamma-amino butyric acid (GABA), glutamate, and endorphins (the endogenous opiates). These substances regulate communication between nerve cells, or neurons, throughout the body, and are associated with a wide range of states associated with stress and relaxation, including: anxiety (GABA); general pleasurable and reinforcing states (dopamine); positive mood, sleep, and pain reduction (serotonin); arousal, excitement, and wakefulness (norepinephrine); and pain reduction and feelings of euphoria (endorphins). Many man-made psychoactive pharmacological agents (Valium, Prozac) that are occasionally used to reduce stress and induce relaxation work through their impact on various neurotransmitters.

The Brain

In tracing the physiology of stress, it is useful to begin with three levels of the brain. First, most people know that we think and feel with the brain. Actually, such advanced "human" abilities are performed by the structures near the surface of the brain just under the skull known as the *cortex*. The cortex is our sophisticated "thinking/feeling" organ. It is most responsible for processing input from the sense organs, communicating with the world, coordinating muscle activities, and engaging in such higher functions as imagination, logic, planning, concept formation, and, of course, worry. It is the cortex that is primarily responsible for identifying what is stressful or relaxing.

Recent research has focused on the front portion of the cortex (behind the eyebrows), the *prefrontal anterior cortex*. The prefrontal cortex controls many higher functions such as thinking, paying attention, controlling impulses, and self-observation or monitoring.

Deep under the surface of the brain, is the brain's primary emotional control center, sometimes known as the limbic system. There are many organs in the brain's interior that are of interest to students of stress and relaxation. We will simply list them for the time being: hypothalamus, thalamus, hippocampus, amygdala, and pituitary gland. Suffice it to say that all are deeply involved in emotion, emotional memory, and basic human drives like hunger and sex.

The deepest level of the brain is responsible for life-sustaining vegetative functions such as heartbeat and breathing, as well as the relay of information from the body to higher brain functions. Two salient features of this part of the brain are the medulla and the reticular activating system (RAS), both involved in the transport of incoming stimuli to the brain. The medulla is involved in many basic functions associated with stress and relaxation, including blood pressure, heart rate, and breathing. The RAS connects the brain with the rest of the body. It keeps us awake and helps activate the brain for dealing tasks and stress.

AUTONOMIC STRESS AROUSAL

Each of us has a stress arousal response that automatically awakens and energizes the body for emergency action in what is traditionally termed the "fight or flight response." A constellation of changes occurs, most of which involve providing energy for fighting or fleeing:

- Fuels, in the form of glucose, fats, cholesterol, and proteins, are released from the liver into the bloodstream.
- Levels of oxygen in the blood increase so fuel can "burn" through metabolism. Breathing rate and volume increases. Bronchial tubes in the lungs dilate to let in more air.
- Enriched with fuel and oxygen, blood must be quickly and efficiently transported. The heart beats more quickly, and more blood is pumped with each beat, so blood pressure increases.
- The muscles responsible for vigorous activity must "open the gates" to take in increased blood supplied by the heart. Blood vessels to the

The Brain and Autonomic Nervous System

The brain's cortex is primarily responsible for the habits and choices we make under stress—to assume stress-related postures, tense up our muscles, hold our breath, and so on. But much of this activity, and the stress arousal response, is supported by a cluster of neurons in the center of the brain known as the hypothalamus.

The hypothalamus is about the size of an almond and resides nearly in the center of the brain. More precisely, it is strategically nestled close to critical areas of the brain responsible for worry and negative emotion, fear, wants and needs, and so on. Given its location, it is easy to see how the stress response can be triggered, not only by outside assaults, but by negative thinking and emotion.

The hypothalamus mediates the stress arousal response in three ways:

1. *Rapid response.* The hypothalamus directly activates the sympathetic nervous system to quickly arouse key organs. The brain tells the heart to beat more quickly, and the lungs to breathe more rapidly, and so on.

2. *Slower response.* The hypothalamus can stimulate the adrenal glands (residing above the kidneys) to secrete a variety of stress hormones, notably epinephrine (sometimes called adrenalin) and norepinephrine. This is where we get the "adrenalin rush." We experiences the diverse effects of stress arousal, delayed by about half a minute and lasting an hour or longer.

3. *Slowest response.* The hypothalamus indirectly triggers the release of corticoid stress hormones (also from the adrenal glands) which evoke a slow-acting stress response that can last for days or weeks, prolonging and aggravating the effects of stress.

ADVANCED MATERIAL: This third process is much more complex. The hypothalamus secretes a hormone called corticotropin-releasing factor (CRF) into the blood, which in turn causes the brain's tiny central pituitary gland to secrete adrenocorticotropic hormone (ACTH). ACTH then activates the adrenal gland to release corticoid stress hormones, including the fuel-producing glucocorticoids. This is often referred to as the hypothamic–pituitary–adrenal, or HPA, pathway.

In sum, much of the autonomic stress arousal response is a massive combination of hundreds of physiological changes, some of which are immediate and short-lived, and some of which can persist for weeks. This constellation of responses is ideally suited for coping with the threats our ancestors may have faced in the wild. They had little time to think about how to awaken

heart and other large muscles expand, providing more fuel to pa
the body that may be involved in emergency action. Tiny blood ve,
near the skin, particularly the palms of the hands and the feet, consti
Blood is not essential here for vigorous action. Our hands and feet fo
cold and clammy.

- Metabolic rate increases as body fuels are burned. Excess heat is carriec
  away through breathing and perspiration.
- Functions not needed for emergency action are reduced: stomach and
  intestinal activity are limited, and blood flow to the stomach, kidneys,
  and intestines decreases.

In addition, secondary changes occur that enhance our mobilization for emergency action:

- The body prepares itself for possible injury. Surface blood vessels
  constrict, reducing the possibility of serious blood loss. Clotting substances are dumped into the bloodstream supporting the formation
  of protective scar tissue. The immune system increases activity in
  anticipation of possible infection, or reduces activity to minimize the
  potentially damaging effects of over infection and to conserve resources
  for fighting and fleeing.
- Natural painkillers, endorphins, are released by the brain, to help us
  keep on going in the face of considerable discomfort.
- Finally, the body readies itself for active involvement with the outside
  world. Pupils of the eye enlarge to let in more light and enhance vision,
  palms and feet become moist to increase grip and traction when running,
  and brain activity increases.

Three things about autonomic stress arousal are important to recognize.
First, it is adaptive, supplying quick energy for fighting off or fleeing attack,
quickly responding to unexpected physical assault, and so on. Second, it can
have a delayed and prolonged effect, important for maintaining stress-fighting
resources at a high level over a long period of time. And third, the response
is automatically integrated. All relevant body systems are energized together—heart, lungs, circulatory system, etc. One does not have to plan for
increased stress arousal, as one might deliberately prepare the proper stance
for striking a golf ball, or running a race. In times of severe crisis, our ancestors
in the jungle needed complete, automatic, quick energy. To understand how
much of this transpires, we begin with the brain.

and energize all body organs to deal with an attacking wild bear. However, the stress response is also triggered by many 21st-century challenges such as deadlines, arguments, school exams, publication deadlines, alarms, worries, physical problems, studying this chapter—the list is endless. As a result, we are often subjected to chronic high levels of stress arousal. Indeed, our stress arousal system may become chronically hypersensitized, increasing the propensity for heightened and prolonged stress arousal.

Getting "Tuned" or "Set" for More Stress

With severe or prolonged stress, the body and brain can actually become increasingly sensitive to or "primed" for stress so that even modest challenges can evoke serious, prolonged, and self-sustained stress arousal. This is the idea underlying "stress tuning." We use the image of an abused vehicle that gets out of tune, and as a result is more likely to wear out and perform poorly. One can also think of a heat-regulating thermostat in an apartment; stress resets the threshold lower so that (unwanted) heat is more likely to be triggered. Gelhorn (1970) has offered one of the earliest views of stress hypersensitivity:

> It is a matter of everyday experience that a person's reaction to a given situation depends very much upon his own mental, physical, and emotional state. One might be said to be "set" to respond in a given manner. In the same fashion the autonomic response to a given stimulus may at one time be predominantly sympathetic and may at another time be predominantly parasympathetic. . . . The sensitization of autonomic centers has been designated "tuning" and we speak of sympathetic tuning and parasympathetic tuning . . . and refers merely to the "sensitization" or "facilitation" of particular centers of the brain. (Gelhorn & Loofbouroow, 1963; pp. 90–91)

Gelhorn (1970) coined the phrase *ergotropic tuning* to refer to a shift toward increased sympathetic nervous system dominance. He postulated that an extremely intense and acute traumatic stressor, or a chronic stressor of less intensity, may cause one to be ergotropically tuned, and therefore more likely to respond with chronic elevations of stress. Ergotropic tuning can be self-perpetuating, that is, may result in self-sustained stress despite the absence of external stressors.

ADVANCED MATERIAL: Impulses from the hypothalamus and limbic system (the brain's emotion center) can stimulate other parts of the brain (leading to increased worry and negative emotion), which in turn can further stimulate the limbic system. Similarly, limbic hypothalamic stimulation can travel through the reticular activating system to the skeletal muscles and other organs, which, when excited, can send stimulating feedback to the limbic system and cortex. The result is continued arousal, and a heightened propensity for future arousal in response to stressful stimulation. Stress can be self-sustaining.

STRESS AND THE RELAXATION ENGINE

Stress and the Benefits of Relaxation

It seems that every 5 years or so the popular media makes an astonishing rediscovery: stress contributes to illness and impaired performance, and relaxation is healthy. Experts are interviewed, television documentaries appear, and once again the public is alerted to the perils of stress and the promise of relaxation. To date I've collected no fewer than two dozen *Time* and *Newsweek* cover articles devoted to these topics. The fact is, the links between stress, illness, and relaxation have been known for centuries and have been recognized and repeatedly documented through research over the past two decades. The results of this research are resoundingly presented in thousands of solid scientific articles. The research will continue until some sort of critical mass of understanding is reached or until a new generation of newly educated editors take charge and once again stress and relaxation become hot news.

First, what is the latest research on the effects of stress, especially on health? Put simply, the latest studies suggest that acute and brief stressors can actually boost parts of the immune system, particularly inflammation. Chronic and uninterrupted stressors, especially those involving loss and bereavement, uncontrollability of the personal environment, and requirements that one make serious changes in one's identity or social role are likely to evoke prolonged stress and have destructive impact on health, especially on all components of immune functioning (Segerstrom & Miller, 2004). Relaxation training may not only deactivate or dampen chronic stress arousal, but may well give one some perceived control over a situation ("I know how to deeply relax and meditate"), provide powerful breaks in a chronic life of stress, provide internally created replacements for loss ("At least I have my meditation"), and may even contribute to subtle changes in how one perceives one's role ("My task is to approach life in the spirit of mindfulness or prayer").

To elaborate, stress arousal appears to make one more vulnerable to, less likely to recover quickly from, and more likely to suffer complications from the following illnesses (and this list is not all-inclusive):

AIDS, angina, arthritis, asthma, back pain, bradycardia, cancer, cardiac arrhythmia, chemotherapy side effects, chronic fatigue syndrome, colitis, common cold, coronary heart disease, diabetes, fibromyalgia, gastrointestinal disorders, hypertension, hyperventilation, inflammation and infection, influenza, injury/healing, insomnia, irritable bowel syndrome, migraine headaches, multiple sclerosis, muscle cramps, myocardial infarction, nausea, peptic ulcer, psoriasis, Reynaud's syndrome, spasmatic dysmenorrhea, tachycardia, and tinnitus.

Intense and chronic activation of the stress response subjects the body to measurable wear and tear. Our organs were not meant to continue in a state of emergency readiness for long periods of time; something usually gives or wears out. Second, although brief stress can boost the body's immune system, too much stress interferes with immune functioning, making one more vulnerable to illness and less likely to heal or recover quickly. Wear and tear as well as impaired immune functioning are two important reasons why stress can be unhealthy.

Severe and prolonged stress can also have a detrimental effect on how well one functions, that is, performs the tasks of living. Eventually attention is reduced and one is likely to let important stimuli go unnoticed. Behavior is more rigid and less flexible; creativity is impaired (one can get "stuck in a rut," trying over and over the same unsuccessful coping strategies). Memory is impaired. Energy reserves are depleted and one is more likely to experience fatigue.

An impressive body of research suggests that relaxation can reduce arousal and mitigate arousal-related problems (Goodkin & Visser, 2000; Jones & Bright, 2001; Sapolsky, 1998; Wolkowitz & Rothschild, 2003). This research has spawned an ever-growing library of health psychology textbooks (Allen, 1998; Brannon & Feist, 2000; DiMatteo & Martin, 2002; Friedman, 2002; Nezo, Nezu, & Geller, 2003; Taylor, 1999). Generally, the scientific literature strongly suggests that relaxation has the potential for:

1. Reducing susceptibility to illness;
2. Relieving the destructive wear and tear of severe and chronic stress arousal on specific body systems and organs as well as on the body's immune system;
3. Speeding healing and recovery from nonchronic conditions (for example, the wounds of physically injured people who are relaxed heal more quickly);

4. Reducing serious complications of chronic conditions (for example, individuals with AIDS or diabetes appear to do better); and
5. Reducing the destructive impact of stress on functioning (attention, flexibility, memory, energy).

The Relaxation Engine

The relaxation engine consists of those body and brain processes associated with stress relief and relaxation. In the early 1970s, Harvard cardiologist Herbert Benson (Wallace, Benson, & Wilson; 1971; Wallace & Benson, 1972) found that practitioners of transcendental meditation show a constellation of physiological changes suggesting deepened relaxation. These include reduced heart rate, blood pressure, respiration rate, brain wave activity, and so on. Benson's research was not only partly responsible for increasing public and scientific interest in meditation, but popularized a definition of relaxation as *generalized reduced arousal*, the *relaxation response*. Here is how he summarized his findings:

> Each of us possesses a natural and innate protective mechanism against "over-stress," which allows us to turn off harmful bodily effects, to counter the effects of the fight-or-flight response. This response against "over-stress" brings on bodily changes that decrease heart rate, lower metabolism, decrease the rate of breathing, and bring the body back into what is probably a healthier balance. This is the Relaxation Response. (Benson, 1975, pp. 25–26)

In other words, the relaxation response is the mirror image of the stress response. It is mediated primarily by the parasympathetic nervous system and automatically results in a protective and recuperative reduction in arousal. The body more or less pauses for rest and recovery.

Just as one can be tuned for autonomic stress arousal, one can also be tuned for relaxation. More precisely, the opposite of *ergotropic* tuning is *trophotropic* tuning. Here, the parasympathetic nervous system (responsible for recovery and rest) becomes more dominant and one is therefore less sensitive to stress.

4

The Six Access Skills of Relaxation

Why do hundreds of relaxation techniques sort into six general families: yogaform stretching, progressive muscle relaxation, breathing exercises, autogenic training, imagery/self-statements, and meditation/mindfulness? There is an underlying order to the universe of relaxation, one that traces back to the very nature of stress. This is an important question. If the division of exercises into six families is arbitrary, then perhaps it makes little difference which, or how many, techniques are taught. However, if there are basic physiological and psychological reasons for a differentiated conceptualization, then different techniques may well have important differences.

In chapter 3 we saw that each of us possesses an emergency response that automatically prepares and coordinates body organs for vigorous emergency activity. This is the body's "stress engine," and includes among its many components the hypothalamus (part of the stress arousal trigger), the autonomic nervous system (conveys arousing messages to key organs), and the adrenal glands (help sustain stress arousal through the release of various hormones). A key characteristic of the autonomic stress response is that it is generally out of our voluntary control. Once the stress response is triggered by the hypothalamus, a constellation of changes occur without deliberation. Fuels are pumped into the bloodstream, heart rate increases, blood pressure increases, blood flows to major muscle groups, palms perspire, and so on. We are energized for fight or flight.

However, there are ways we can indirectly control stress arousal. Six *self-stressing processes* (Smith, 2004) (a) augment and sustain arousal and (b) indirectly contribute to arousal by producing aftereffects that interfere with full relaxation. These same processes hold a remarkable secret—they suggest six fundamental relaxation access skills, six families of relaxation that give us voluntary access to the relaxation response and those aspects of relaxation deeper than reduced arousal. In terms of our vehicle metaphor, relaxation access skills enable us to control the engine of relaxation, something like the various control panel devices (accelerator, breaks, power switches, etc.) in the driver's cabin. Three of these skills are predominantly centered in the body and three are in the brain.

SELF-STRESSING AND THE BODY

Let us return to the primitive basics of fight or flight. Picture an unlucky distant ancestor who has encountered an angry bear in the forest. In response to this perceived threat, our subject experiences a quick rush of energy. As we have seen, his hypothalamus initiates a series of bodily changes that provide blood and oxygen to organs for vigorous action. In addition, various *self-stressing* actions serve to augment and sustain arousal. He crouches in a defensive position and holds his arms very still so as not to arouse the bear. His muscles tighten, ready to flee at a moment's notice. He holds his breath tightly, breathing in through his expanded chest, and takes an occasional deep sigh. Even after the threat is over, various aftereffects may interfere with relaxation. He may maintain an awkward posture, experience muscle fatigue, and continue breathing in a tight, shallow manner. Here we see three forms of self-stressing that involve the body: (a) posture and position, (b) skeletal muscle tension, and (c) breathing.

Posture and Position

Stressed Posture and Position

When confronted with stress, we often assume a variety of defensive or aggressive postures or positions, including crouching in preparation to run, cringing and bracing for attack, extending our chests, raising our shoulders, or even standing or sitting in a fixed position for an extended time. In the office or classroom we may sit still watching the lecturer, bend our necks to hear more clearly, lean over our desks, hold our elbows in a raised position over the computer keyboard, or curl our fingers in a rigid typing position.

In sum, stressed posture and position can be defined primarily in terms of joint stress, which indirectly contributes to skeletal muscle tension as well as muscle and nerve fatigue and decreased energy. To elaborate:

STRESSED JOINTS

- Joints connecting to tendons and muscles are bent, pinched, and subjected to strain.
- Nerve tissue around the joints become cramped, increasing pain and discomfort or numbness.
- Renewing flow of blood and lubricating fluid to the joints is restricted, limiting movement, healing, and recovery.

SECONDARY TENSION, FATIGUE, AND REDUCED ENERGY

- Moderate levels of skeletal muscle tension and fatigue are created and maintained. Awkward stress-related postures take effort to maintain and contribute to skeletal muscle tension. For example, if you sit hunched over a desk it takes some effort to keep from falling over; you may have to prop your chin on your hands, lean on your elbows, and so on. In contrast, it takes little effort to sit comfortably upright, with each bone in your back restfully aligned like a stack of bricks. It should be noted that often the distinguishing feature of muscle tension associated with stressed posture and position is not its intensity but its duration and absence of movement. Sitting still in a car for four hours may not evoke the same degree of muscle tension as, perhaps, clenching one's jaw in anger. Indeed, the act of sitting may require little exertion at all. However, such a sustained and unchanging posture can create fatigue as well as the effects described below.
- Fatigue-related waste products, including carbon dioxide and lactic acid, build up and are not readily carried away through constricted blood and lymph vessels.
- Blood tends to collect or pool in inactive areas, less oxygen gets to muscles, increasing fatigue and reducing energy.
- Muscle and connective tissue fibers become less coordinated (with some areas more tense than others, or muscles working against each other).
- One becomes numb to stress and less aware of the body and where it may be stressed.

Relaxation Access Skill: Stretching Postures and Positions

I propose that the primary and secondary effects of stressed posture and position can be addressed through various stretching exercises such as those found in Hatha yoga. Hatha yoga may have many effects and work through many mechanisms. However, from our perspective, a stretch is achieved through a posture or position that centers around some form of joint extension. You bend over backwards, and the spine is stretched and the back is gently relaxed. You reach to the sky, and the shoulder and arm joints are stretched and lightly relaxed. These effects can be summarized:

THE JOINTS

- The muscles and ligaments that surround the joints are relaxed and the joints themselves are no longer tightly bent or constricted.
- Pressure on joint-related nerve tissue is relieved.
- The flow of blood and lubricating fluids to the joints are increased.

REDUCED SECONDARY TENSION AND FATIGUE; INCREASED ENERGY AND KINESTHETIC STIMULATION

- Skeletal muscles are gently relaxed. Postural and muscular imbalances associated with stress are corrected. When muscles are relaxed, bones are no longer held in a posture or position that takes effort or strain to maintain.
- Fatiguing and energy-sapping waste products are washed away as the movement of blood and lymph increases.
- Muscles are energized with increased oxygen from blood.
- Muscle and connective tissue fibers are stretched into coordinated alignment.
- The stretching of muscles, ligaments, blood vessels, and nerve tissue creates intense and sustained kinesthetic stimulation. This is experienced as an energizing and awakening effect.

Hatha yoga as traditionally practiced is truly a complex mixture of approaches. Even the effects of relatively pure stretching postures are not simple. However, we can summarize the highlights. Stretching: (1) unstresses the joints, (2) evokes mild muscle relaxation, (3) reduces fatigue, and (4) increases energy and provides intense internal attention-directing stimulation.

Skeletal Muscles

Stressed Muscles

The skeletal muscles are those muscles over which we have voluntary control (and are connected to various bones in our skeleton). They include the muscles of our hands, arms, legs, feet, chest, jaws, and mouth. When threatened, we tighten our skeletal muscles to prepare for attack or escape. One clenches and raises one's fists and arms, stands ready to run, and so on. If stress is severe or chronic, skeletal muscle tension can become self-perpetuating and continue even after a threat is over. Jacobson (1938) has speculated that continued tension creates additional arousing stimulation to the brain, which then contributes to even more muscle tension. Furthermore, the brain tends to tune out continuous and unchanging stimuli, such as the background drone of traffic, air conditioners, and skeletal muscle tension. As an aftereffect, tension may persist; one may habituate to its effects and lose awareness of being tense.

Relaxation Access Skill: Letting Go

With progressive muscle relaxation one deliberately identifies a tensed or clenched skeletal muscle and lets go. This directly reduces striated muscle tension, and reduces arousing stimulus input to the brain. Muscle relaxation can also be cultivated through autogenic training, yoga stretching, breathing exercises, meditation, and mindfulness.

Stretching vs. Letting Go

It is important to distinguish between the effects of stretching and the effects of progressive muscle relaxation. First, stretching exercises have an impact on joints and tendons; progressive muscle relaxation generally does not. Indeed, one can accomplish virtually every PMR exercise without bending a single joint. Stretching reduces sustained high levels of tension to moderate baseline levels of tension characteristic of simple inactivity; PMR has the potential for reducing muscle tension (moderate–to–high levels) to profound levels of relaxation, below everyday baseline levels. One might stretch before taking a leisurely walk; one might practice PMR in order to feel completely limp.

The actual postures and movements of popular Hatha yoga exercises make clear that stretching is not targeted to evoking deep muscle relaxation. Many hatha yoga exercises can be done in a standing position; very few PMR exercises can be done while standing. In contrast, only a few Hatha yoga exercises can be done while resting on the floor; virtually all PMR exercises can be done in this position. Standing, even when relaxed, requires at least a minimal level of muscle tension (otherwise one would fall over). Resting on the floor requires virtually no skeletal muscle tension.

Second, PMR is characterized by restricted focus, on isolated skeletal muscle groups such as the hands or biceps. The focus of yoga stretching is typically (but not always) diffuse and on posture rather than any particular muscle. One attends to slowly and gracefully executing a movement (bending forward, for example), or maintaining a challenging posture (standing on one leg) with calm poise.

Third, PMR cultivates the voluntary act of releasing tension, often very abruptly. Images such as "turning off a light switch" or 'cutting the stings of a puppet" are often used to convey this action. In contrast, there is nothing quick and abrupt about yoga stretching, and as already mentioned, the emphasis is not so much on attending to and releasing tension as it is on gracefully achieving various postures, which may indeed require some muscle tension.

Finally, yoga stretching, and not PMR, can require high levels of focused coordination. Advanced postures (such as standing on one's foot, or one's head) require substantial focus. However, even simple stretches can be presented as meditative focusing exercises. When done so, the instructions emphasize the importance of achieving a slow, smooth, and graceful stretch, and maintaining attention on a particular posture. When presented as a focusing exercise, yoga stretching targets both the access skills of stretching posture and position, and of sustained effortless simple focus discussed later.

Breathing

Stressed Breathing

Breathing is normally involuntary. However, we can deliberately modulate the pace of our breathing. Stressed breathing maintains arousal and can continue as a relaxation-impeding aftereffect. First we need to consider the process of breathing.

The process of breathing is complex and involves more than simply breathing in and out. We shall consider only the highlights. First, at least three groups of muscles are involved: the chest muscles in the ribcage (intercostal muscles), the shoulder muscles (trapezius muscles), and the diaphragm. The diaphragm is like the skin of a kettle drum, and separates the stomach from the lungs. Generally, when we inhale, the diaphragm pulls down, like a piston, and the lungs expand with air. When we exhale, the diaphragm muscles relax inward, move up, and forcing air out.

When we breathe in, oxygen-rich air enters the lungs, and life-giving oxygen transfers to the bloodstream. The "exhaust" gas, carbon dioxide (CO_2) is transferred from the blood to the air in the lungs and exhaled. This transfer of oxygen takes place in tiny air sacks (bubbles) of tissue called alveoli, near the bottom of the lungs, closest to the diaphragm.

Stressed breathing is often rapid, shallow or deep, and uneven, a pattern that may have some value in fight or flight emergencies. Rapid and deep breathing can bring in an immediate infusion of oxygen for action. Shallow breathing makes us less noticeable to attackers, and is associated with effortful active concentration (on a potential threat, for example). Uneven breathing results when our breathing is shallow; we occasionally sigh and gasp to take in an overdue breath. However, in time, a stressed pattern of breathing creates additional stress. Spending more time on the inhalation phase of breathing, while rapidly breathing out, triggers stress arousal. Shallow breathing eventually results in a buildup of CO_2 and deficits in oxygen, which in itself can create symptoms.

Rapid and deep breathing can itself create a stress-related condition termed hyperventilation. In hyperventilation too much CO_2 is expelled, resulting in low levels of CO_2 in the blood. Low blood CO_2 causes the small blood vessels leading to the brain and spinal cord to constrict, reducing blood flow to the central nervous system. This is termed hypocapnia, a condition associated with anxiety-related symptoms, panic, dizziness, and eventually unconsciousness.

Stressed breathing is more likely to incorporate the ribcage and collarbone, the intercostal and trapezius muscles. Note the defensive attack position of expanding one's chest (the gorilla pounding his or her pumped up chest). However, in chest/shoulder breathing, air is drawn into the upper part of the lungs, away from the oxygen-transferring alveoli near the bottom of the lungs. As a result, one has to breathe harder and more rapidly for an adequate amount of oxygen.

Chest/shoulder breathing is also associated with another stress-related breathing condition, paradoxical breathing. Here one breathes in through the chest while pulling in one's abdomen, i.e., puffing up the chest while sucking in the stomach. Note what happens to the diaphragm during this process: because the stomach is pulled in, it pushes the diaphragm up into the chest cavity, reducing lung capacity. As a result, breathing is even more stressful and it takes more effort to take in adequate quantities of air.

In sum, stressed breathing is likely to be rapid, uneven, and shallow or deep. It is more likely to involve the chest and shoulder muscles. All of these may persist as aftereffects and interfere with recovery and relaxation.

Relaxation Access Skill: Relaxed Breathing

Relaxed breathing is more likely to involve the diaphragm and has a pace that is slow and even, and at times deep or shallow (depending on whether one is relatively active or inactive). Such breathing is diaphragmatic and is less likely to involve the trapezius or intercostal muscles. During inhalation, the diaphragm muscle moves down, drawing air into the lungs and pushing the stomach out. During exhalation, the diaphragm relaxes and moves up drawing the abdomen in. Diaphragmatic breathing is relaxed because it is most efficient. Most of the lung's alveoli, those tiny air sacks through which oxygen is transferred to the blood, are near the bottom of the lungs, close to the diaphragm. When we breathe diaphragmatically, we draw air down to the highest concentration of alveoli, where the "work" of oxygen-transfer takes place. Thus, diaphragmatic breathing uses the least amount of energy.

In addition, relaxed breathing has a special rhythm. Exhalation is slow and even. Initially it may be deep, and later (when one is relaxed and needs less oxygen) effortlessly shallow. Although muscle tension is generated during inhalation, the chest muscles and diaphragm relax while air is quietly expelled. When air has been exhaled, there is a pause until the need for oxygen prompts an automatic and relaxed inhalation. The inhalation phase occurs quietly and easily. Generally relaxed exhalation takes twice as long (6 seconds) as inhalation (3 seconds).

Slow, shallow breathing, may contribute to relaxation by increasing blood carbon dioxide (CO_2) levels. Moderate CO_2 elevation can lower heart rate, dilate peripheral blood vessels, depress arousing cortical brain activity, and evoke a general sense of mild somnolence (Lichstein, 1988). Indeed, early stages of sleep, when one moves from wakefulness to drowsiness, are associated, in part, with increments of CO_2.

SELF-STRESSING AND THE BRAIN

Cognitive Autonomic Processes

Stressed Body Focus

Most direct manifestations of increased autonomic arousal occur outside of awareness and voluntary control. We are rarely aware of increases in glucose discharge rate or blood pressure. However, simply attending to and evoking thoughts and images about a specific body part or process can evoke related physiological changes. This is a process frequently deployed in hypnosis. A hypnotist may utter body-directed suggestions, such as "attend to your body and how it feels warm," and most participants will experience the suggested effect.

Frequently we evoke stress-related physical changes on our own. If someone were to describe a disgusting meal experience, you might notice your own stomach feeling a bit queasy, a sensation triggered by simple thoughts and words. If a friend were to describe a recent case of fleas she caught during camping, you might find yourself attending to your arms and legs, and feel a bit itchy.

You can see this self-stressing process in a simple experiment:

Think of an incident in which you were seriously angered or frightened. For the next two minutes, fantasize this incident, including all of the details. What was happening? Who was there? What did you think and do? What did you feel? Get into the fantasy with your whole body. If you imagined arguing with your boss about an unfair demotion, think about how it made you feel. Feel the anger rising in your belly, the burning or butterflies in your abdomen, your heart beating. Imagine what you want to do and what you say. There, now relax for a few seconds.

In this fantasy you may well have experienced such bodily changes as increased heart rate, queasiness, or burning in your stomach—all manifestations of autonomic arousal. Flushing and heart rate are linked to the sympathetic nervous system, and abdominal sensations are linked to nerve activity in the gut's enteric nervous system. In your fantasy you demonstrated a type of self-stressing, an ability to stir the sympathetic and enteric nervous systems. You did this by directing your attention to your body, and thinking thoughts and images about the body. As an aftereffect, cognitive autonomic arousal may persist as a habit. One may overreact to minimal stress with self-induced increased heart rate, queasiness, and so on.

Relaxation Access Skill:
Physically Targeted Relaxing Words and Images

Cognitive autonomic arousal processes enable us to voluntarily evoke autonomic relaxation. For example, a fantasy of doing nothing at a quiet lake while soaking in the sun actually warms the skin. We think of biting into a delicious orange, and our mouths water. We imagine a sensuous back rub, and the mind stirs feelings of warmth and tingling.

Through autogenic training one attends to and thinks of (through words or pictures) suggestions such as heaviness and warmth in the hands and arms, relaxed heart rate, and abdominal warmth, thereby targeting sympathetic and enteric nervous system arousal. With suggestions of "heaviness" skeletal muscle tension may also decrease. Reductions in autonomic arousal can also occur as a byproduct of PMR, breathing exercises, and to some extent, all approaches to relaxation.

Cognitive (Verbal/Nonverbal) Affective Processes

Stressed Emotion

We often motivate and energize ourselves for a stressful encounter with affect-arousing cognitions. We may think about the supervisor who cancelled the raise, and as a result we feel angry. We may think about what is causing the mysterious midnight thumping sound in the attic and then feel anxiety and fear. These negative emotions can persist as an aftereffect even when there is no threat. And such emotions can stir us into action.

Self-stressing, emotion-stirring cognitions (thoughts) are primarily verbal and secondarily nonverbal. Worry primarily consists of words and self-statements, and secondarily (if at all) fantasies of visual images, sounds, touch sensations, and smells. Before an argument, we may contemplate how we have been provoked, of how unfair the provoker is, or of how we have been victimized. This may at times be accompanied by fantasies of the provoking person frowning and shaking his fist.

Relaxation Access Skill: Imagery/Relaxing Self-Talk

I hypothesize that relaxation imagery and self-talk have the greatest potential for evoking relaxing emotions (see relaxation states in chapter 5). However, unlike self-stressing cognitions, relaxation cognitions are primarily nonverbal and secondarily verbal. Relaxing imagery and fantasy primarily involve things we see, hear, touch, and smell. These are supported by relaxing verbal thoughts (self-statements).

Positive relaxation states can emerge indirectly from the practice of any relaxation technique. Simply, one might feel Joyful or Thankful/Loving after a good session of nearly any activity. One might feel Prayerful after meditation.

The physiological mechanisms underlying cognitive affective arousal are extremely complex and often unclear. Verbal thoughts are often loosely associated with the right cortex (for left-handed people) and the left cortex (for right-handed people). Many have proposed significant involvement of the limbic system (thalamus, amygdala, and hippocampus), and for positive emotion, the left prefrontal cerebral cortex.

Attentional Processes

Stressed Attention

When dealing with a threat, we actively and effortfully concentrate on attacking, defending, or running. We deliberately and effortfully concentrate on an exam, an interview, a difficult job, or an attacking dog. Such stressed attention is effortful and prolonged. In addition, it is often directed to multiple targets, including competing tasks (as in multitasking), a targeted task versus worried preoccupation, or self-stressing efforts (thinking about how one is breathing, maintaining a stressed posture or position, thinking about related fantasies or negative emotions, etc.) rather than the task at hand. Put simply, when attention is stressed, we have a lot on our minds.

Researchers at the Roosevelt University Stress Institute suggest that simple attention deficits (not to be confused with Attention Deficit Hyperactivity Disorder [ADHD]; see Piiparinen & Smith, 2003) may be a common consequence of stressed attention. The Smith Stress Symptoms Inventory (Piiparinin & Smith, 2003; Smith, 2004) has identified six common stress attention deficit symptoms: losing one's concentration, becoming easily distracted, losing memory and forgetting things, becoming confused, feeling disorganized, and feeling restless and fidgety. Stress attention deficit symptoms are quite prevalent, at least as common as striated muscle tension, autonomic arousal, or negative emotions.

Relaxation Access Metaskill:
Sustained Effortless/Passive Simple Focus

The skill of sustained effortless/passive simple focus is the opposite of stressed attention. Stressed attention is effortful, not passive or effortless. It is often divided, not sustained, with regard to one simple target or task.

I propose that such focus is an access skill in and of itself, a *metaskill* basic to all other access skills. For example, in order for a yoga stretch to work, it must be completed with minimal effort and with sustained focus.

Likewise, one must with the least effort sustain a simple focus on letting go, breathing in a relaxed way, thinking "warm and heavy," and entertaining a relaxing image or phrase. We have already seen that stretching postures have as a main secondary effect increased awareness and energy. In addition, they can evoke intense and sustained kinesthetic stimulation, which can serve to capture and sustain attention.

However, in it most pure and challenging form, sustaining effortless/ passive simple focus is the definition of *meditation*. For concentrative meditation, the focus is tightly narrow, whereas for mindfulness meditation it is openly diffuse.

At a very crude level, sustaining effortless/passive simple focus can simply involve actively diverting attention from sources of stress, simply changing one's situation or the object of our attention. One may choose to leave the crowded restaurant, or think about the vacation rather than work assignments. Such diversion reduces stimuli that can trigger and maintain arousal. All approaches to relaxation, including causal leisure activities, deploy this skill. Engaging physical techniques such as overt PMR, yogaform stretching, and all breathing exercises perhaps offer the easiest, fastest, and most direct form of diversion.

When sustained, such diversion from sensory input becomes a form of self-imposed sensory deprivation. To the extent stress arousal processes are maintained by stimulus input, restricted input should lessen stress arousal. This may occur at many levels. We have already seen that progressive muscle relaxation may reduce stimulation of the brain, resulting in less worry and negative thought. This in turn may lead to further muscle relaxation. Similarly, sustaining effortless/passive simple focus restricts stimulation from those brain structures responsible for analytic thought and worry. As these structures rest, sustained focus becomes easier. Nonanalytic thought activity, that is, dreamlike imagery, may actually increase. At one time, this process was described as a shift in brain functioning where the usually dominant left cortical hemisphere becomes less active, and the nondominant right hemisphere becomes more active (Naranjo & Ornstein, 1971). To summarize, through meditation the very processes that support self-stressing become less dominant. One learns to deactivate all forms of self-stressing.

There is much debate about other brain mechanisms that may be involved in calm and focused attention. Some believe it is important to consider brain wave activity, slow beta, alpha, and theta in particular. Others consider the synchronization of brain activity. Still others argue the importance of the brain's decision center, the prefrontal cortex. Such considerations are beyond the scope of this book.

Whatever the physiological reasons, sustained effortless/passive simple focus is a difficult and special skill, one most people do not possess. This complex issue merits elaboration.

Most people have experienced brief moments of sustained effortless/passive simple focus. Imagine you are resting on the beach at a quiet vacation spot. The sun is setting and everything grows quiet. Your mind easily attends to the beautiful sunset and nothing else. You feel very quiet and peaceful. Or, imagine you are listening to a very beautiful and peaceful piece of music. The music reaches one section that is especially serene. You are completely and quietly focused. Nothing is on your mind but the music. Or imagine you are resting in a tent at a campsite. It is evening, and everything is very quiet. There is nothing on your mind and you are doing nothing. All the cares of the day are distant memories. Unexpectedly, you hear the gentle sound of a bird. It comes and goes, and again everything is silent. A quiet breeze stirs and touches your skin. Again, everything becomes still, and you simply rest, thinking nothing. You notice the wonderful clean scent of pine. And the scent comes and goes. In each of these situations, you have experienced a moment of passive/effortless simple focus. These moments are part of life's treasures. But they are moments that come and go. One goal of relaxation is to sustain the moment, sustain our effortless/passive simple focus.

In its most pure and challenging form, sustained passive/effortless simple focus is meditation. For concentrative meditation, the focus is limited to a single target, for mindfulness meditation is open to the flow of all stimuli.

Meditation and the Skills of Relaxation

Meditation is the most direct way of evoking the access metaskill of sustained effortless/passive simple focus. However, the precise nature of the skills of meditation, mindfulness, and relaxation have been the subject of some discussion (Dunn, Hartigan, & Mikulas, 1999; Davidson & Kabat-Zinn, 2004). Because this discussion is highly relevant for our presentation of access skills, we will offer our thoughts. Are meditation and mindfulness unique approaches to altering consciousness or are they forms of relaxation? In my opinion, we need to look at all access skills of relaxation.

First, concentrative meditation can be seen as a tool for developing the "simple focus" component of the general skill of sustained passive/effortless simple focus. Mindfulness develops nonattachment, a stance of effortlessness and passivity concerning distraction, the "effortless/passive" part of our defined skill. Both forms of meditation require the "sustained" component of the definition. With this conceptualization, the complete development of sustained effortless/passive simple focus involves both types of complementary meditation.

In contrast, all approaches to meditation involve a bit of relaxation. No meditator is able to sustain effortless/passive simple focus indefinitely without distraction. In order for meditation to work and deepen, the meditator often must briefly and often unconsciously employ other relaxation access skills to deal with distraction. While meditating, one may be distracted by an awkward posture, a tense muscle, tight breathing, and so on. The meditator can put the distraction aside by briefly and automatically (if the skill has been mastered) adjusting posture, letting go, taking a gentle breath, noticing warmth and heaviness, or noting a pleasant affirmation or fantasy—and then move on.

Conversely, all approaches to relaxation involve a bit of meditation. As previously suggested, the meditative act of sustaining effortless/passive simple focus is a part of every family of relaxation, especially (when so emphasized) yoga stretching and breathing exercises. We cannot deliberately maintain a yoga posture, release muscle tension, breathe deeply and slowly, or engage in relaxing autonomic or emotional imagery unless we sustain attention. Before we can adjust a stressed posture, we must attend to and notice that our posture is indeed stressed. Before we can let go of a clenched fist, we must first notice our fist is clenched.

Continuing with this point, we can view all families of relaxation as different types of meditation. Each approach combines the act of focusing (on a posture, muscles, the breath, etc.) with an additional tension/distraction-reducing activity (adjusting posture, letting go, breathing deeply, etc.). These additional activities can be seen as assists or aids to maintaining focus. Here, concentrative and mindfulness meditation are unique, in that they can be done for prolonged periods of time without assists. They are purely attentional strategies. In concentrative meditation, one just attends to a target stimulus, a mantra for example; additional "relaxation" activities such as stretching, tensing and letting go, and thinking suggestions become unnecessary and distracting. In this progression, mindfulness becomes the next step, one of directing calm, undistracted, and focused attention to all the world. Here, even the target focus of concentrative meditation, the mantra, the sensation of breathing, etc., themselves become distracting assists, to be gently put aside. Mindfulness represents the simplest application of the lessons of all of relaxation to all of life. One goes on living, mindfully aware of the present, fully involved in what one is doing, and unattached to passing sensations, emotions, thoughts, or judgments.

SIX FAMILIES OF ACCESS SKILLS

The logic of six families of relaxation may well be traced to six skills of relaxation and six voluntary self-stressing processes. At times, this link provides a justification for applying relaxation techniques. For simple posture, striated muscle tension, and breathing difficulties, direct application of a technique to a symptom is justified and supported by research. For carpal tunnel syndrome, one might apply PMR, yogaform stretching, or autogenic exercises targeted to the hands and wrist.

However, beyond a concrete level of technique-symptom specificity, it is risky to apply families of techniques directly to apparently similar symptom patterns associated with arousal and arousal aftereffects. For example, even though we list autogenic training as a cognitive autonomic technique, we cannot assume it is always best for autonomic arousal. Nor can we assume that cognitive-affective imagery techniques are best for negative and positive affect, in spite of their surface similarity. Let me explain.

I find it useful to think of each family of relaxation as a way of fostering an access skill. Of course, by definition, each access skill is also an effect. After performing a stretch (an access skill), one's joints are stretched (an effect). After releasing muscle tension (an access skill), muscle tension is released (an effect). After breathing slowly (an access skill), one breathes slowly (an effect). For each access skill and family of relaxation there is a defining effect. However, the defining effect may not be the only, or even the most important, effect. Relaxation access skills also give us access to other dimensions of relaxation and enable us to voluntarily (a) cultivate the relaxation response, (b) reduce other forms of self-stressing (e.g., joint-targeted stretching may relax skeletal muscles, letting go of muscle tension through progressive muscle relaxation may cultivate slow breathing, imagery may help foster positive emotion as well as relaxed breathing and reduced muscle tension), (c) contribute to the discovery of relaxation states, and (d) help us achieve goals beyond stress reduction.

TABLE 4.1   Self-Stressing, Relaxation Access Skills, and Relaxation Families

SELF-STRESSING PROCESS	SELF-STRESSING AREA OF MANIFESTATION	RELAXATION ACCESS SKILL/ DEFINING EFFECT	PARALLEL RELAXATION FAMILY
Stressed Posture and Position	Stressed joints; Secondary tension, fatigue, and reduced energy	Stretching	Stretching exercises/Hatha yoga
Stressed Muscles	Skeletal Muscles	Letting Go	Progressive muscle relaxation
Stressed Breathing	Breathing	Relaxed Breathing	Breathing exercises
Stressed Body Focus	Sympathetic Nervous System Arousal	Relaxing Body-Directed Suggestions and Images	Autogenic training
Stressed Emotion	Emotion	Imagery and Self-Talk Focusing on Positive Emotion	Imagery and positive self-talk
Stressed Attention	Attentional Focus (strained, divided, preoccupied, worried)	Sustained Effortless/Passive Simple Focus	Meditation/ Mindfulness

5

The Paths and Landscapes of Relaxation

To fully understand relaxation, we must consider both body and mind. In chapters 3 and 4 we looked at what might be called the engine of relaxation and how we control it. In this chapter we examine the psychological paths and landscapes through which we travel when practicing relaxation.

R-STATES AND THE BENEFITS OF RELAXATION

Research strongly suggests that positive states of mind contribute to greater health, increased immune system competence, enhanced perseverance and problem solving, work success, popularity, recovery from surgery, and longevity (Seligman & Csikszentmihalyi, 2000).

The positive states associated with relaxation can be termed R-States (relaxation states). What are they? If you ask around, you will find many answers. Some claim relaxation helps them feel "peaceful," or "rested." Others feel "sleepy" after practicing and still others feel "energized." Some report feeling "thankful" or even "prayerful." Clearly people feel much more than just "relaxed" when they practice relaxation. I have devoted over a decade of research to sorting and mapping R-States. I started with an exhaustive catalog of 400 words used in core textbooks of progressive muscle relaxation, autogenic training, yoga, breathing exercises, imagery, creative visualization, tai chi, self-hypnosis, meditation, contemplation, and prayer.

Several dozen studies, involving over 10,000 participants, revealed an interesting map of 15 R-States:[1] (Most R-States are comprised of groups of words identified through factor analysis. Generally, for each factor grouping the highest loading word or words were selected as R-State labels.)

- Sleepiness
- Disengagement
- Rested/Refreshed
- Energized
- Physical Relaxation,
- At Ease/Peace
- Joy (Happy)
- Mental Quiet
- Childlike Innocence
- Thankful/Loving
- Deep Mystery
- Awe/Wonder
- Prayerful
- Timeless/Boundless/Infinite/At One
- Aware (meta R-State)

THE R-STATE PYRAMID

The R-State pyramid is a tool for helping us understand the relationships among R-States. It consists of horizontal and vertical dimensions, columns, and levels).

Three columns of R-States reflect a cycle of healing and growth set into motion by relaxation. The three phases of this *cycle of renewal* are: (1) *withdrawal* from sources of stimulation, stress, and arousal, (2) *recovery* from fatigue, effort, and tension, as well as *release* from the constraints and burdens of adult, analytic, verbal thinking and ordinary everyday expectations, and (3) *opening up* to the world, renewed and refreshed. Each phase or column has its own R-States. For example, R-State Disengagement is defined as *withdrawal from and reduced awareness of external stimuli*; it clearly

---

[1]To earn placement on this list, an R-State had to emerge as an orthogonal dimension in at least one factor analysis or (in the case of Rested/Refreshed and Childlike Innocence) appear as an independent predictor or correlate in at least one study (Lewis, 2001; Smith & Sohnle, 2001). I chose a liberal inclusion strategy given the persistent reductionistic bias of relaxation research.

fits within the column, Withdrawal. Rested/Refreshed is a manifestation of Recovery/Release, and Energized reflects Opening Up. We explore more subtle distinctions later.

In addition, R-States can be organized into five levels:

Level 1—Stress Relief
Level 2—Pleasure and Joy
Level 3—Positive Selflessness
Level 4—Spirituality
Level 5—Transcendence

Each level is more abstract (conducive to philosophical interpretation) and encompassing (it can incorporate lower levels). In addition, higher levels reflect increased sustained effortless/passive simple focus. (Please refer to Figure 5.1 to see how columns and levels build a pyramid.)

Level 1: Stress Relief includes relatively concrete and limited R-States associated with stress relief. These states are easy to identify, even by those not skilled at relaxation.

Column 1, Withdrawal, is represented by two R-States, Sleepiness (feeling "drowsy," "napping off") and Disengagement ("far away," "indifferent," "distant"). Most relaxation instructors recognize that people who relax sometimes feel sleepy and even slip into a nap. Although sleep can be a distraction to completing an exercise, sleepiness is perhaps an important component of most, if not all, forms of relaxation. It may represent withdrawal at a concrete and undifferentiated level. Beginning relaxers may lack the ability to differentiate the subtleties of higher R-States and experience most of relaxation in terms of napping and sleep.

Disengagement also involves withdrawal from, and reduced awareness of, the world. Three types of statements illustrate this concrete level of withdrawal, spatial, attitudinal, and somatic. States such as feeling "distant," "far away," or "in my own world," are primarily spatial. In contrast, statements such as feeling "detached," "indifferent," "not caring about anything," or "unmoved or unbothered" represent an attitude of withdrawal. Finally, as relaxation progresses, one may display a type of disengagement in which one becomes less aware of one's limbs and parts of one's body. A person may realize that he or she has completely lost awareness of hands, arms, legs, or feet. More dramatically, a person may have an "out-of-body experience" in which he or she feels as though, or hallucinates that he or she is, floating above and observing the physical body. All of these experiences, although often dramatic, are usually quite normal and reflect another manifestation of

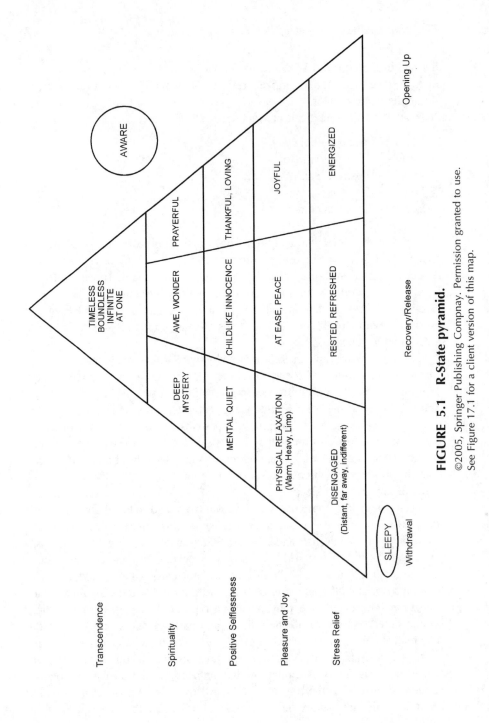

FIGURE 5.1   R-State pyramid.

©2005, Springer Publishing Compnay. Permission granted to use.
See Figure 17.1 for a client version of this map.

disengagement. Clinically, one might view R-State Disengagement at least in part as low-level, potentially adaptive dissociation.

Our research (Smith, 2001) has frequently found that individuals under high levels of stress or pain, or displaying above-average levels of diverse forms of psychopathology, including anxiety, depression, and hostility, report a constricted range of R-States. When asked to describe their most effective way of relaxing, and to think about their most recent attempt at relaxing, Disengagement consistently emerges as the R-State evoked by this activity. Apparently, troubled individuals think of relaxation in terms of withdrawal from, or reduced awareness of, a source of distress. In contrast, individuals not under stress or pain or not displaying high levels of psychopathology are much more likely to report a rich variety of R-States, notably At Ease/Peace and to some extent Joy and Energized.

Continuing at Level 1, Stress Relief, Column 2, Recovery and Release, we find the R-State, Rested/Refreshed. Concretely, one feels rested and refreshed when effort and fatigue are reduced. These are the feelings one has after a nap. They are readily identified and expressed by beginning practitioners of relaxation.

Column 3, Opening Up, is defined concretely by the R-State, Energized. When stress and fatigue are gone, and one is refreshed, one can open up to full involvement in the world. Other words associated with this R-State are "strengthened" and "confident." A substantial literature has developed on the dimension of "self-efficacy," a dimension of perceived personal competence. The R-State, Energized may underlie a sense of personal self-efficacy.

Level 2: Pleasure and Joy includes positive states of sustained effortless simple focus that have a rich and intense affective and sensory component. These states are also relatively concrete and easily identified by beginners.

One withdraws (Column 1) into a world of pleasant Physical Relaxation ("limp," "warm," "heavy," "sensuous, pleasant body feelings"). Surprisingly, the R-State, Physical Relaxation, has been difficult to define. The full lexicon of words people use to describe physical relaxation (determined through factor analysis) includes: "dissolving, elastic, light, limp, listless, liquid, heavy, massaged, melting, motionless, sensual, sinking, slack, slow, supple, throbbing, tingling, and warm." The experience of Physical Relaxation reflects withdrawal from everyday discursive pursuits into the pleasures of the body associated with relaxation. This is most obvious in simple activities such as sitting in a hot tub or sauna, sunbathing, or receiving a massage. One might feel pleasantly "limp, warm, heavy," and so on.

One must be careful interpreting words such as "limp," "warm," and "heavy." They can also refer to R-States other than Physical Relaxation.

Clients may feel "warm" while feeling "Joy," "Thankful/Loving," and even "Timeless/Boundless" or they may feel "heavy" or "far away" when Disengaged. Conversely, when sick, anxious, angry, or even depressed, one might also feel "limp," "warm," or "heavy." To minimize misunderstanding, it is important to make sure a person is indeed referring to positive states and that these states are associated with relaxation. For example, I ask, "Are you feeling *relaxed* and warm?" rather than simply "Are you feeling warm?"

I recommend not thinking of R-State Physical Relaxation and physical stress as direct opposites or end points on a single continuum. I find that in relaxation training, R-State Physical Relaxation typically emerges early, whereas reductions in symptoms of physical stress may emerge several sessions later.

Recovery/Release (Column 2) is strongly represented by the R-State, At Ease/Peace. Initial item content (Smith, 1999a) for this factor is revealing: "at ease, calm, carefree, contented, laid back, peaceful, relaxed, restored, soothed." Dictionary definitions of these items reveal that they all connote an absence of tension ("calm, relaxed"), conflict ("peaceful"), threat ("carefree"), desire and frustration ("contented"), fatigue ("rested, restored"), pain ("soothed"), or effort ("at ease, laid back"). Factor analytic research suggests that diverse expressions of recovery and release are most generally conveyed by the terms "At Ease and Peace, the title of this R-State.

One opens up (Column 3) in relaxation to stimuli that evoke R-State Joy (happiness). Much of research in positive psychology has focused on joy to the exclusion of other R-States. Indeed, this is my biggest criticism of this area of research.

Joy accounts for much of what nonclinical individuals report during relaxation. And joy is diverse and forms the central feature of feelings of beauty, optimism, fun, mirth, humor, harmony, and so on. When clients use these words in relaxation, they are elaborating on their feeling of Joy. In addition, joy may be a consequence of sustained, undistracted awareness. Once the window is free of dust, one can attend clearly. In time, as one sustains attention, one opens up to a world of beauty and joy.

Level 3: Positive Selflessness includes R-States that reflect reduced self-referent, analytic, goal-directed thinking, not necessarily in a spiritual context. The key feature is reduced self-reference, a notion that can be difficult to understand.

First, when people think of selflessness, they often think of elimination of a negative, an undesired "ego." There are many types of negative selflessness, including humility, obedient surrender to authority, painful renunciation of things the ego may desire, and self-inflicted penance for perceived sins. Negative selflessness may have its place; however, it can be a source of tension. We consider positive selflessness, or simply reduced self-referent thought, to be intrinsically reinforcing.

To begin, needless tension often has a "selfish" or self-directed component. Consider the following statements:

> "I am fearful of speaking in public places. I am concerned about what people might think of me."

> "I am deeply frustrated that I am single and do not have a lover. One of my important needs is not being met."

> "I am very angry at my lover. She always wants her way and never thinks of me. I am left out of the picture."

> "I feel depressed and hopeless. There is nothing in life for me. I am empty."

Obviously, these are expressions of distress. Let's consider another set of states that reflect self-induced tension, if not distress:

> "I am a perfectionist. It is important to me that everything fit my personal exacting standards, even if they are more rigorous than the standards of other people."

> "I want to win that game. I push myself to the max. 'Come on, you can do it!' I say."

> "I must get rid of that awful pain. I just can't go on without banishing it from me."

If you examine these two sets of statements very carefully, you will realize that in each statement the person has a serious concern *about him- or herself.* He or is she is self-aware (of his or her pains, desires, frustrations, needs, threats, losses, and so on). In each case, the individual is the star, the center of attention, of a tiny story about him- or herself, a small soap opera. The importance of self-involvement or self-directed attention may be made clear if you come up with a descriptive title for each story. The titles might sound like this:

My Fear of Public Speaking
My Life as a Single Person
My Complaint About My Lover

My Empty Life
My Pursuit of Perfection
My Determination To Win
My Terrible Pain

Each is a story about "me"; each is self-directed. In each, part of one's attention is diverted from the outside world and pointed to oneself, that is, one's personal hurt, desire, frustration, fear, and so on.

Level 3 of the pyramid, Positive Selflessness, simply involves reduction of self-directed focus. When this key element is reduced, tension in general lessens. We can now consider the three columns under Positive Selflessness.

The R-State, Mental Quiet, involves withdrawal from the world into inner silence and quiet. All thought and emotion are minimized. Positive emotions like joy and happiness are also absent. Even R-States such as At Ease/Peace are no longer present. The mind is completely quiet and silent. It is important to note that in the state of Mental Quiet one is not "asleep," "blank," "dazed," or "numb." One remains quietly awake. In the state of Mental Quiet, even self-referent thinking is stilled (along with all other thoughts). Even positive or negative feelings about oneself are stilled (along with all other feelings). In this sense, Mental Quiet is very much a selfless state.

The R-State, Childlike Innocence, is selfless in a different way, one that reflects Recovery/Release, of which it is a part. The key questions to ask about Childlike Innocence are: What is being released? How is one selfless? It is here that one lets go or releases certain burdens of adulthood, burdens that call for a degree of self-directed attention. Consider what it means to be a responsible adult in today's complex world. *You* are responsible for finding *your* own housing, *you* are responsible for getting *your* own food, *you* are responsible for supporting *your* own family, *you* are responsible for taking care of *your* health, and so on. Generally, none of these are provided for *you*. *You* have to do much of it by *yourself*. This is the self-focused burden of adulthood, "I am responsible for a lot." In the R-State, Childlike Innocence, we temporarily let go of the normal burdens of the adult role, the adult self, and become carefree. The most complete image for such release is Childlike Innocence, and it is very much a type of positive selflessness.

Opening Up at Level 3 is displayed by the R-State, Thankful/Loving. The selfless quality of this R-State is easy to describe. Self-directed concern diminishes as one experiences thankfulness, possibly for the R-States evoked through relaxation. Such concerns also lessen as one wishes to share the rewards of relaxation with others, sharing being an act of love and care. Note that when you are in the R-State Thankful/Loving you are less aware of yourself and more aware of the recipient of your thankfulness and love. Such loving appreciation reflects a type of opening up. Clearly, in love we open up to understanding and appreciating another person. Thankful appreciation connotes an openness to all of that for which we are thankful: "I genuinely appreciate all that you have done for me."

To summarize, at the level of Positive Selflessness, the defining feature of each R-State is a reduction in self-directed worry, concern, desire, and so on. Such thoughts are stilled (Mental Quiet), released as adult burdens (Childlike Innocence), or supplanted by other-directed thought (Thankful/Loving).

Level 4: Spirituality incorporates and goes beyond Positive Selflessness. One is less concerned about oneself and aware of a larger, greater reality beyond oneself. It is beyond the scope of this book to specify what this reality may be; the reader has both supernatural and natural options: God, Allah, the unconscious, the flow of being, the higher power, or perhaps just the night sky. Suffice it to say that atheists (those who do not accept the notion of an unprovable, supernatural/paranormal entity that answers personal prayers by altering the laws of physics and changing the course of history) can have deeply authentic spiritual experiences.

The spiritual R-State, Deep Mystery ("I sense the Deep Mystery of things beyond my understanding") reflects an appreciation of a deeper and greater reality that is beyond comprehension. As such, Deep Mystery suggests a certain distance, or withdrawal, from a deeper reality. This reality may itself be "far away" from one's understanding ("The universe is so big I can't possibly understand it all"). Or one might experience a withdrawal from concepts and appraisal processes that had provided a false sense of understanding of the incomprehensible. ("Now that my mind is quiet, I realize I never fully appreciated how big the universe actually is").

The R-State, Awe and Wonder, reflects a nonanalytic and goal-less awareness of a larger and greater reality that is new, awesome, beyond ordinary expectations; it is "extra-ordinary." Put simply, one releases everyday and familiar expectations. This can occur several ways. One might feel profoundly free and detached from the preoccupying burdens and expectations of daily life, and see the world freshly through different eyes. The R-State, Awe and Wonder, can reflect a childlike and innocent release from adult, verbal, analytic thinking; one might feel like a small child facing a wonderful, larger world. Awe and Wonder can also result from momentary "decommissioning" of adult analytic thinking. The Grand Canyon can leave one "struck with awe." Here the intensity and immensity of an external stimulus leave one temporarily "shocked" or "blinded." Our language provides many phrases that convey this notion: "shock of the new," "blinding truth," "dumbstruck," "speechless," "far out," "mindblowing," "knocks one's socks off," or simply "Wow!" or "Amazing!" However expressed, one's adult, verbal, analytic thinking cap has been knocked askew; one is temporarily freed or released from these constraints and sees things anew.

The R-State, Prayerful, is an affective response to a perceived larger, greater reality. One opens up and feels reverent, spiritual, and worshipful. In a religious context, one might express opening up through expressions of profound love or surrender. Additional words that reflect this R-State are "worshipful, spiritual, blessed, reverent, thankful, answered, reborn, cleansed, and surrendering."

The three spiritual R-States often appear together; one may well feel Deep Mystery, Awe and Wonder, and Prayerful at the same time. However subtle, distinctions can be made. Awe and Wonder is not quite the same as Deep Mystery. For example, a master painting, an elegantly designed automobile, or an unexpected achievement from a child may evoke awe and wonder, yet not be mysterious; they can remain fully understandable. In contrast, a premonition that occurs with some reliability every night in a dream is not unexpected; however, it might be quite mysterious. Perhaps it is useful to view spiritual R-States as different facets of a spiritual response, one that can be expressed in three simple statements: Deep Mystery—("I do not understand this"), Awe and Wonder—("I do not expect this"), and Prayerfulness—("I feel reverence towards this").

Level 5: Transcendence is defined by the R-State, Timeless/Boundless/Infinite/At One (or simply, Timeless/Boundless/Infinite). Here, too, one is aware of something larger or greater than oneself. But for the first time one forgets oneself as much as is absolutely possible and becomes completely aware of a transcendent "other."

How is transcendence different from spirituality? In one simple way. Spirituality always involves awareness of a relationship between oneself and some larger, greater other. *You* feel Deep Mystery when *you* cannot figure out this reality. *Your* expectations are challenged when facing what is awesome. *You* relate to a larger, greater other in prayer. It is always you and the larger, greater other. In Transcendence, you forget yourself as much as is absolutely possible and are just aware of the larger, greater other, in and of itself. At this level of abstraction, obviously everything is included ("infinite, boundless"); therefore, there is no fundamental distinction between any conceivable component, including oneself and the world and past and future. One therefore might feel "Timeless" or "At One."

The component descriptors of the R-State, Timeless/Boundless/Infinite loosely parallel the dimensions of Withdrawal, Recovery/Release, and Opening Up on the pyramid. "Timeless" suggests withdrawal from moment-to-moment, day-to-day temporal awareness. One forgets time itself. "Boundless" reflects a release from conceptual boundaries, distinctions, and limits. "Infinite" reflects an experience of opening up, not just to a specific experience, but also to all that is. "At one" combines all three.

Aware: The meta R-State. Our fifteenth R-State, Aware, is a meta state that can appear at any level, in any column of the pyramid. One can be Aware and Disengaged, Aware and Physically Relaxed, Aware and Mentally Quiet, and so on. Or one might be just Aware, and not particularly cognizant of any other R-State. However, our research has found that the state of being Aware most often appears with being Energized, but somewhat less so with Mental Quiet, suggesting that Awareness can be manifest at two levels. At a basic level of stress relief, reports of feeling Aware reflect strength, energy, and confidence, a readiness to open up to the world. At a higher level of selflessness, Aware may reflect a basic quality of Mental Quiet, an experience that remains when affective, somatic, and cognitive content have stilled. Thus, feeling Aware can depict opposite experiences, one of increased cognitive content, or one of reduced content.

Paths of R-States

R-States can be experienced in sequence, even in a single session. In this sense, R-States can define a relaxation path. To give an obvious example, a napper may first experience Sleepiness, then become Rested/Refreshed, and then Energized, possibly experiencing Joy, thus defining the following "napping path":

Sleepiness → Rested/Refreshed → Energized → Joy

Generally, I find this progression of effects for those practicing techniques involving progressive muscle relaxation or autogenic training:

Sleepiness → Disengagement → Physical Relaxation →At Ease/Peace; Joy; Mental Quiet → Other R-States

As mentioned earlier, I find that individuals scoring high on tests of clinical anxiety, depression, and hostility (Smith, 2001) tend to report Sleepiness and Disengagement. They seem to lack the ability to achieve significant sustained effortless simple focus or to detect and differentiate R-States. They have not traveled far along any relaxation path.

The paths for individuals not experiencing severe stress or psychopathology are a bit more differentiated. Early in training, practitioners typically are able to experience, identify, and differentiate R-States at the first two levels, first Stress Relief and then Pleasure and Joy. As training progresses, Mental Quiet and Thankfulness and Love are often the first higher-level R-States to emerge. Mental Quiet reflects the absence of thought and emotion directly associated with significantly reduced discursive effort. Thankfulness and Love reflect the appreciation one may have for experiencing R-States. It should be noted that any R-State may emerge spontaneously at any time in training, providing a glimpse of relaxation's potential. Such moments should not be ignored, but reinforced. Indeed, they may prompt serious thinking about one's life philosophy, which can, in turn, have an impact on relaxation.

Finally, individuals usually experience several R-States in combination. The patterns can be hard to predict. One might feel "Happy" (Joyful) and Rested/Refreshed, Disengaged, Aware, and so on. Perhaps it is more useful to consider our pyramid not so much as a rigid map as a palette of pigments which different artists may mix in a variety of ways.

The Value of R-States

R-States are powerful reinforcers to continue practicing a relaxation technique. Indeed, I predict that practitioners who experience valued R-States in relaxation are more likely to continue practicing and benefit from their techniques. By explaining, measuring, and discussing R-States, one sensitizes clients to the potential rewards of continued practice. Second, society often discounts R-States as distractions to true productivity, as laziness or a needless indulgence to be enjoyed only after work, or at best as good feelings as inconsequential as a passing memory of a good meal. Positive psychology, in spite of its limited focus on "happiness," has shown clearly that positive states have a direct impact on health, immune system functioning, and even longevity. They are central to the very physiological benefits clients may seek. Perhaps the most important task of a relaxation trainer is to persuade a client that R-States are not trivial and passing moods, but a fundamental and powerful part of all of relaxation.

Finally, R-States help clients articulate their relaxation goals, and integrate relaxation with the rest of life. If relaxation is simply viewed as physical stress relief, then it is little more than a nap—one practices a technique and returns to work. By considering the full rainbow of R-States, clients can appreciate the value of relaxation for goals beyond stress relief.

6

The Destinations of Relaxation:
Ten Great Goals

We have nearly completed our survey of relaxation basics and have considered a variety of families of techniques and perspectives. We looked at the vehicle and underlying engine of relaxation and basic access skills, and surveyed the psychological paths and landscapes of relaxation, the map of 15 R-States. This chapter examines where the vehicle of relaxation travels, its destination. In other words, why relax?

Professional deep relaxation has been applied to 10 overall goals (Figure 6.1). Techniques have been used to enhance sleep, alleviate unwanted states, achieve states that may be desired, and explore the possibilities beyond everyday frustrations and joys. In more formal terms, these are the sleep-related, negative, positive, and transcendent goals of relaxation. Of these, sleep-related and negative goals are adequately supported by research, whereas positive and transcendent goals are reflected in numerous anecdotal accounts and form the basis of centuries of promotional claims for various relaxation and meditation techniques. However, it is not the purpose of this chapter to review supportive research, but simply to articulate goals that have been expressed over thousands of years.

SLEEP-RELATED GOALS OF RELAXATION

People untrained in professional deep relaxation often think relaxation is sleep. Indeed, combating insomnia as well as enhancing sleep and mastering

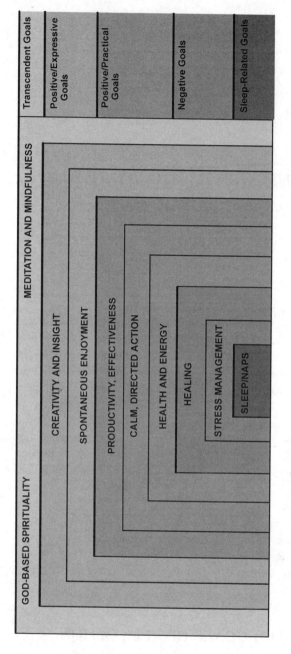

FIGURE 6.1   The 10 great goals of relaxation.

the skill of "catnapping" or "power napping" can be important preliminary goals of relaxation. Insomnia is one of several specific sleep disorders, the treatment of which is beyond the scope of this book. Suffice it to say that most treatments incorporate professional relaxation as a way of preparing for sleep. We have found that clients, through trial and error, may select any of the six families of relaxation.

For individuals not displaying a specific sleep disorder, the goal of enhancing sleep may have several objectives, ranging from increasing the ability to sleep through interruption to enhancing dreams. A catnap or power nap is a 10–25 minute sleep session, practiced usually in the middle of the day for renewed energy. A "boosted power nap" is a nap session preceded by a 5-minute relaxation session (see chapter 20, "spot and mini-relaxation").

THE NEGATIVE GOALS OF RELAXATION: STRESS MANAGEMENT/HEALING

A Review

One relaxation goal has defined professional training for over a century. Overall and targeted reductions in stress arousal can alleviate physical symptoms, fatigue, pain, discomfort, physiological arousal, negative emotions, and worry. These same processes can enhance recovery from illness and injury. We can formally name these *the goals of stress management and healing.* Both are *negative* goals in that they involve reducing or minimizing something one does not want, a negative. Four key points of chapter 3 are worth repeating. Relaxation appears to have the potential for:

1. Reducing susceptibility to illness;
2. Relieving the destructive wear and tear of severe and chronic stress arousal on specific body systems and organs as well as on the body's immune system;
3. Speeding healing and recovery from nonchronic conditions (for example, the wounds of physically injured people who are relaxed heal more quickly);
4. Reducing serious complications of chronic conditions (for example, individuals with AIDS or diabetes appear to do better); and
5. Reducing the destructive impact of stress on functioning (attention, flexibility, memory, energy).

It is likely that the negative goals of relaxation have saved many lives and contributed substantially to the health and wellbeing of thousands. It would take another set of volumes to explain the precise physiological mechanisms underlying the impact of relaxation on AIDS, diabetes, hypertension, peptic ulcers, psoriasis, and the like.

In this chapter we go beyond traditional negative conceptualizations of stress management and healing, and consider additional goals of relaxation. We begin by considering what has been the most serious roadblock to such an encompassing vision, the bias that has defined the field for over a century.

The Medical-Model Bias

For over a century, negative goals have defined the professional study and practice of relaxation. Most health professionals and clients think of relaxation only as a bodily response or some alteration in brain functioning, as nothing more than the relaxation engine. Too often, bodily changes are assumed to be more basic, perhaps "more real," than other processes. Relaxation's impact on feelings, thoughts, and behaviors are of secondary importance, "grounded" only to the extent that "basic, underlying physiological processes" can be identified.

Such thinking reflects a medical-model bias because it is analogous to how physicians conceptualize illness. Diseases are understood in terms of symptoms that can be traced to underlying physical problems in the body or brain. Your cough may be caused by inflamed lungs. Your legs may hurt because of arthritis. The inflammation or arthritis are basic, underlying physiological causes. Indeed, the underlying pathology is no less real or important even when symptoms of distress are absent. At first it may seem that this is an academic issue, not relevant for the real-world practice of relaxation. However, I suggest that the prevailing medical-model bias has actual and measurable costs on how relaxation has been taught and how relaxation goals have been selected, for example:

- The medical model of relaxation promotes a "one size fits all" strategy in which all clients are taught the same family of practices. This, in turn, increases the risk that clients will receive families that are not ideally suited for them.
- The medical model of relaxation offers little advice for practitioners who have mastered the relaxation response and want more.

• The medical model of relaxation risks making relaxation training a mechanical health chore, something like a prescribed fitness routine one does and puts aside. The possibility of integrating relaxation with work, sports, study, and leisure is reduced. Relaxation becomes a boring exercise not tied to what deeply interests or motivates clients. Potential clients may not be sufficiently motivated to try relaxation, and clients may quit practicing out of lack of interest

Let me elaborate. First, those who define relaxation in terms of the medical model have difficulty identifying important and consistent differences between families of approaches. Progressive muscle relaxation, autogenic training, imagery/relaxing self-talk, and meditation may all have more or less similar physiological effects, primarily the relaxation response. And if different families basically have the same effect, it makes little sense to teach more than one family. It doesn't really matter which family one chooses because they are all more or less interchangeable, like different versions of an anxiety medication. At best, astute textbooks may caution that some clients may have "special needs" that rule out or call for some techniques over others (for example, avoid teaching deep breathing exercises to someone who has just had lung surgery). However, these special needs are either obvious caveats or untested guesses. The dominance of the medical model is most readily apparent in how relaxation is actually taught in clinics, hospital, businesses, and stress-reduction programs. Here the near universal practice is to present exercises from a single family.

Second, it is a little known but well researched finding that most clients can learn the relaxation response in about a month (Lehrer & Woolfolk, 1993; Smith, 1999a). This is the time it takes for most people to learn how to effectively release tension. According to the medical model of relaxation, a desired physiological change has occurred and relaxation training is over (except for possible booster sessions). Yet, many continue their approach to professional deep relaxation for more than a month, often for years and even decades. It is easy to find practitioners of yoga, stretching, meditation, imagery, and the like who have incorporated their preferred family of practices into their daily routine. Furthermore, if you ask these long-term practitioners why they continue, few say "to evoke the relaxation response." Most can articulate more encompassing psychological and even spiritual goals. The medical model says little about what long-term practitioners might get from such extended practice.

Third, the medical model of relaxation can prompt trainers and practitioners to miss important and subtle psychological and behavioral effects that may augment and deepen the effects of relaxation (even physiological changes). Let me share with you the example of Ernie, a young student of progressive muscle relaxation (PMR):

> Ernie has been practicing PMR for three months to alleviate his headaches. After the first month, his headache problem abated, but Ernie continued practice. One session was particularly good. During the session he felt nicely loose and relaxed. This was not particularly unusual. However, he was surprised by a completely unexpected experience that occurred an hour after training, while driving home. "I was filled with a very deep sense of inner silence, love, and thankfulness, stronger than I had ever felt before. The feeling was very wonderful. I was overjoyed and amazed."

A traditional trainer of progressive muscle relaxation might smile, acknowledge Ernie's report, and do nothing. He or she may well accept payment and discharge Ernie as "cured." From a medical-model perspective, PMR indeed did its work. The headache was gone and Ernie learned to become nicely loose and relaxed. However, if we look at his report carefully, you may detect that Ernie has reported four R-States: Mental Quiet, Thankfulness and Love, Joy, and Mental Quiet. These R-States emerged an hour after the session, "while driving home." Such delayed aftereffects seem to be characteristic of practitioners who are progressing well. Furthermore, the four R-States Ernie reported are advanced, high-level states on the pyramid (chapter 5). Beginners (especially males) rarely experience states at this high level, and rarely experience this number of R-States together. In sum, whereas a medical-model perspective might conclude that Ernie has mastered the relaxation response and eliminated an unwanted symptom, his reports suggest that he is doing so well at developing his relaxation skills that he may be ready for deeper and more advanced interventions and goals beyond tension reduction—goals not considered by his trainer.

The following is an alternative ending to this brief relaxation story. In it, the trainer has read and applies the ideas of this book:

> Ernie reports, "I'm enjoying my PMR and it seems to do more than get rid of my headaches. It gives me enthusiasm and hope for the day. I feel like I have tapped into energy I never knew I had. I would like to explore this further. After considerable discussion, my trainer and I decided I might

consider breathing exercises and meditation. My new goal for relaxation is to develop my skills at focusing and enjoying what relaxation has to offer. Perhaps relaxation will enhance my creativity and stamina at work. I would sure like something to help me recover quickly from a tough day. And perhaps I can find new meaning when reading my religious books."

Proponents of the medical model of relaxation claim that their perspective is more basic because any possible psychological or behavioral benefit, even those reported by practitioners such as Ernie, must have some physiological basis. Every R-State on the pyramid must be caused by something in the body and the brain. However, many of the physiological processes presumed to form the basis of R-States and relaxation goals have yet to be discovered, and may well not be discovered for decades, if at all. Saying that a physiological process "could theoretically be discovered" is not the same as saying the process "is already known." One cannot base a credible system of relaxation, or even a workable theory, on such promissory notes.

There is a place for the medical model. However, let me suggest that as trainers we should exercise a bit of humility when tempted to proclaim one perspective "more basic" or say that we are "grounded" in another. In a journey, one does not speak of a vehicle engine, or control panel, or path and landscape, or end destination as the "most basic part." All parts are equally important. Those who focus excessively on the medical model risk missing the richness of relaxation, including the many skills, paths, landscapes, and destinations that are available. They risk spending their entire vacation polishing and tuning the engine.

Standing back, let me say that contemporary psychology is one of the great success stories of modern science. With limited or no reliance on medical-model variables, psychology has made major and profoundly useful discoveries concerning a myriad of psychological and behavioral variables—aggression, love, and grief, to name only three. It is not particularly informative or helpful to speak of a medical model of aggression, love, or grief. If anything, psychology has taught us that aggression is more than a clenched jaw. Love is more than a heartbeat. Grief is more than a tear. Likewise, relaxation is more than the relaxation response.

Stress management and healing are real and worthy goals of professional deep relaxation. However, it is important to realize that additional goals are available. And as we shall see, these additional goals may well enhance relaxation's negative potential.

THE POSITIVE PRACTICAL GOALS OF RELAXATION: HEALTH AND ENERGY/CALM DIRECTED ACTION/ PRODUCTIVITY AND EFFECTIVENESS

The negative goals of relaxation involve getting rid of something one does not want. The positive goals involve getting what one wants. Given the dominance of the medical model, empirical research on positive goals is in its infancy; so let me share my hypotheses.

The goal of *health and energy* seeks to maintain health and resistance to disease, and increase energy reserves and stamina. Those who use relaxation as a tool for enhancing health and energy have acquired a healthy habit, not unlike good diet, exercise, sleep, and proper hygiene. For them, the practice of relaxation limits extremes of stress arousal, enhances routine recovery from the stressors of daily living, and helps support a positive frame of mind. Energy is enhanced by limiting unnecessarily draining stress and worry, thus enabling the body to recover from sustained discursive effort, and opening sources of energy by enhancing breathing and cardiac functions.

The goal of *calm directed action* (or more briefly, "calm direction") is to continue with a chosen task in spite of distraction or the urge to do something else or quit. It is the application of the relaxation access meta skill of sustained effortless/passive simple focus to the tasks and challenges of active living. Calm direction is the opposite of excessive self-stressed attention in which one strains to focus on a task, wastes energy through inefficient multitasking, and divides attention between self-directed worries and concerns and the task at hand. Calm direction has the additional emphasis of sustaining attention on a desired course of action, and returning to this course of action after internal or external distraction.

Calm directed action can be misunderstood. It does not refer to a stern, self-conscious overcontrol of thoughts and feelings. It is not the fierce and deliberate concentration one might display in the last phases of a competitive game. Instead, calm direction involves carrying the effortless simple focus of the relaxation session into active life. Unnecessary sources of tension, worry, and negative emotion, as well as boredom and distracting desire, are lessened so that one can pursue one's chosen activities with fewer distractions.

The skill of calmly letting go of a distraction and returning to a relaxation task is rehearsed in a relaxation practice session and can be generalized to active life. For example, a practitioner of yoga stretching learns to maintain focus on a simple stretch. Irrelevant thoughts, both positive and negative, interfere with completing a good, focused stretch (a distracted stretch becomes "jerky," "forced," or "uneven"). The practitioner learns to put such distractions aside and continue with his or her yoga stretch. Similarly, in active life, he or she puts distraction aside to continue with the task of the moment.

Such calm direction can apply to addictions. Any craving can be seen as a disturbing distraction. A cigarette smoker craves a cigarette. She is upset until she gets a smoke. Feelings of craving interfere with what she wants to do. The skill of relaxation involves learning to (1) reduce overall tension, so that the disturbance of craving is less intense, (2) put aside distracting impulses, including the craving impulse, or (3) calmly and nonjudgmentally (mindfully) tolerate a continuing craving while devoting one's primary focus to the task at hand. Furthermore, relaxation provides the addicted individual with a tool for dealing with life's demands, lessening the need to resort to addictive behavior.

Finally, relaxation can be used to enhance effectiveness at work, school, or sports. This goal is partly a combination of the previous two goals, and is also a goal in and of itself.

THE POSITIVE EXPRESSIVE GOALS OF RELAXATION: SPONTANEOUS ENJOYMENT/CREATIVITY AND INSIGHT

Relaxation becomes an expressive activity when it is done because it is fun or meaningful, and does not necessarily have any immediate pragmatic use.

The simplest expressive goal is simple *enjoyment*, practicing a relaxation exercise because it is fun or because it contributes to the unstructured, unplanned, and spontaneous enjoyment of another fun activity. Any of the six families can be presented in the spirit of play and pleasure. PMR and yoga become dance, imagery becomes storytelling, meditation becomes an adventure, and so on. Furthermore, one can deliberately introduce relaxation before a pleasurable activity, for example, by practicing breathing exercises before dancing, meditating before a concert, etc.

The goal of *creativity and insight* involves nurturing an expressive source of ideas. Of course, creativity and insight may be required for highly pragmatic goals, for example, deciding on a job, a term paper topic, a new business strategy, a course of action in a crisis, or a proper gift for a friend. However, the act of brainstorming, of actually generating potential ideas, involves temporarily putting aside pragmatic concerns and freely entertaining all ideas, good and bad, sane and silly. To this end, relaxation can very much enhance creativity and insight.

A different type of creativity and insight is far less structured. One might put aside one's logical thinking cap and accept whatever experiences or insights may emerge in a practice. Here one begins not so much with a goal but with an open mind, a willingness to accept whatever relaxation may bring.

THE TRANSCENDENT GOALS OF RELAXATION: GOD-BASED SPIRITUALITY/MEDITATION AND MINDFULNESS

Transcendent goals involve going beyond one's everyday wants, both negative and positive. Self-directed concerns are minimized. *God-based spirituality* focuses on celebrating and relating to a theistic entity, one's God or Higher Power. This may or may not be in the context of organized religion. And the goal of *meditation/mindfulness* has as its goal the cultivation of calm and focused awareness and action in the world as it is, undistracted by irrelevant personal concerns or biases. For God-based spirituality, one transcends self-centered negative and positive motivations and expectations in service of God or one's Higher Power; for mediation/mindfulness, one transcends such distracting personal motivations and expectations in order to see and act in the world as it really is. We consider these two goals more extensively in the final chapter of this book.

The goal of meditation/mindfulness can be distinguished from the goal of calm directed action considered earlier. Calm direction is concerned primarily with pursuing and completing a desired and chosen course of action. You want to complete an important work assignment in the next two hours, but have the urge to snack, get a drink, quit, and so on. The skill of calm direction enables you to complete what you want to do. You want very much to learn to play the drums, but are tempted to interrupt your practice to call your friends, go out for coffee, or read a comic. Calm direction involves staying on the task you want to do. For meditation/mindfulness, your desires are not the main concern. Primary is the philosophical commitment to seeing the world as it actually is, and acting honestly and realistically in the real world—in spite of your personal biases, wishes, habits, and so on. Meditation/mindfulness involves in part cultivating something of a personal philosophy, one that values selfless awareness, calm, and honesty. It is not a means to an end but an end in and of itself.

OVERLAPPING GOALS

Taken together, the ten goals of relaxation are not isolated, but overlapping. Some goals can be components of another. You may want to learn relaxation to enhance your performance at sports (health and energy, calm direction). In addition, a chronic backache interferes with how much energy you have for sports. So, you may also want to include relaxation exercises to target back pain (stress management). Or you may wish to enhance your creativity and insight as a student, artist, or entrepreneur, recognizing that your creativity is at times limited by lack of energy and excessive stress, and that this combination calls for its own relaxation strategy.

The ten goals of relaxation form a tentative and fluid hierarchy, in which each goal is increasingly abstract and encompassing. In the messy real world, many hierarchies are possible. In our hierarchy, transcendent goals are the most encompassing. One can pursue any lower goal in service of a personal God or meditation/mindfulness. Similarly, one might learn to manage stress, develop calm direction, and enhance health and energy in service of the higher goal of creativity. And one might learn to sleep and nap effectively, management stress, deal with illness in order to pursue the goal of increased work productivity.

Hierarchies can be fluid and change over time. A cancer patient may decide that heath and energy are top goals, and the goals of stress management, creativity, and God-based spirituality are subservient goals, means to the end of dealing with cancer and hopefully living longer. After sincere pursuit of her identified goals, she may come decide that the goal of God-based spirituality doesn't work unless it is the most important goal, and all other goals, including health, are secondary. Hierarchies can grow and change.

7

Summary of ABC₂ Relaxation Theory: Psychological Relaxation Theory

The ideas we have just considered constitute ABC₂ Relaxation Theory, which I alternatively call "Psychological Relaxation Theory." They represent a significant revision of original ABC Theory (Smith, 1999a, 1999b, 2001, 2004). This chapter summarizes the similarities and differences between these perspectives and the relaxation response hypothesis.

Herbert Benson's (1975) popularized relaxation response hypothesis proposes that relaxation techniques evoke a state of reduced nonspecific physiological arousal, a relaxation response. The relaxation response is responsible for the many benefits associated with relaxation. His hypothesis can be summarized:

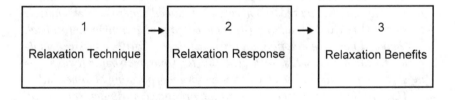

ORIGINAL ABC RELAXATION THEORY

The first version of ABC Relaxation Theory (Smith, 1999a, 1999b, 2001) proposed that all approaches to relaxation evoke the relaxation response and

71

15 relaxation states, or R-States, both of which are prerequisites to any experienced benefit of relaxation. Key elements of the original ABC Theory can be summarized:

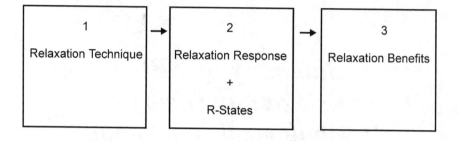

SUMMARY OF ABC$_2$ RELAXATION THEORY

ABC$_2$ Relaxation Theory introduces two variables: relaxation access skills and initial specific effects. The following is a formal summary of ABC$_2$ Theory:

Most forms of relaxation training can be grouped into one or more of six families of exercises: (1) stretching/yoga postures and positions, (2) progressive muscle relaxation, (3) autogenic training, (4) breathing exercises, (5) imagery and relaxing self-talk, and (6) meditation/mindfulness. These families require and develop six parallel relaxation access skills, each with an associated initial specific effect: (1) reduced joint and skeletal muscle stress associated with sustained stressful posture and position; reduced fatigue and increased energy; (2) reduced general skeletal muscle tension, (3) relaxed breathing, (4) reduced cognitive autonomic arousal, (5) reduced negative emotion, and (6) sustained effortless/passive simple focus. Of the access skills, sustained effortless/passive simple focus is the most encompassing and has the potential for incorporating all other skills.

The initial specific effects of relaxation practice contribute to an overall relaxation response and psychological relaxation states (R-States). Fifteen R-States include:

- *Sleepiness*
- *Disengagement*
- *Rested/Refreshed*

- *Energized*
- *Physical Relaxation,*
- *At Ease/Peace*
- *Joy (Happy)*
- *Mental Quiet*
- *Childlike Innocence*
- *Thankful/Loving*
- *Deep Mystery*
- *Awe/Wonder*
- *Prayerful*
- *Timeless/Boundless/Infinite/At One*
- *Aware (meta R-State)*

The goals and benefits of relaxation are mediated by initial specific effects, the relaxation response, and R-States. All six components of this theory are potentially interactive and mutually reinforcing.

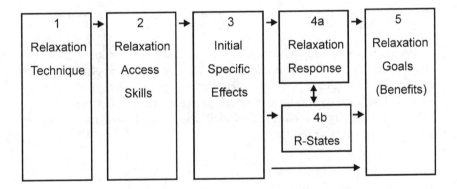

This theory can be applied to progressive muscle relaxation:

Illustration: progressive muscle relaxation and back pain.

Deploying the skill of tensing up and releasing tension (2) eventually reduces skeletal muscle tension (3) and evokes the relaxation response (4a) and the R-States, Disengagement and Physical Relaxation (4b). These R-States (4b), as well as the initial effect of reduced skeletal muscle tension (3) contribute to an enhanced relaxation response (4b), which, in turn, deepens the experienced R-States (4b). Reduced skeletal muscle tension

(3), the relaxation response (4a), and R-States (4b) contribute to enhanced recovery from back pain (5).

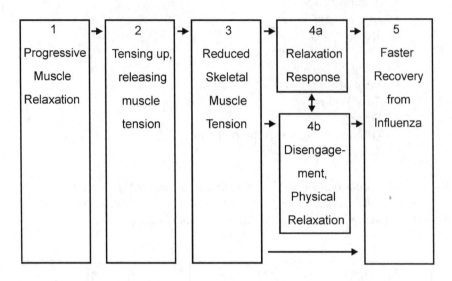

For purposes of simplicity, we have presented a linear path with components acting in one direction. However, all components are potentially interactive. For example, experiencing Disengagement (4b) may make it easier to detect and correct hidden postural problems (2), which may increase stamina for the day's activities (5), which may facilitate sustaining a relaxed posture or position in the future (2):

$$4b \rightarrow 2 \rightarrow 5 \rightarrow 2$$

Mastering sustained effortless/passive simple focus (2) may enhance the development of other relaxation access skills (2), evoking both a relaxation response (4a) and a variety of R-States (4b):

$$2 \rightarrow 2 \rightarrow (4a + 4b)$$

In addition, components can be mutually reinforcing. Achieving sustained relaxed posture (3) while feeling the R-State, Aware (4b), may together increase stamina (5) and facilitate future attempts at yoga stretching (2):

$$(3 + 4) \rightarrow (5 + 2)$$

Part II

The Relaxation Instruction Manual

8

General Instructions
for All Approaches to Relaxation

This chapter presents overview of instructional elements common to all families of relaxation, For every approach to relaxation, I recommend the following general preparatory and instructional steps:

PREPARATION (before teaching any technique):

1. *Selection of Training Format* (chapter 15)
2. *Orientation* (chapter 16)
3. *Assessment* (chapter 17)

This book presents chapters that consider preparatory material (chapters 15–17) after actual technique instructions (chapter 9–14) for instructor convenience and in recognition that many instructors may already have a preferred format, orientation and preparation routine, and assessment protocol.

INSTRUCTION (when teaching a specific approach):

1. *Exercise Rationale.* Explain the rationale for the specific family of techniques to be taught. When appropriate, explain how a specific family of techniques contributes to overall relaxation or the goal selected.
2. *Demonstration/Warmup.* Demonstrate and teach the technique, focusing on (a) the general procedure and (b) specific parts that may

prove troublesome. The demonstration also serves as a useful warmup exercise. Imagery and meditation may require additional warmup.

3. *Practice.* Practice the entire sequence with the client, observing how they practice and interrupting to correct mistakes. If an audio recording is available, play it.

4. *Assessment postsession.* Explain and give the Smith Relaxation States Inventory Brief Version (SRSIbv; Table 17.7 or SRSIabv, Table 17.9). The SRSIbv (or alternatively the SRSIabv) asks clients to describe how the exercise affected them, which R-States they experienced.

5. *Process technique.* Discuss responses to the SRSIbv (or alternatively the SRSIabv). Review any problems encountered.

6. *Revision.* Delete or modify any exercises that caused problems.

7. *Discuss aftereffects.* Before terminating the session, ask clients "How do you feel now? What words on your questionnaire (SRSIbv or alternatively the SRSIab) fit now?" Explain that often the major effects of a technique may not be immediately apparent after practice and may take a few minutes to emerge.

All cognitive exercises presented here offer several technique options. For example, the autogenic sequence presents warmth, heaviness, evenly beating heart, and warmth in the solar plexus; imagery introduces travel, outdoor/ nature, water, and indoor themes; and mediation presents techniques of the body, mind, and senses, as well as mindfulness. For any cognitive approach, if a client does not select a preferred exercise in the first practice session with a trainer (they rarely do), have them practice a full sequence once a day (usually 3 days) until it becomes apparent to them what their preference is. Then they may simply continue with their preference.

The procedures in this book may be used with coordinated prerecorded audio instructions. There are two ways to obtain these recordings.

1. Record your own set using the scripts at the end of each chapter.

2. Utilize the SMITH AUDIO RELAXATION INSTRUCTION SERIES (SARIS). For information, contact www.springerpub.com or www.roosevelt.edu/stress. The roosevelt.edu Web site has a free version of the RELAXATION SAMPLER, a 25-minute demonstration comprising exercises taken from each of the six families of relaxation (www.roosevelt.edu/stress/sampler.htm).

9

Yogaform Stretching

Yoga stretching is a popular approach to relaxation, with ancient roots. Traditional yoga exercises number in the thousands and have deep ties to religion and philosophy. We focus on simple and relatively easy stretching postures, mostly "static stretches." Our general instructions are to systematically, slowly, smoothly, and gently stretch various muscle groups and correct stressful postures and positions.

HYPOTHESIZED EFFECTS OF STRETCHING

Physical/Autonomic Effects
(see chapter 4 for more details on physiology)

Yoga stretching exercises define the intersection between physical fitness, rehabilitation, and relaxation. The effects of stretching on relaxation are relatively direct. For a chronically tense individual, tension is manifest in posture and position, specifically in stressed joints and joint tissue. Secondarily, tension and fatigue may be manifest in the skeletal muscles (arms, legs, face, etc.) Stretching exercises correct joint stress and secondarily evoke mild to moderate levels of muscle relaxation. Importantly, yoga stretching also reduces fatigue and loss of energy, and evokes and sustains intense kinesthetic stimulation, which in turn contributes to sustained focus. In sum, yoga stretching: (1) unstresses the joints, (2) evokes mild muscle relaxation, (3) reduces fatigue and energy loss, and (4) provides intense internally generated and attention-direting stimulation.

Attentional Effects

Stretching provides an effective diversion from external stimuli. It can contribute to a limited reduction in deliberate physical activity and thought; however, the act of stretching in and of itself is a type of physical activity. Although yoga instructors tell practitioners to focus on the stretch and not engage in thought, in fact stretching is an activity that can proceed (against the advice of instructions) even while engaging in related thought ("This stretch feels good." or "Am I stretching slowly enough?").

Stretching exercises differ in the level of required sustained effortless/ passive simple focus. For most exercises, one attends to the resulting sensations of stretching and maintaining a posture. For beginning exercises, this is relatively easy. The activity level, complexity of the exercise, and vividness of kinesthetic stimuli evoked through stretching make focusing relatively easy. However, for advanced exercises, stretching becomes more of a focusing exercise in which one maintains and attends to a posture for a sustained period of time.

R-States

In my experience, yogaform stretching appears to enhance the R-States, At Ease/Peace and Energized, and should be used when greater alertness and awareness is desired (Smith, 2001). Stretching exercises may be fairly effective for reducing modest levels of skeletal muscle tension to an "average" baseline. Because many beginning exercises require sustained skeletal arousal to maintain a posture or stretch, they are perhaps less effective for evoking the R-State, Disengagement, and deep reductions in physiological arousal below the resting level baseline. Thus, the simple stretches in this book may be insufficient for serious stress management. It remains to be demonstrated if the more strenuous, demanding, and occasionally risky stretches and postures presented in popular Hatha yoga programs are more effective. Unlike the six families of instructions of this book, such training is difficult and requires considerable professional supervised practice.

FORMAL CONSIDERATIONS

Exercise Placement

I recommend placing yogaform stretching at the very beginning of an exercise sequence as preparation, or at the very end in order to ease the transition out of relaxation. Stretching exercises may be combined with breathing and progressive muscle relaxation exercises. Historically, yoga stretching exercises are often placed before meditation/mindfulness.

Duration

When stretching is the only approach to relaxation that is practiced, a session should last at least 30 minutes. When combined as a preparatory or ending segment, a few minutes are sufficient.

Portability

Advanced Hatha and Prana yoga postures and stretches (not considered in this book) are not particularly portable, and often require a special practice place and supervision. The simple stretches in this text vary considerably in portability. Hand and neck stretches can be done nearly anywhere. The face stretch (the "lion") is probably best practiced alone, or with a group of other practitioners. The remaining stretches (arms, back, legs) are considerably more vigorous, limiting their application to confined places, in a vehicle, or in public.

APPROPRIATE CLIENTS

The stretching exercises in this book are most appropriate for clients experience mild to moderate muscle tension and strain and fatigue associated with sustaining a posture or position for prolonged periods of time (driving, sitting at a desk, standing in front of class). They are also useful for combating fatigue and evoking energy. And of course humans, like cats, find a good set of stretches useful for waking up after a nap.

Although a moderate amount of research has considered the impact of yoga, much of it is of questionable value (Funderburk, 1977). The most frequently cited studies (Patel, 1993; Vahia, Doongaji, Jeste, Ravindranath, Kapoor, et al., 1973) have combined stretching, sustained postures, breathing, imagery, meditation, philosophical discussion, and even PMR, a technique that tends to evoke a different pattern of R-States. Thus, it is difficult to assess the source of any effects obtained. In addition, many studies have considered Hatha yoga and related stretching exercises for physical fitness or rehabilitation and measured flexibility, respiratory capacity and efficiency, circulation, and the like. The impact of yoga stretching on such variables is, of course, beyond the consideration of this book. Finally, occasional lifelong practitioners of yoga stretching have demonstrated dramatic abilities to lower heart rate, breathing rate, and the like. Impressive as such feats of self-control may appear, their generalizability to most practitioners, and their implications for relaxation, are unclear.

The exercises of this book may be applied on a trial-and-error basis with relative safety. However, any client who has an injury, weakness, or any problem associated with any muscle group should either not practice the stretching exercise targeted to that group, or practice very gently. If an exercise is not physically practiced, it can be imagined ("Just imagine you are stretching your shoulders").

Clients who are professionally trained in Hatha yoga, dance, or a variety of sports may have substantial experience with advanced stretching exercises. They often find the exercises we present insufficiently challenging. I recommend that such practitioners continue with whatever stretching routine works for them. Alternatively, some advanced practitioners find our stretches to be a very simple and quick way of evoking the same effects associated with more advanced exercises.

OUR VERSION OF YOGAFORM STRETCHING

Although Hatha yoga is derived from a rich philosophical tradition, the exercises we present are simple stretches and postures; for this reason we call our approach yogaform stretching. I have attempted to include relatively "pure" stretches, not mixed with breathing or imagery. This enables the practitioner to detect the effects unique to stretching.

Generally, our approach incorporates only those exercises that are mentioned most frequently in introductory yoga texts and have a record of ease, safety, and enjoyability. Spiritual, religious, and metaphysical references have been avoided. Potentially dangerous and superfluous exercises have not been included. We do not emphasize sustaining challenging postures, twists, or contortions—for these are exercises that require direct professional supervision. A client who finds our yogaform stretching rewarding may well wish to pursue advanced training in a qualified yoga program.

We present eleven stretching exercises. Full yogaform stretching includes instructions with repetitions for the left and right sides; in abbreviated yogaform stretching, the left and right sides are stretched simultaneously. The full instructions are appropriate in most circumstances. Abbreviated instructions are for individuals who have mastered the full instructions or for cases when there is insufficient time for full practice.

TRAINING

Step 1: Select Format, Provide Overall Orientation, Conduct Assessment

Step 2: Exercise Rationale

It is perhaps appropriate to avoid excessive claims often found in popular yoga manuals ("yoga will . . . stimulate your liver, clean your spleen, give you superhuman powers," etc). Instead, I recommend describing yoga stretches as one approach to relaxing "stressed muscles and posture," reducing muscle tension and stiffness, combating fatigue, and generating energy. Here is one rationale I use:

> When tense, our muscles and joints can be likened to a tightly bent and coiled spring (or a crumpled scarf). If we wanted to straighten out and loosen the spring (or smooth out the scarf) and reduce its stiffness, we could easily stretch it out and then release the stretch. Similarly, in the yogaform exercises, we slowly, smoothly, and gently stretch out each muscle, stretch our joints, and then easily release the stretch. This is relaxing and energizing.

Step 3: Demonstration/Warmup

First, demonstrate a full, correct, slow stretch on the hands and fingers. Then quickly "walk through" each stretch to ensure proper form. After this quick demonstration, both you and your client perform the rapid walk through together. Emphasize that in actual practice, one proceeds much more slowly and gracefully, and that this rapid walkthrough is only to demonstrate procedure. Practice in an alert, seated position (feet flat on floor, spine and neck erect) or standing up. Explain that each stretch is to be done slowly, smoothly, and gently, in contrast to PMR. For each exercise, take about 20 seconds to stretch the indicated muscle group. When a muscle is stretched, have the client hold the stretch and attend to the pleasant sensations for a few seconds. Then take about 20 seconds to unstretch. Have the client move as slowly, smoothly and gently as possible, keeping the mind focused on the movement and the sensations produced.

When presenting yogaform stretching, moderate your voice to suggest the act of slowly stretching and unstretching. Elongate vowels ("Sloooowly stretch"). Speak as if you were stretching yourself. Avoid at all costs speaking in a dull monotone. The yoga voice should be relaxed, calm, and refreshed, suggesting calm alertness.

Step 4: Practice

Practice the entire sequence.

Steps 5 and 6: Review, Revision, and Special Problems

The stretching exercises here are relatively easy and enjoyable, and rarely cause problems. At times clients want to speed up (or perhaps slow down) the pace of presentation. Try to maintain a slow pace that the client can tolerate. Emphasize that the point is to create a pleasurable stretch, not an athletic or heroic stretch, or a stretch that is painful.

It is important to stretch slowly, and hold a stretch for a short period of time. Rapid stretching sends signals to the spine, resulting in a reflexive contraction of the stretched muscle. This is called the "stretch reflex" and is the body's attempt to protect itself from possible injury from excessive stretching. Slowly stretching and holding a stretch helps prevent triggering the stretch reflex and permits the body to habituate to stretching.

Clients vary considerably in how far they can stretch. Emphasize that the value of a stretch is not how far one can move, but the degree to which one creates a smooth movement and a pleasurable "stretch sensation." Thus, a small stretch and a large stretch can be equally effective. Bowing and touching the floor with one's nose is in itself no better than bowing a few inches. Never bounce and stretch.

Some clients show concerns that their movements are not completely smooth. Reassure clients that such "rusty, jerky movement" is a natural sign of being a beginner. Movement generally smoothes out with practice. Indeed, smoothness of movement is an internal sign of stretching skill mastery.

Go gently with the neck stretches; they can create discomfort. And finally, there is the matter of the face stretch, or as it is called among Hatha yoga trainers, the "lion." In group practice, clients invariably break out in laughter when everyone fully opens their jaws (with extended tongue), mouths, eyes, and so on in public. Some yoga instructors treat such mirthfulness with solemn admonitions to "practice seriously." This is regrettable. A little humor is very good, and can contribute to an attitude of letting go in relaxation, and the R-States of Joy, At Ease/Peace, and Energy. After the laugh, try the exercise again, this time with everyone looking toward the sky. Or, you might try to avoid the issue entirely by having practitioners look to the sky before starting this exercise.

If the full sequence of PMR exercises has already been taught, the very same muscle groups are presented in yogaform stretching. This gives the client the opportunity to compare and contrast the effects of these very different approaches.

ENHANCING YOGAFORM STRETCHING

- Freely incorporate breathing exercises
- Introduce phrases and images suggestive of Energized and Aware R-States, typically evoked through yoga stretching and imagery. For example, when stretching one's arms to the sky, an accompanying image of "imagine you are a tree, with branches reaching high into the sky" would be appropriate.
- Avoid PMR and AT, given that these approaches foster R-States that are different from those associated with yogaform stretching.
- End with imagery or meditation.

TABLE 9.1 Yogaform Stretching Instruction Scripts

FULL YOGAFORM STRETCHING

In this exercise we are going to relax by slowly, smoothly, and gently stretching various muscle groups. First make sure you are seated upright in a comfortable position. Place your feet flat on the floor. Close your eyes.

(continued)

TABLE 9.1 *(continued)*

Hand Stretch

We'll begin with the right hand.
Slowly, smoothly, and gently open your fingers and easily stretch them back and apart.
[PAUSE]
Try not to stretch so it hurts.
[PAUSE]
Focus on the good feelings of stretching.
[PAUSE]
Take your time.
[PAUSE]
Stretch every muscle fully.
[PAUSE]
Then hold the stretch.
[PAUSE]
And slowly, smoothly, and gently release the stretch.
[PAUSE]
Let your fingers very slowly return to their original relaxed position.
[PAUSE]
Notice the sensations as the muscles unstretch.
[PAUSE]
Take your time, there is no need to hurry.
[PAUSE]
[REPEAT ONCE FOR RIGHT HAND AND TWICE FOR LEFT HAND]

Arm Stretch

Now move to your right arm.
[PAUSE]
Slowly, smoothly, and gently slide you hand down your leg.
[PAUSE]
Extend your arm farther and farther.
[PAUSE]
Reach out and extend your arm in front of you.
[PAUSE]
Very gracefully, like you are balancing a feather on your hand.
[PAUSE]
And hold the stretch and become aware of the sensations.
[PAUSE]
Then slowly, smoothly, and gently release the stretch.
[PAUSE]

TABLE 9.1 *(continued)*

Gently rest your hand on your leg and slide your arm back to its resting position.
[PAUSE]
Take your time.
[PAUSE]
Slowly and gently unstretch your arm.
[REPEAT ONCE FOR RIGHT ARM AND TWICE FOR LEFT ARM]

Arm and Side Stretch

Now let both your arms fall limply to your sides.
[PAUSE]
Slowly, smoothly, and gently circle your right arm and hand up and away from your body like the hand of a clock or the wing of a bird.
[PAUSE]
Let your arm extend straight, and circle higher and higher.
[PAUSE]
Let it circle to the sky.
[PAUSE]
And then circle your arm over your head so your hand points to the other side . . . and arch your body as you reach and point farther and farther, like a tree arching in the wind.
[PAUSE]
Become aware of the invigorating feelings of stretching.
[PAUSE]
Now gently and easily . . .
[PAUSE]
Like the hand of a clock or the wing of a bird . . .
[PAUSE]
Circle your arm back over your head . . . to your side . . .
[PAUSE]
Finally to the resting position . . .
[PAUSE]
And let your arm hang.
[REPEAT ONCE FOR RIGHT ARM AND SIDE AND TWICE FOR LEFT ARM AND SIDE]

Back Stretch

Now focus your attention on your back, below your shoulders.
[PAUSE]
Slowly, smoothly, and gently relax and bow over.
[PAUSE]

(continued)

TABLE 9.1 *(continued)*

Let your arms hang limply.
[PAUSE]
Let your head fall forward, as you bow forward farther and farther in your chair.
[PAUSE]
Do not force yourself to bow over . . . let gravity pull your body toward your knees . . . farther and farther. It's OK to take a short breath if you need to.
[PAUSE]
Feel the stretch along the back.
[PAUSE]
Let gravity pull your body forward, as far as it will go.
[PAUSE]
Then gently and easily sit up.
[PAUSE]
Take your time.
[PAUSE]
Inch by inch, straighten your body . . .
[PAUSE]
Until you are seated comfortably in an upright position.
[REPEAT]

Shoulder Stretch

Now lift both arms straight ahead in front of you and let your fingers touch.
[PAUSE]
Slowly, smoothly, and gently circle them around together, as if you were squeezing a big pillow.
[PAUSE]
Let your hands cross, pointing in opposite directions.
[PAUSE]
Squeeze farther and farther, so you can feel a stretch in your shoulders and back.
[PAUSE]
Hold the stretch.
[PAUSE]
Become aware of the good sensations of stretching.
[PAUSE]
And gently release the stretch.
[PAUSE]
Gradually return your arms to your sides.
[PAUSE]

TABLE 9.1 *(continued)*

Take your time, there is no need to hurry.
[PAUSE]
Let your arms relax.
[REPEAT]

Back of Neck Stretch

Now, while sitting erect, let your head tilt easily toward your chest.
[PAUSE]
Try not to force it down.
[PAUSE]
Simply let gravity pull your head down . . .
[PAUSE]
Farther and farther.
[PAUSE]
Focus on the stretch in the back of your neck . . .
[PAUSE]
The refreshing and renewing energy it releases . . .
[PAUSE]
As the force of gravity easily and slowly pulls your head down.
[PAUSE]
When you are ready . . .
[PAUSE]
Gently and easily lift your head.
[PAUSE]
Lift it until it is again comfortably upright.
[REPEAT]

Face Stretch

Now attend to the muscles of your face.
[PAUSE]
Slowly, smoothly, and gently open your jaws, mouth, and eyes while lifting your eyebrows.
[PAUSE]
Open wide.
[PAUSE]
Feel every muscle of your face stretch more and more.
[PAUSE]
Hold the stretch.
[PAUSE]

(continued)

TABLE 9.1 *(continued)*

Then gently and easily release the stretch.
[PAUSE]
Let the muscles smooth out as they relax.
[PAUSE]
Let your face settle into a comfortable position.
[REPEAT]

Front of Neck Stretch

Now, like before, let your head tilt, this time backward.
[PAUSE]
Let gravity pull your head back, but not too far, just enough to feel the stretch.
[PAUSE]
Do not force it back.
[PAUSE]
Let gravity do the work for you as it pulls the heavy weight of your head back, farther and farther.
[PAUSE]
Gently and slightly open your mouth, and let your head relax and fall back.
[PAUSE]
Focus your mind on the front of the neck stretch as it stretches.
[PAUSE]
Gently hold the stretch.
[PAUSE]
Then gently and easily lift your head.
[PAUSE]
Gradually return it to its upright position.
[PAUSE]
Take your time. There is no need to hurry.
[REPEAT]

Stomach and Chest Stretch

Now lean back comfortably in your chair.
[PAUSE]
Slowly, smoothly, and gently arch your stomach and chest out.
[PAUSE]
Do this slowly and gently.
[PAUSE]
Feel the stretch along your torso . . .
[PAUSE]

TABLE 9.1 *(continued)*

Arch and stretch.
[PAUSE]
Then gently and easily release the stretch.
[PAUSE]
Slowly and easily return to an upright position.
[PAUSE]
Take your time. There is no reason to hurry.
[REPEAT]

Leg Stretch

Now focus your attention on your right leg.
[PAUSE]
Slowly and easily stretch the leg out in front of you.
[PAUSE]
Stretch so you can feel the muscles pulling.
[PAUSE]
Do this easily and gently.
[PAUSE]
Feel a good energizing stretch all along your leg.
[PAUSE]
Then gently release the stretch.
[PAUSE]
Slowly let your leg return to its original resting position.
[PAUSE]
Take your time.
[PAUSE]
Gently unstretch your leg.
[PAUSE]
And let it rest.
[REPEAT ONCE FOR RIGHT LEG AND TWICE FOR LEFT LEG]

Foot Stretch

Now focus your attention on your right foot.
[PAUSE]
While resting your heel on the floor, gently pull your toes and foot up, as if they are being pulled by strings.
[PAUSE]
Let the foot and leg stretch more and more.
[PAUSE]
Feel the full and comfortable stretch in every muscle fiber.
[PAUSE]

(continued)

TABLE 9.1 *(continued)*

Stretch all the way.
[PAUSE]
And hold the stretch.
[PAUSE]
Now easily and gently release the stretch.
[PAUSE]
Let the foot slowly and smoothly relax.
[PAUSE]
Inch by inch, let the foot return.
[PAUSE]
Unstretch the foot until it is resting again on the floor.
[REPEAT ONCE FOR RIGHT FOOT AND TWICE FOR LEFT FOOT]

Ending

Let go of what you are attending to. Slowly open your eyes all the
way. Take a deep breath and stretch. This completes our exercise.

ABBREVIATED YOGAFORM STRETCHING

The instructions are the same as those for full yogaform stretching, except combine left and right sides for:

Hand Stretch
Arm Stretch
Arm and Side Stretch
Leg Stretch
Foot Stretch

10

Progressive Muscle Relaxation

Progressive Muscle Relaxation (PMR) is the most popular relaxation technique among health professionals in the United States. The basic strategy of PMR is to detect, attend to, and systematically tense up and then release tension in various muscle groups (Alternate forms involve just releasing tension without first creating tension.) One does this while learning to distinguish sensations of tension and relaxation and isolate specific muscle groups.

HYPOTHESIZED EFFECTS OF PMR

Physical/Autonomic Effects
(see chapter 4 for more details on physiology)

Initially tensing up a muscle is typically claimed to set the stage for a relaxation rebound effect when one releases tension. This enables the muscle to relax more. (Note: the "rebound effect" is a useful explanatory metaphor; however, its existence has yet to be confirmed.) Also, deliberately inducing muscle tension, followed by relaxation, teaches the client to detect subtle and often hidden sources of tension and to differentiate muscle tension from relaxation. PMR is perhaps the most effective technique for evoking rapid reductions in skeletal muscle tension.

Attentional Effects

PMR is an effective diversion from external stimuli and a tool for reducing deliberate, competing physical and thought activity. Of all families of techniques, PMR requires the least skill at sustained effortless/passive focus. The trainer is always talking, presenting a continuous stream of instructional patter, which helps keep the distracted client focused. In addition, PMR is relatively active and varied, making it easier to focus. Finally, the muscle sensations generated by PMR are vivid, providing a focal target that is easy to detect and attend to.

R-States

PMR is particularly well-suited for evoking the R-States of Disengagement and Physical Relaxation. Clients frequently report feeling distant and far away. As training progresses, they may report sensations of somatic disengagement involving loss of awareness of parts of the body, or even "out-of-body" experiences. Later in training, perhaps after 4 or 5 weeks, Energized (personal experience) as well as Mental Quiet and Joy may emerge (Matsumoto & Smith, 2002; Ghonchec & Smith, 2004) for individuals not in therapy. These R-States may be noted as an aftereffect rather than an immediate post-session effect (chapter 17). That is, in addition to asking clients how they feel immediately after training, I recommend asking again after a 5-minute delay (after they have first discussed the immediate effects). Often such appraised aftereffects are more pronounced.

It should be noted that for individuals under high levels of stress, or in psychotherapy for depression or anxiety, Physical Relaxation and Disengagement may be the only R-States that are evoked. The finding that more intensely rewarding R-States may take time to emerge, or may not emerge at all, limits the extent to which PMR is intrinsically reinforcing. Considerable attention must be paid to motivating clients and adding reinforcing features to enhance compliance. This may include any of the enhancement suggestions offered at the end of this chapter.

FORMAL CONSIDERATIONS

Placement

I recommend placing PMR near the beginning of an exercise sequence. It may readily be combined with passive breathing and autogenic training, and some somatic imagery.

Duration

When PMR is the only approach practiced, sessions for beginners should last at least 25 minutes. For advanced practitioners, sessions may be reduced to 10 minutes.

Portability

PMR exercises are not particularly portable because of the effort and time required to achieve an effect. Letting go exercises (which omit the "tense up" phase) are more portable than overt "tense-let go" exercises. Of all PMR exercises, perhaps the hand, arm, neck, and shoulder exercises are applicable in the widest range of places.

Appropriate Clients

PMR is relatively easy, familiar, and unthreatening. It is an appropriate beginning technique for those inexperienced with relaxation, children, and those displaying high levels of somatic tension, worry, and negative emotion. Both PMR and breathing exercises may be appropriate in anger management.

The most direct clinical application of PMR is for disorders with a clear muscle-tension component. The initial, specific effects of PMR (chapter 4) suggest the value of targeting PMR to skeletal muscle groups that may be sources of tension.

Stress Institute research and clinical experience clearly suggests that PMR is the relaxation treatment of choice for individuals experiencing psychopathology who wish a tool for evoking physical relaxation and reducing physical stress symptoms, worry, and negative emotions such as anxiety, anger, and depression. PMR is also valuable for clients who have difficulty relaxing or maintaining focus on a relaxation task because of anxiety (Weinstein & Smith, 1992), impulsivity, or cognitive impairment.

Clients who have an injury, weakness, or any problem associated with any muscle group should either not practice the PMR exercise targeted to that group, or practice very gently. If an exercise is not physically practiced, it can be imagined ("Just imagine you are squeezing and letting go of tension in your shoulders").

OUR VERSIONS OF PMR

This book presents two versions of overt PMR ("Tense up—let go") and one version of covert PMR ("Just let go without first tensing up"). No instructions are offered for Minimal PMR, a rarely used approach. All instructions are designed to be as "pure" as possible and incorporate only tensing and letting go (or simply letting go) without potentially confounding breathing, stretching, or imagery exercises. The objective is to help the client identify the unique effects of PMR. Full PMR, is a complete version comparable to how PMR is taught in other programs.

Our sequence targets 11 muscle groups, selected and presented in a logical and easily remembered order. The selected muscles are similar to the eleven presented for yogaform stretching (chapter 9). The first three proceed from the hand, up the arm (hand, arm, arm, side). These three are easy to remember. The remaining eight start at the lower back, move up the back, over the head, and down the front of the body to the feet. For these I find the following image a useful memory tool.

> Think of a warm spot of light starting at the lower back. Slowly this light moves up the back to the shoulders, up the back of the neck, over the top of the head to the face, down the front of the neck to the stomach and chest and to the legs and feet.

Abbreviated PMR, contains the same 11 exercises; however, practice time is cut by a third by combining left and right side practice ("Tense up both left and right hands, now"). Letting Go, is a pure version of covert PMR in which one lets go without first tensing up. This sequence is about half the length of Full PMR and further combines the eleven muscle groups into nine.

Our three versions of PMR are appropriate for different clients. Full PMR is the standard sequence for beginners. Abbreviated PMR is appropriate for clients who (1) do not have the time, patience, or focusing skill for Full PMR, or (2) have mastered Full PMR and are ready to combine exercises and graduate to a shorter sequence. Similarly, Letting Go is for those who (1) do not have the time for Full or Abbreviated PMR, or (2) have graduated from both Full and Abbreviated PMR and are ready to apply their skills in a highly abbreviated format.

TRAINING

Step 1: Select Format, Conduct Assessment, Provide Overall Rationale

Step 2: Exercise Rationale

Explain the importance of muscle tension in stress and anxiety. One goal of PMR is to induce muscle relaxation by creating its opposite; one first tenses up, and then releases tension. Because clients may find this paradoxical, explain how initially tensing up may actually help the process of tension release through something of a "rebound effect." The image of a pendulum can help.

> To make a pendulum swing in one direction, one could push it in that direction. Another way would be to pull it in the opposite direction, building up tension, and then letting go. The built-up energy is released as the pendulum swings in the opposite direction.

Other metaphors can be used to illustrate the hypothetical "rebound effect," including pushing a sled up a snowy hill and letting go so it can slide down; pulling an arrow back on the string of a bow, and then releasing tension, letting the arrow soar, and so on.

The following sequence illustrates the overt tension-release act on the shoulder muscles:

> Here is how we will tense up and let go. Let me demonstrate on the shoulders. First, let's shrug our shoulders and create a good squeeze. Do this now, with me. Let the tension build. Do not tense so much that it hurts. This is not a fitness exercise. Now let go. Let the tension flow. Simply let the tightness dissolve and begin to melt away. There is nothing you have to do but relax. There, how was that? We will be tensing up and releasing all the major muscle groups in the body.

A second goal of PMR is to help clients identify hidden sources of muscle tension so such tension can be more readily identified and released. Eventually, one learns to isolate and relax specific targeted muscle groups.

Step 3: Demonstration/Warmup

I recommend fully demonstrating tensing up and letting go for every muscle group. An acceptable abbreviation is to focus on these selected groups:

- Demonstrate to the client the basic idea of tensing up and letting go, usually with the shoulder muscles. Perform a full shoulder muscle exercise.
- Quickly note the 11 muscle groups to be targeted. Name each muscle group while briefly tensing and letting go that group. Use the image of the "warm spot of light" previously described.
- Explain that clients sometimes have difficulty with certain muscle groups. Present the full instructions for the following and demonstrate how each is tensed up. Then practice along with the client, observing and making sure they practice correctly.

> *Arm and Side*. Press your arm against your side as if you were squeezing a sponge in your armpit . . . or squeezing a lemon . . .
>
> *Lower Back*. Tense up your lower back in whatever way feels comfortable, such as pressing your back against the back of the chair, rubbing your back against the back of your chair, trying to push the back of your chair away by pressing against it, and so on. (*Alternative:* Pull your shoulders and elbows back behind you; try to touch your elbows behind your back. Notice your back tensing up.
>
> *Face*. Tense up all the muscles in your face, forehead, eyebrows, eyes, nose, cheeks, mouth, tongue, and jaws . . . all at once. Make an ugly face! Scrunch up your face as if you were biting into something awful!
>
> *Stomach and Chest*. Tense up the muscle in your stomach and chest very tightly. You might try pulling your abdomen in as if you were trying to fit into some very tight jeans. Or try making your abdomen 'rock hard' like the muscle builders do.

When demonstrating and practicing overt PMR, I find these *procedural rules* helpful:

1. *Tense up.* Do not tense up so much that your muscles feel uncomfortable or hurt. Emphasize that this is not an "isometric" fitness exercise. This is a particularly important caution for clients (especially males) engaged in sports or fitness training.

2. *Let go.* The tension release part of each tense-let go cycle must be sufficiently long to permit tension to actually dissipate. Generally, this is between 20–50 seconds. Beginning clients often expect the release of tension to be instant; emphasize that this process is gradual and takes about half a minute. Again, PMR is not a fitness exercise.

3. *Posture.* It is preferable to practice with eyes closed (except when looking at a trainer modeling). Avoid an upright alert position that fosters R-States related to opening up. Also, avoid crossing or extending the arms or legs, positions that can generate distracting tension. PMR can be practiced while seated in a soft, comfortable lounge chair. One might assume a position often recommended by autogenic trainers. Here, a client sits comfortably with arms resting easily in the lap and head slightly bowed (not so much as to cut off breathing). This position resembles that of a seated string puppet, with strings cut, so that the puppet is seated relaxed, limp, and slightly slouched. PMR can be practiced in a reclining position, although such a position can foster the R-State Sleepiness.

4. *Double practice.* For each muscle group, present a complete tense–let go cycle twice ("Make a fist . . . let go . . . make a fist . . . let go").

5. *Separate practice for left and right side.* For arms, hands, legs, and feet, practice a complete cycle ("tense–let go . . . tense–let go") twice on the right side, and then on the left side of the body.

6. *Frequent relaxation checks.* After presenting a "tense–let go" cycle twice, and before moving on to the next muscle group, ask the client if he or she is relaxed (by gently shaking head "yes" or "no." If not relaxed, repeat the exercise up to three more times. A special arm exercise relaxation check can be a useful demonstration of the idea of muscle relaxation. Here, after a client has tensed and relaxed the right arm, simply lift the relaxed arm about 5 inches and let it drop. If the arm stays in the air, or descends slowly, then it is not relaxed. A relaxed arm should drop with an audible thud, like a dropped piece of meat. Use these instructions for the arm exercise relaxation check:

```
In a minute I'm going to do a simple little check. What I will
do is gently hold your wrist like this (demonstrate on your
own wrist) and lift your arm a few inches, and let it drop.
That's all. Ready? Make sure your arm is completely relaxed.
```

Now I gently hold your wrist. [HOLD CLIENT'S WRIST] I lift it
up. [LIFT ARM] And I let go. [LET IT DROP. IF ARM DROPS SLOWLY,
OR STAYS UP, EXPLAIN HOW THIS ILLUSTRATES THAT THERE IS STILL
MUSCLE TENSION. DEMONSTRATE HOW THE ARM SHOULD DROP, AND TRY
AGAIN ONE OR TWO TIMES.]

7. *The "keep talking rule."* PMR works well for clients who are very
tense and have a hard time focusing. The trainer makes focusing easier
through continuous and monotonous relaxation talk or chatter.

8. *The 2–4 rule.* Trainer patter either instructs a client to "tense up"
or "let go." Generally, speak two "tense up" phrases followed by four "let
go" phrases. This will result in a properly timed sequence, that is, 5 or
so seconds for the "tense up" phase and at least 20–30, and no more than
50, seconds for the "let go" phase. In the "let go" phase, a 3- to 5-second
pause should precede each statement.

9. *Adjust pauses.* Beginning trainers frequently fail to pause between
each PMR phrase. It is extremely important to introduce a sufficient pause
between each of the two tense-up phrases and each of the four let-go
phrases. It is equally important to introduce a longer pause between each
complete 2–4 segment. It takes time for each suggestion to "settle in."
Determining the length of the pauses depends on the degree to which
clients have developed relaxation access skills, particularly the skill of
sustained effortless/passive simple focus. For easily distracted and very
tense clients, use a short, two-second pause (think "one thousand one, one
thousand two") between each 2–4 phrase and a four-second pause at the
end of each 2–4 sequence. A skilled trainer should be able to detect from
a client's body relaxation when a pause is too long (see chapter 17 for a
discussion of behavioral signs of relaxation). It is appropriate to try out
different pause lengths (starting with four-second pauses) during Step 3,
Demonstration Warmup:

Tense up your shoulders. Let the tension grow. And let go.
[4-SECOND PAUSE]. Let the tension flow away. [4-SECOND
PAUSE]. Let yourself become more and more limp [4-SECOND
PAUSE]. Enjoy the pleasant sensations of relaxation. [4-SEC-
OND PAUSE]. There, what was that like? Did you have any diffi-
culties. Did I pause too long, or not long enough? [WAIT FOR
ANSWER. IF CLIENT INDICATES THE PAUSE WAS TOO LONG, THEN USE
SHORT, 1- or 2-SECOND PAUSES IN THE ACTUAL PRESENTATION OF
EXERCISES]

10. *The PMR voice.* Pay very close attention to voice speed, volume, and quality. ***Beginning instructors talk too fast, and do not introduce enough pauses***. Cultivate a different voice for speaking "tense-up" and "let-go" phases. "Tense-up" talk should be relatively loud and tense, as if you were a gym coach gently urging your students to put forth more effort. "Let-go" talk should communicate letting go. The first "let-go" phrase (of the four) should be spoken with a sigh, almost as if you were letting go—("And let go-o-o-o"). The remaining phrases should be spoken slowly and softly, in a rather gentle and uninteresting monotone.

It can be difficult for beginning instructors to deploy an appropriately slow and monotonous PRM "let-go" voice. Because most have been well-trained in speaking clearly and quickly, for the instructor the proper PMR voice will sound very strange, like a tape recording that has been deliberately slowed down, or the voice of someone who is dozing off or perhaps a little inebriated. Trainers should be reminded in a training session that their state of mind will be quite different from that of their clients. A trainer will be quite alert and actively focused; in contrast, a relaxing client will be much less alert and less focused. The trainer will be in "fast, active mode" whereas a client will be in "slow, passive mode." Speak to the mind of the client, not another trainer. In sum, strive for a slow, monotonous, and boring tone of voice. Avoid sounding dreamy, serene, interesting, alert, refreshed, or lively.

11. *What to say.* No PMR script ever won a literary award. Because of the requirement to keep talking, PMR is necessarily uninteresting and repetitive. There are five topics that let-go phrases can reflect: (a) the process of releasing tension; (b) reassurances of control; (c) suggestions of the R-States, Disengagement and Physical Relaxation, and, to some extent in later sessions, Mental Quiet; (d) suggestions to keep muscles other than those targeted relaxed; and (e) detecting tension. Beginning instructors find it very difficult to remember what to say. I suggest creating a simple "cheat sheet" of PMR let-go phrases that can be easily placed on one's lap or a nearby table (Table 10.1). Simply read through the list, four statements at a time, starting again at the beginning when the list is completed. It is not particularly important to present let-go phrases in the order suggested.

12. *Suggest muscles "smoothing out" when appropriate.* For clients who are self-conscious about appearance, especially wrinkles, substitute "muscles smooth out" for "muscles go limp," especially for the face and neck. Note that there is absolutely no evidence that PMR either decreases

TABLE 10.1   List of "Let-Go" Phrases

General Phrases (may be placed anywhere in script)

> Let the tension go.
> Release your tension.
> Let yourself go limp.
> Let tightness go.
> Tension smoothes out (FACE AND NECK}.
> Sink into relaxation.
> Let tension dissolve and flow away.
> Let yourself become more and more relaxed.

Later Phrases (In any "2–4" sequence, use these as phrase "3" or "4")

> Notice the difference between tension and relaxation.
> Let go of any feelings of tightness you may feel.
> Your muscles feel heavier.
> Sink deeper and deeper into relaxation.
> Enjoy the feelings of muscle relaxation you have created.
> Let the rest of your body remain relaxed.
> Tension melts into liquid.
> Sink deep into relaxation, far away from the world.
> Notice the control you have over tension and relaxation.
> Let your entire body become loose and limp.
> Let your muscles become more deeply relaxed.

---

or increases wrinkling. Of course, a relaxed face and neck are less likely to show fatigue and frown lines.

13. *Avoid emphasizing R-States higher on the R-States Pyramid.* Avoid emphasizing words suggesting the R-States, Energized, Aware, Joy, Childlike Innocence, Thankful/Loving, Deep Mystery, Awe and Wonder, Prayerfulness, or Timeless/Boundless/Infinite. PMR appears to foster Disengagement and Physical Relaxation. In addition, avoid words suggesting At Ease/Peace that can also indirectly suggest awareness, peaceful, rested, refreshed, contented, and restored. For beginners and very tense clients, PMR is a good exercise for evoking Disengagement and Physical Relaxation. However, once relaxation advances, other R-States may be considered (as well as other families of relaxation).

14. *Avoid negative phrases.* Do not use phrases that suggest getting rid of a negative ("Sink far away from your worries, cares, and concerns," "Forget your troubles and pain," "Let yourself feel less and less anxious").

Simply mentioning potentially aversive topics can stir disruptive worry and rumination or remind clients of the problems they are trying to forget.

15. *Suggest increased generalization of relaxation as session progresses.* Early in the session, restrict your instructions to specific body parts. However, when the session is at least half over, begin to introduce phrases suggesting generalization to the entire body.

Of these suggestions, let me repeat: beginning trainers are most likely to have difficulty with the "2–4 rule," application of the "PMR voice," and inserting pauses of sufficient length. Students invariably present instructions too quickly, with too few pauses, and in a voice that is inappropriately articulate, energized, dreamy, or peaceful. I have yet to find a beginning trainer who presented instructions too slowly. And I have yet to find a beginner whose voice is too monotonous or colorless. A seasoned trainer should be able to read a phone book and, using the "PMR voice," evoke R-States Disengagement and Physical Relaxation.

Step 4: Practice

Present instructions for the entire PMR sequence from beginning to end. Live presentation is more effective than listening to a recording. I recommend not reading a PMR script. Instead, you should (1) memorize the 11 muscle groups targeted in PMR (this is easy if you use the "warm spot of light" memory tool described earlier), and (2) place a list of "let-go phrases" (Table 10.1) on your lap or a nearby table to suggest patter. Remember: it is important to continue talking; boring repetition is okay.

Practice along with your client. Invite them to close their eyes, if they wish, and to briefly check with you to see if they are practicing correctly. You should keep your eyes open and check the accuracy of your client's procedure. Pause instructions whenever you note that a client is practicing incorrectly. Correct the technique, and continue practicing.

Steps 5 and 6: Review, Revision, and Special Problems

Check for any problems that emerged. Some of the more common problems include the following.

Cramps. Clients may complain of cramps. If a muscle cramps repeatedly, do not include it in the sequence. The trainer should not show alarm or upset when a cramp occurs. Wait patiently, and the cramp will most likely go away. It is alright for a client to massage or rub a cramped muscle, or simply shift to a comfortable position in which little strain is placed on the muscle (the trainer should not touch the client). A very slow and gentle stretch can help a cramp.

Giggling/crying/tears. A client may giggle or appear to cry in a relaxation session. Such reactions are often a sign of tension release. The trainer should simply ignore them, not displaying any concern or upset. If necessary, reassure the client, "Tears may come to your eyes, that's OK. We can continue."

Difficulty tensing up. A client may complain of an inability to create muscle tension. Try alternative methods of tensing up until an effect is created. If this doesn't work, isolate separate muscles within a larger muscle group and target each separately. For example, if a client has difficulty creating tension in the face, try dividing the face into regions by focusing on the forehead, then the cheeks and nose, and then the lower face. Note that exercises targeting the lower back and abdomen are less likely to create vivid feelings of tension.

Difficulty letting go. A client may complain of an inability to release tension. In these cases repeat the tense-let go cycle, for no more than five times total.

Sleepiness. Clients may report drowsiness or fall asleep in training. Drowsiness is normal, and can be an indication of the R-States, Sleepiness or Disengagement. However, frequent sleep during practice should be avoided. If you suspect that a client has fallen asleep, and is not displaying the usual obvious signs (snoring), check for consciousness. Bernstein and Borkovec (1973) suggest repeating the relaxation check, "Let me know if you are relaxed." If the client does not respond, repeat a tense-let go cycle. If a client does not respond, wait 10 seconds and repeat it again, louder. Continue, until the client wakes up. See chapter 18 for more suggestions.

LETTING GO

Instructions for Letting Go parallel those for Full and Abbreviated PMR, except all references to "tensing up" are omitted. Perhaps the greatest change is in the exercise rationale. Instead of explaining the importance of the "tense-release cycle" and the "relaxation rebound effect," focus on the importance of detecting and releasing subtle and often hidden sources of tension.

ENHANCING PMR

- Breathe in before tensing up; exhale while releasing tension. For Letting Go exercises, first breathe in, and then breathe out while letting go.
- Introduce one complete deep breathing cycle (see Breathing Exercises, chapter 11) after the following exercises: Hand, Arm and Side, Shoulder, Legs, and Feet. Coordinate exhaling with instructions to let go ("And let go as you breathe out . . . ")
- Follow each tense-let go cycle with a stretch of the same muscle group ("Tense and let go of your right hand; stretch and unstretch your right hand"). This may make PMR more pleasant for beginners (enhancing compliance), but limit depth of relaxation.
- Incorporate autogenic "warm, heavy" suggestions.
- Incorporate imagery suggestive of Physical Relaxation, or the release of tension ("Let tension unwind like a tight wad of paper" or "melt away like candle wax").
- Precede PMR with a Body Mindfulness meditation. That is, before overtly tensing up and letting go, simply have a client attend to the sensations of:
  - Hands touching the chair (or legs)
  - Buttocks against the chair
  - Legs against the chair
  - Feet on the floor

Such preparation can serve to direct focus toward muscle groups.

TABLE 10.2 Progressive Muscle Relaxation Scripts

FULL PROGRESSIVE MUSCLE RELAXATION

In this exercise, we are going to relax by gently squeezing and letting go of various muscle groups.

First make sure you are seated upright in a comfortable position. Place your feet flat on the floor. And close your eyes.

[NOTE: INSERT APPROPRIATE PAUSE AFTER EACH PHRASE—SEE INSTRUCTIONS]

(continued)

TABLE 10.2 *(continued)*

Hand

 Let's begin by focusing on the right hand.
 Squeeze the fingers together by making a fist, now.
 Tighten up the muscles.
 Let the tension grow.
 And let go.
 Release the tension.
 Let your muscles begin to go limp.
 Let the tension begin to flow out . . .
 As your hand sinks into relaxation.
 [REPEAT ONCE FOR RIGHT HAND AND TWICE FOR LEFT HAND]

Arm

 This time, focus on your right arm.
 Squeeze your lower and upper arm together . . .
 Touching your wrist to your shoulder.
 Do this now.
 Press tighter and tighter.
 Notice the feelings of tension.
 And let go.
 Let the tension go.
 Let the rest of your body remain relaxed.
 The tension melts away.
 Let the muscles become more deeply relaxed.
 [REPEAT ONCE FOR RIGHT ARM AND TWICE FOR LEFT ARM]

Arm and Side

 This time, rest your hands in your lap.
 Focus your attention on your arm and side and press them together, now.
 Tighten up the muscles.
 Let the tension grow.
 And let go.
 Let the muscles go completely limp.
 Let tension flow away.
 Let yourself relax.
 [REPEAT ONCE FOR RIGHT ARM AND SIDE AND TWICE FOR LEFT ARM AND SIDE]

Back

 This time focus your attention on the back muscles that are below the shoulders.
 Tense up your lower back, now.

TABLE 10.2 *(continued)*

Let the tension build.
Let the muscles get nice and hard.
And let go.
Let the tension go.
Feelings of tightness melt and flow away.
Let yourself feel more relaxed.
Let feelings of tightness go.
[REPEAT FOR BACK]

Shoulders

This time, focus on your shoulder muscles.
Squeeze your shoulders, now.
Create a nice good shrug.
Let the feelings of tightness grow.
And let go.
Let the tension flow out.
Let your tension begin to unwind.
Let the muscles begin to smooth out.
Let the muscles become more deeply relaxed.
[REPEAT FOR SHOULDERS]

Back of Neck

Focus on the muscles in the back of the neck.
Gently tilt your head back and gently press the back of your head against your neck, now.
Tighten up the muscles.
Squeeze the muscles more and more.
And let go.
Let the muscles become more deeply relaxed.
Let your entire body become loose and limp.
Let yourself sink deeper and deeper into relaxation . . .
Far away from the world.
[REPEAT FOR BACK OF NECK]

Face

This time, focus on the muscles of your face.
Squeeze them all together, now.
Squeeze your jaws, tongue, lips, nose, eyes, eyebrows, and fore-head . . . all together.
Squeeze your entire face together.
Let the feelings of tightness grow.
And let go.

(continued)

TABLE 10.2 *(continued)*

Feel calm and relaxed.
Let the tension smooth out.
You begin to feel more and more calm.
As you relax, you feel more at ease.
[REPEAT FOR FACE]

Front of Neck

Focus on the muscles of the neck.
Bow your head and gently press your chin down to your chest, now.
Tighten up the muscles.
Let the tension grow.
And let go.
Let tension begin to melt into liquid.
Let the rest of your body remain relaxed.
Let yourself sink deeper and deeper into relaxation . . .
Like a tight wad of paper, slowly opening up.
[REPEAT FOR FRONT OF NECK]

Stomach and Chest

Focus on the muscles of your stomach and chest.
Tighten them up, now.
Tense your stomach and chest in whatever way feels best . . .
By pulling your stomach in . . . pushing it out . . .
Or tightening it up.
Let the muscles get nice and hard.
And let go.
Feelings of tension dissolve.
Let yourself feel more detached.
Tension begins to melt into liquid . . .
Far away from the world.
[REPEAT FOR STOMACH AND CHEST]

Legs

Focus on the muscles in your right leg.
Tense the muscles in the leg, now.
Push your leg against the leg or back of your chair . . .
Or press your leg tightly against the other leg.
Tighten up the muscles.
Let the tension grow.
And let go.
Relax.

TABLE 10.2 *(continued)*

Let yourself feel more at ease.
Your muscles become heavier and heavier . . .
As you sink deep into relaxation.
Tighten up the muscles.
[REPEAT ONCE FOR RIGHT LEG AND TWICE FOR LEFT LEG]

Feet

Focus on your right foot.
Tense up the muscles of the right foot and toes, now.
Curl your toes into the floor while pushing down.
Tighten up the muscles.
Tense up only the muscles of your right foot.
And let go.
Let the tension flow out.
And you become more completely relaxed, at ease.
Completely passive and indifferent.
Far away from the world.
[REPEAT ONCE FOR RIGHT FOOT AND TWICE FOR LEFT FOOT]

Review

Quietly attend to how you feel.
Your hands and arms.
If you feel any leftover tension, just let go. Go limp.
Your back and shoulders.
If you feel any leftover tension, just let go. Go limp.
Sink deeper and deeper into relaxation.
Your shoulders and neck.
If you feel any leftover tension, just let go. Go completely
limp.
Relax more and more.
Far away from the world.
The muscles of your face.
If you feel any leftover tension, just let go. Go completely
limp.
Sink into a state of deep relaxation, indifferent to the world.
The muscles of your legs and feet.
If you feel any leftover tension, just let go. Go completely
limp.
Distant and far away.
Deep into relaxation.
And your entire body.

(continued)

TABLE 10.2 *(continued)*

Is there any part of your body where you feel even the slightest
bit of tension?
   Just let go. Go completely limp.
   Sink deeper and deeper, far away into relaxation.

Ending

   Let go of what you are attending to.
   Slowly open your eyes all the way.
   Take a deep breath and stretch.
   This completes our exercise.

ABBREVIATED PMR

THE INSTRUCTIONS ARE THE SAME AS FOR FULL PMR. TENSE UP AND RELEASE

BOTH LEFT AND RIGHT SIDES FOR:
   HANDS
   ARMS
   ARMS AND SIDES
   LEGS
   FEET

LETTING GO

Quietly attend to how you feel.
Direct your attention to your hands and fingers.
If you feel any tension, just let go, and go completely limp.
[PAUSE 5 SECONDS]
Let the tension melt and flow away.
[PAUSE 5 SECONDS]
Attend to both arms.
If you feel any tension, just let go.
Go completely limp.
[PAUSE 5 SECONDS]
Let the tension dissolve and flow away.
[PAUSE 5 SECONDS]
Attend to both arms and sides.
If you feel any tension, just let go.
Go completely limp.
[PAUSE 5 SECONDS]
Let the tension dissolve and melt away.

TABLE 10.2 *(continued)*

[PAUSE 5 SECONDS]
Attend to your lower back.
If you feel any tension, just let go.
Go completely limp.
[PAUSE 5 SECONDS]
Let the tension dissolve and flow away.
[PAUSE 5 SECONDS]
Attend to your shoulders.
If you feel any tension, just let go.
Go completely limp.
[PAUSE 5 SECONDS]
Let the tension melt away.
[PAUSE 5 SECONDS]
Attend to the back of your neck.
If you feel any tension, just let go.
Go completely limp.
[PAUSE 5 SECONDS]
Let the tension flow away.
[PAUSE 5 SECONDS]
Attend to the muscles of your face. Your jaws, mouth, lips, eyes, and forehead.
If you feel any tension, just let go.
Go completely limp.
[PAUSE 5 SECONDS]
Let the tension dissolve and flow away.
[PAUSE 5 SECONDS]
Relax more and more.
Far away from the world.
[PAUSE 5 SECONDS]
Attend to the muscles of your stomach and chest.
If you feel any tension, just let go.
Go completely limp.
[PAUSE 5 SECONDS]
Let the tension dissolve and flow away.
[PAUSE 5 SECONDS]
You feel distant and far away.
[PAUSE 6 SECONDS]
Deep into relaxation.

(continued)

TABLE 10.2 *(continued)*

[PAUSE 6 SECONDS]
Attend to the muscles in your legs.
If you feel any tension, just let go.
Go completely limp.
[PAUSE 6 SECONDS]
Let the tension flow away.
[PAUSE 6 SECONDS]
Sink deeper and deeper.
Far away into relaxation.
[PAUSE 6 SECONDS]
Attend to the muscles in your feet.
If you feel any tension, just let go.
Go completely limp.
[PAUSE 6 SECONDS]
Let the tension dissolve and flow out through your toes.
As you become more and more relaxed.
[PAUSE 6 SECONDS]
And attend to your entire body.
Is there any part of your body where you feel even the slightest
bit of tension?
Just let go. Go completely limp.
[PAUSE 7 SECONDS]
Let tension melt and dissolve.
[PAUSE 7 SECONDS]
Let tension flow out through your fingers.
And out through your toes.
[PAUSE 10 SECONDS]
Sink deeper and deeper.
Far away into relaxation.
[PAUSE 10 SECONDS]

Ending

Let go of what you are attending to.
Slowly open your eyes all the way.
Take a deep breath and stretch.
This completes our exercise.

11

Breathing Exercises

The goal of breathing exercises is to foster diaphragmatic breathing and a breathing pace that is slow and even. Initially, relaxed breathing is deep, and later (as relaxation increases) it is effortless and shallow. One also learns to detect and differentiate relaxed and tense breathing.

HYPOTHESIZED EFFECTS
OF BREATHING EXERCISES

Physical/Autonomic Effects
(see chapter 4 for details on physiology)

Relaxed breathing increases involvement of the diaphragm (chapter 4) and lessens activity of the chest (intercostal) and shoulder (trapezius) muscles. In addition, relaxed breathing has a special rhythm. Exhalation is slow and even. Slight muscle tension is generated during inhalation. The chest muscles and diaphragm relax automatically while air is quietly expelled. Although air is flowing through the lungs and out, there is a sinking movement associated with the automatic relaxation of the breathing muscles. When air has been exhaled, there is a pause until the need for oxygen prompts automatic and relaxed inhalation. The inhalation phase occurs quietly and easily. Generally relaxed exhalation takes twice as long (6 seconds) as inhalation (3 seconds). In contrast, the rhythm of tense breathing is more active and forced.

Attentional Effects

Breathing exercises are appropriate diversions from external stimuli and useful for reducing competing physical activity and thought. The may evoke immediate but modest reductions in autonomic arousal, and to a lesser extent, skeletal muscle tension. However, I hypothesize that their impact here is less than what might be achieved through PMR or AT, and is comparable in degree to yogaform stretching. Beginning breathing exercises require and develop relatively low levels of skill in focusing/refocusing.

R-States

In our own research, we have found a strong connection between breathing exercises and the R-States, At Ease/Peace and Energized. In contrast, autogenic breathing suggestions ("My breathing is free, easy, and effortless") and variations of van Dixhoorn's (1994) "breathing awareness" technique ("Do the technique in a 'lazy,' or indifferent, almost careless, way," without conscious effort to breathe in any particular way) may foster Disengagement. This speculation has yet to be explored in research.

FORMAL CONSIDERATIONS

Placement

Breathing stretching exercises can be placed near the beginning of a relaxation sequence, or at the very end. Passive exercises can be woven in anywhere, and successfully integrated with PMR, AT, imagery, and meditation.

Duration

Beginning and ending breathing stretching exercises can be less than 5 minutes long. When breathing is the primary or only approach practiced, it should include no more than 15 minutes of breathing stretches, 10 minutes of diaphragmatic breathing, and 10 minutes of passive breathing.

Portability

Breathing exercises may well be uniquely effective in their portability and ability to produce a quick effect. One can take a deep breath, or breathe slowly through the lips, nearly anywhere and feel some relaxation. This portability makes breathing exercises valuable in stress situations. Some passive breathing exercises (practiced with eyes open), can be practiced while driving or during activity.

APPROPRIATE CLIENTS

Passive breathing exercises are brief and easy, and can be used by most clients. Their portability makes them ideal for candidates who need low levels of "relaxation on the go," or brief relaxation at work, school, or transit. Breathing (and PMR) may be appropriate in anger management.

Passive breathing is an obvious intervention for hyperventilation syndrome. A hyperventilating client simply breathes too rapidly and deeply under stress, and as a result, exhales too much carbon dioxide. This can trigger a variety of symptoms (cramping in the abdomen, dizziness, fatigue, hot flashes, loss of consciousness, panic, pains in chest, rapidly beating heart, nausea, tension, trembling), which may be misinterpreted by the client as anxiety or panic. The passive breathing exercises in this book, when practiced slowly and deliberately, can interrupt hyperventilation syndrome by decreasing oxygen intake. The increasing levels of carbon dioxide in the blood might also have a mildly soothing effect (such as when one feels "groggy" in a stuffy room).

I must note that the literature frequently promotes various breathing exercises as a rapid way to combat situational stress. Consistent with this consensus, Everly and Lating (2002) begin their chapter on breathing by stating:

> Controlled respiration is one of the oldest and certainly the single, most efficient acute intervention for the mitigation and treatment of excessive stress. (p. 215)

Although in some circumstances this may well be the case, in careful comparative studies our research generally finds PMR to be much more effective in reducing somatic stress, worry, and negative emotion (Ghonchec & Smith, 2003).

Excessive use of breathing stretches or diaphragmatic breathing can evoke hyperventilation. Also, one should take the same precautions with breathing stretches as one would with yogaform stretches. Clients suffering from a severe respiratory disorder should avoid breathing exercises, unless they are part of a properly supervised program of rehabilitation or under a physician's support. Active, diaphragmatic breathing exercises should be avoided by clients who have any abdominal or chest injury or weakness, or are recovering from abdominal or chest surgery. Breathing stretches and active diaphragmatic breathing can also contribute to rapid blood oxygenation, an abrupt change that could be stressful for cardiac patients. Breathing may also not be appropriate for clients with temporal lobe epilepsy or who suffer from psychosis (Fried, 1993).

Fried (1993) suggests that diaphragmatic breathing should be attempted only with a physician's approval for patients who display a tendency toward metabolic acidosis; these include those having severe hypoglycemia, kidney disease, heart disease, or diabetes.

OUR APPROACH TO BREATHING EXERCISES

This book offers a total of twelve breathing exercises (five breathing and stretching exercises, three active diaphragmatic exercises, and four passive breathing exercises). Each can be presented separately or in sequence.

TRAINING

Step 1: Select Format, Provide Overall Rationale, Conduct Assessment

Step 2: Exercise Rationale

Explain that the way we breathe reflects our level of tension and relaxation.

> We breathe quickly and choppily when angry, momentarily hold our breath when afraid, gasp when shocked, and choke when in despair. In contrast, we sigh deeply when relieved. When we are relaxed, our breathing is initially full, even, and unhurried. When deeply relaxed, full breathing becomes more effortless and shallow. Breathing exercises teach us to breathe in a more relaxed way.

To understand breathing and relaxation, clients need to understand something about the process of respiration. Explain the role of the lungs, ribcage, collarbone, and diaphragm. It is useful to demonstrate that diaphragmatic breathing is most efficient:

First sit up comfortably with your feet flat on the floor. Place your hands gently over your stomach, so your thumbs are below your lowest rib. Now, breath in through your chest. Keep your stomach as still as possible. Breathe in and out only through your chest. [PAUSE FOR 3 OR 4 INHALATIONS]. Now relax. This time we will breathe in a different way. Keep your hands over your stomach. When breathing in, hold your ribcage and collarbone as still as possible and breathe in through your stomach as slowly as you can. Imagine you are filling your stomach with air. Can you feel your stomach move as you inhale? Breathe in and out this way for about a minute or so. {PAUSE FOR 3 OR 4 INHALATIONS].

Most people find they can breathe more slowly and with less strain "through the stomach" than "through the chest. " This is because stomach breathing involves primarily the diaphragm and is more efficient.

Step 3: Demonstration/Warmup

Clients can try three types of breathing exercises: breathing stretches, active diaphragmatic breathing, and passive breathing. Breathing stretches are designed to deliberately, but somewhat indirectly, foster diaphragmatic and slow, deep, even breathing. Exercises include:

- Slight Bowing and Breathing (Exhale has you bow forward a few inches.
- Leaning Breathing (Lean back while breathing in.)
- Bowing Breathing (Bow all the way forward while breathing out.)
- Stretching Breathing (As you breathe in, slowly lift and circle your arms in front of you.)
- Slow Bowing Breathing (Take three breaths while bowing forward.)

The general idea of these exercises is to exhale while bowing, and inhale while stretching. Such pacing automatically fosters appropriate movement of the diaphragm. Beginning instructors can have difficulty timing the pace of stretching, bowing, and breathing. It can be useful to keep several points in mind. Observe the client. Look for nonverbal clues that a client is ready to inhale or exhale before suggesting inhalation or exhalation. When a client needs to inhale during bowing, simply suggest "It is OK to pause and take a breath." When exhaling during stretching, suggest "It is OK to pause and exhale." Then continue. This enables a client to breathe naturally, without anxiety, and to emphasize exhaling during bowing, and inhaling during stretching.

Active diaphragmatic breathing exercises also deliberately foster diaphragmatic, slow, deep, even breathing. These include:

- Stomach Squeeze Diaphragmatic Breathing
- Stomach Touch Diaphragmatic Breathing
- Book Breathing

Passive breathing exercises foster a relaxed breathing pattern that is slow, even, and deep-to-effortlessly shallow. They include:

- Inhaling through nose
- Exhaling through Lips
- Deep Breathing
- Focused Breathing

You may present all exercises in sequence, or select those that appear most appropriate.

A special voice quality is appropriate for breathing exercises. You may wish to pattern instructions after your own inhalations and exhalations. That is, as you instruct a client to "inhale," you yourself would inhale (before the instruction). As you instruct a client to "exhale," you would breathe out (while saying "exhale"). In addition, add a touch of "breathiness" to your speech, increasing the flow of air as you speak each word. Your voice should not convey the slow monotony of PMR and AT. Instead, cultivate a voice that sounds refreshed, relaxed, and alert.

Step 4: Practice

The entire breathing sequence presented here may be practiced under supervision. Otherwise, I recommend selecting and practicing specific exercises.

Steps 5 and 6: Review, Revision, and Special Problems

Care should be taken not to present too many breathing exercises in sequence. The active diaphragmatic exercises are most likely to present problems. From

5 to 15% of clients may display "paradoxical breathing," a pattern that involves extending the stomach (diaphragm down) while exhaling, and pulling the stomach in (diaphragm up) while inhaling. To such clients, this may seem natural, perhaps because the chest also extends out while breathing in. However, explain that this goes against the pattern of relaxed breathing; extending the stomach out should help inhalation, rather than exhalation. It is useful to illustrate this with a diagram. Clients may need to experiment with "book breathing" (resting a book over the abdomen and observing its movement during breathing) to discover how to pull the stomach in while exhaling. This exercise can be most effective when the client rests with back on the floor, legs slightly apart, and hands on the abdomen.

Another strategy for fostering diaphragmatic breathing is the standing, side-to-side stretch. Here one simply stands upright in a comfortable position with feet slightly apart and arms hanging to each side. As you inhale, slowly and simultaneously raise your arms to your sides (like the hands of a clock) until your hands and arms are pointing straight away from your body, horizontal to the floor. Do not force a stretch. Breathe naturally. Yoga instructors claim this position naturally encourages diaphragmatic breathing (Coutler, 2001).

A second problem some clients may have is anxiety and self-consciousness during breathing. Directing attention to the very process of inhaling and exhaling can prove troublesome. Most clients adapt to this discomfort and can proceed with little additional concern. For clients who remain anxious or self-conscious about breathing, try presenting the active breathing stretches, avoiding all references to breath, inhalation, exhalation, and air. The stretches, when done alone, can foster a relaxed and diaphragmatic pattern of breathing, even when breathing is not mentioned. If the problem continues, simply discontinue breathing exercises and try something else.

Some clients are self-conscious about appropriately pacing their inhalations and exhalations with instructional patter. First, note that the instructions are written in such a way that one can breathe in and out at one's own pace. There is no need to coordinate breathing with the instructor's pace, because the instructor actually offers no pace. After two or three sessions of practice, such self-consciousness typically habituates.

Some clients may experience signs of hyperventilation, including dizziness, faintness, and nausea. Shorten the exercise sequence or discontinue the exercise.

Finally, when a large number of breathing exercises are combined in sequence, clients may report sleepiness. In that case, I recommend presenting fewer exercises.

ENHANCING
BREATHING EXERCISES

- Incorporate PMR tensing up after inhaling, exhaling while letting go.
- Incorporate yogaform stretches.
- Incorporate imagery suggesting the relaxing flow of breath, wind, or air.
- End with meditation.

TABLE 11.1 Breathing Exercise Scripts
___

BREATHING STRETCHES

Slight Bowing and Breathing

In this exercise we are going to relax by breathing in a way that is full and deep and even. For each exercise that follows, I will first explain how it's done, and then you can practice.

Begin by making sure you are seated in an upright position. Place your feet flat on the floor. And close your eyes.
[PAUSE 3 SECONDS]
Let the tensions of the day flow away.
[PAUSE 3 SECONDS]
Let yourself breathe in a natural and easy way.
In and out, let your breathing become more relaxed.
Let yourself breathe in a natural and easy way.
[PAUSE 3 SECONDS]
We are ready to begin.
Now, let your arms hang by your sides.
[PAUSE 3 SECONDS]
Make sure you are seated in an upright position.
[PAUSE 3 SECONDS]
Here is how we will do our first exercise. Gently exhale as you bow forward a few inches. Pause. And then gently inhale as you slowly sit up. Make your movements be smooth and effortless.

Let's begin, take in a deep breath. And bow forward a few inches while breathing out. Pause, then breathe in.

Do this at your own pace a few times for the next minute or so.
[PAUSE 15 SECONDS]
Slowly and smoothly.
[PAUSE 15 SECONDS]
Take your time.
[PAUSE 15 SECONDS]
Do not force yourself
[PAUSE 15 SECONDS]
___

TABLE 11.1 *(continued)*

And when you are ready, resume sitting up for the next exercise.
Let both arms hang by your sides
[PAUSE 5 SECONDS]

Leaning Breathing

Here is how we will do this exercise. First, here are the instructions. Let your arms hang by your sides. Then lean back while taking in a slow, full breath, and then slowly sit up while breathing out.
[PAUSE]
We can begin. Slowly, smoothly, and gently, lean back and breathe in, and gently sit up while breathing out. Continue breathing this way for about a minute.
[PAUSE 15 SECONDS]
Let the air flow very smoothly and gently.
[PAUSE 15 SECONDS]
Take your time.
[PAUSE 15 SECONDS]
There is no need to hurry.
[PAUSE 15 SECONDS]
And gently return to an upright position for the next exercise.
Let your arms hang by your sides.
[PAUSE 10 SECONDS]

Bowing Breathing

Let me first describe our next exercise. In this exercise bow all the way forward while breathing out. Bend at your waist, letting gravity pull your torso closer and closer to your knees. And when you are ready to breathe in, sit up.
Let's begin.
Let your arms hang to your sides.
Take in a slow deep breath, and begin to bow forward, very easily.
[PAUSE 7 SECONDS]
Smoothly and easily at your own pace.
When ready, very easily sit up while breathing in.
[PAUSE 3 SECONDS]
Continue bowing and breathing for about a minute. Move very easily, at a pace that seems comfortable for you.
[PAUSE 15 SECONDS]
Do not force yourself.
[PAUSE 20 SECONDS]

(continued)

TABLE 11.1 *(continued)*

When you are finished, return your arms to your sides, simply sit and breathe naturally.
    [PAUSE 5 SECONDS]

Breathing Stretches

For our next exercise, as you breathe in, slowly lift and circle your arms in front of you, and reach higher to the sky. And lower your arms to your sides as you breathe out.
    And now begin.
    Breathe out.
    Reach up while breathing in, and return to a relaxed seated position while breathing out, for the next minute or so.
    [PAUSE 10 SECONDS]
    Notice the smooth flow of air.
    [PAUSE 10 SECONDS}
    Very easily and gently.
    [PAUSE 25 SECONDS]
    And when you are ready, simply return to a comfortable upright position and let your arms hang to your sides.
    And breathe naturally.

Slow Bowing Breathing

In this exercise take three breaths while bowing forward. And three breaths while sitting up.
    First let your arms hang by your sides. Take a deep breath. I will count one to three so you can keep pace.
    One. Very slowly and smoothly begin to bow forward, just a few inches, until you have exhaled. When ready, pause and inhale. Stay in your position.
    [PAUSE 6 SECONDS]
    Two. Continue bowing over a bit farther while letting the air flow out.
    When ready, pause and inhale.
    [PAUSE 7 SECONDS]
    Three. Continue bending over, all the way, letting gravity pull you down as you breathe out.
    When ready pause, and breathe naturally if you need to.
    [PAUSE 5 SECONDS]
    And when ready, exhale.
    One. Breathe in while slowly sit up a few inches,
    When ready, pause and slowly exhale.
    [PAUSE 5 SECONDS]

TABLE 11.1 *(continued)*

Two—Continue and pause.
[PAUSE 5 SECONDS]
Three—Continue
[PAUSE 5 SECONDS]
And remain seated in a comfortable position while breathing
naturally.
Continue breathing this way for about a minute, pausing three
times while bowing over and pausing three times while sitting up.
[PAUSE 40 SECONDS]
And now comfortably sit upright with your arms hanging to your
sides.

ACTIVE DIAPHRAGMATIC BREATHING

Stomach Squeeze Breathing

Sit up in your chair and open your hands and fingers and place
them over your stomach.
[PAUSE 3 SECONDS]
Spread your fingers comfortably apart so they cover your entire
stomach, with your thumbs touch the bottom part of your chest.
[PAUSE 3 SECONDS]
In this exercise gently press your fingers into your stomach as
you breathe out, and release your fingers as you breathe in.
[PAUSE]
Now, very easily, take a full breath, filling your stomach and
chest completely. And when you are ready to exhale, firmly press
in with your hands and fingers, squeezing in as if you were squeez-
ing the air out of your stomach.
[PAUSE 3 SECONDS]
And when you are ready to inhale, gradually release your fingers
and let your stomach relax and breathe in as if your stomach were
filling with air.
[PAUSE 3 SECONDS]
Breathe easily and completely.
[PAUSE 3 SECONDS]
Now continue breathing this way, squeezing your stomach as you
are breathing out, and relaxing your fingers as you breathe in.
[PAUSE 3 SECONDS]
Do not force yourself to breathe at a hurried pace.
[PAUSE 3 SECONDS]
Take your time.
[PAUSE 3 SECONDS]

(continued)

TABLE 11.1 *(continued)*

Breathe very gently and very easily.
[PAUSE 3 SECONDS]
Focus on what it feels like to breathe completely and fully.
Notice the awareness breathing brings.
[PAUSE 3 SECONDS]
At your own pace, continue breathing evenly in and evenly out.
Do not hurry. Take your time.
[PAUSE 3 SECONDS]
Focus on the even flow of air as it rushes in and out of your lungs.
[PAUSE 3 SECONDS]
Now, when you are ready, exhale and relax your fingers.

Stomach Touch Breathing

Sit up in your chair and make sure your hands and fingers are placed over your stomach.
[PAUSE]
This time, let your hands and fingers remain relaxed. Do not press in. And gently breathe in, as if you were filling your stomach with air, and exhale, so you can feel the rise and fall of your stomach.
[PAUSE]
We are ready to begin. As you breathe in, let the air come in on its own, as if it were filling your stomach.
[PAUSE]
Feel the stomach filling, like a large, soft balloon, filling completely.
[PAUSE]
And when you are ready to exhale, keep your fingers and hands relaxed. Let the air flow out on its own, gently and slowly.
[PAUSE]
When you have breathed out, pull your stomach in gently toward your backbone.
[PAUSE]
Continue breathing this way, slowly and easily.
Notice your stomach filling and emptying with air.
[PAUSE]
Notice the air coming in and out.
[PAUSE 5 SECONDS]
Very smoothly and easily
[PAUSE 5 SECONDS]

TABLE 11.1 *(continued)*

Book Breathing

This exercise is optional. You can skip it if you desire. And you might want to practice this exercise while lying on your back on the floor. And you need a book.

[PAUSE 5 SECONDS]

And now gently place a book over your abdomen.

Adjust your book so it does not fall off.

[PAUSE]

And let yourself breathe easily and naturally.

[PAUSE]

In and out.

[PAUSE]

There is no hurry to breathe in any particular way.

[PAUSE]

Very smoothly and easily.

[PAUSE]

And now, very gently breathe in, filling your abdomen with air. Breathe in such a way that you can notice the movement of the book resting on your abdomen. You may adjust your book so you can see its movement more clearly.

[PAUSE]

The up and down movement of your book shows if you are breathing using your abdomen.

[PAUSE]

And when you have taken a full breath of air, gently and slowly exhale.

[PAUSE]

Let the air flow out very slowly and smoothly.

[PAUSE]

See if you can notice the movement of the book.

[PAUSE]

And when you are ready, try this again.

[PAUSE]

If you need to, adjust the position of your book.

[PAUSE]

Keep you chest still. Try not to fill your chest with air.

[PAUSE]

And let air flow into your abdomen, so you notice your book moving.

[PAUSE]

(continued)

TABLE 11.1 *(continued)*

Slowly and gently.
[PAUSE]
And when you have inhaled all the way, pause, and slowly exhale.
[PAUSE]
Continue breathing this way for about a minute.
[PAUSE]
See if you can breathe in such a way that you can gently move your book when breathing in and out.
[PAUSE 30 SECONDS]
And now, gently let go of what you are attending to.
We have completed our exercise.

PASSIVE BREATHING

Sniffing

Rest your hands comfortably in your lap.
[PAUSE]
Let yourself relax.
[PAUSE]
As you breathe in, imagine you are sniffing a very delicate flower. Breathe in slowly with many gentle little sniffs. We can begin.
[PAUSE]
Let the sniffing flow of breath into your nose be as smooth and gentle as possible, so you barely rustle a petal.
[PAUSE]
Take a full breath.
[PAUSE]
And when ready, relax, letting yourself breathe out slowly and naturally, without effort.
[PAUSE]
Continue breathing this way, breathing in and out, quietly and evenly at your own pace.
[PAUSE]
Calmly focus on the clear inner calm that comes when you breathe in a way that is slow, full, and even.
[PAUSE]
Notice the refreshing and energizing rush of air as it quietly move in and out of your lungs.
[PAUSE]
See how far you can follow the inward flow of air.
[PAUSE]
Can you feel it move past your nostrils?
[PAUSE]

TABLE 11.1 *(continued)*

Can you feel the air in the passages of your nose?
[PAUSE]
Can you feel the renewing and refreshing air flow into your body?
[PAUSE]
Take your time.
[PAUSE]
Breathe easily and fully.
[PAUSE]
Let yourself be fully aware of your breathing.
[PAUSE 10 SECONDS]

Blowing

Take a slow deep breath and pause.
[PAUSE]
In our next exercise, breathe out slowly though your lips, as if you were blowing at a candle flame just enough to make it flicker, but not go out. Breathe in through your nose.
[PAUSE]
Start by taking a deep breath. And when you are ready, gently exhale, making the stream of air that passes through your lips as you exhale as smooth and gentle as possible.
[PAUSE]
Let tension flow out with every breath.
[PAUSE 4 SECONDS]
Let the gentle movement of air dissolve any feelings of tension you might have.
[PAUSE 5 SECONDS]
Focus on the easy flow of air in as it refreshes and renews.
[PAUSE 5 SECONDS]
Let each breath fill you with peace and calm energy.
[PAUSE 5 SECONDS]
Let yourself breathe fully and evenly.
[PAUSE 10 SECONDS]

Occasional Deep Breaths

Let yourself breathe easily and naturally.
[PAUSE]
In our next exercise, simply take in a full deep breath, filling your lungs and abdomen with good, refreshing air. Do this now.
[PAUSE]

(continued)

TABLE 11.1 *(continued)*

And when you are ready, relax.
[PAUSE]
And slowly let the air flow out, very smoothly and gently.
[PAUSE]
And now, just continue breathing normally for a while, without taking in deep breaths.
[PAUSE]
Do not attempt to force yourself to breathe in any particular way.
[PAUSE]
Just let the air come in and out on its own.
[PAUSE 10 SECONDS]
And again, when you are ready, take in another full deep breath, filling your lungs, with good, energizing air. Feel the calm and strength it brings.
[PAUSE]
And, when ready, gently and smoothly exhale.
[PAUSE]
Then resume breathing in a normal way, easily in and out.
[PAUSE 10 SECONDS]
And again, when you are ready, take in a full deep breath, filling your lungs, with good, energizing air. Feel the calm and strength it brings.
[PAUSE]
And, when ready, gently and smoothly exhale.
[PAUSE]
Then resume breathing in a normal way, easily in and out.
[PAUSE 10 SECONDS]

Focused Breathing

Simply breathe in a relaxed manner, in and out through your nose.
[PAUSE]
Try not to force your breathing.
[PAUSE]
Become fully aware of the air as it rushes in and out, flowing into and out of your lungs.
[PAUSE]
Filling your body with refreshing and renewing air.
[PAUSE]
Calmly focus on the unhurried rhythm of your breathing. Let yourself breathe effortlessly, without strain.
[PAUSE 10 SECONDS]

TABLE 11.1 *(continued)*

Focus on the even flow of air as it moves in and out of your lungs through your nose.

[PAUSE 10 SECONDS]

Notice how the easy flow of air energizes and relaxes you.

[PAUSE 5 SECONDS]

The flow of air brings peace and inner strength.

[PAUSE 5 SECONDS]

Let go of what you are attending to. Slowly open your eyes all the way. Take a deep breath and stretch. This completes our exercise.

12

Autogenic Training

The fundamental strategy of our version of autogenic training (AT) is to mentally repeat phrases or images suggestive of, and associated with, somatic relaxation, specifically reductions in autonomic arousal.

HYPOTHESIZED EFFECTS OF AUTOGENIC TRAINING

Physical/Autonomic Effects
(see chapter 4 for more on physiology)

Whereas PMR and Yogaform Stretching work primarily on the skeletal muscles as well as posture and position, AT works on mechanisms of autonomic arousal, particularly smooth muscles (muscles surrounding blood vessels to the skin and muscles, heart muscles, abdominal muscles) and various nerve clusters or "plexes," specifically the enteric nervous system in the abdomen. Thoughts targeted to specific aspects of autonomic arousal reduction may well foster targeted changes. We think about salivating while eating a lemon, and indeed we salivate (an autonomic response). We think about warm blood flowing into our fingers, and our fingers become warm. In autogenic training, we think of words and images that reflect the immediate effects of specific desired reductions in autonomic arousal.

To elaborate, when relaxation clients report that their hands and legs feel "heavy" and "warm," this is likely a relaxation response effect of increased blood flow to the extremities. Muscles engorged with blood are literally "warm and heavy." Through simple autogenic suggestion, one can suggest the dilation of these same blood vessels. Reductions in skeletal muscle tension may ensue as a sideeffect. Of course, stretching exercises and the tense-release cycles of PMR may evoke reductions in autonomic arousal as a side effect of reduced skeletal muscle tension. Indeed, after Yogaform Stretching and PMR, one may feel flushed, warm, and perhaps initially heavy.

Attentional Effects

For some clients, AT is effective for diverting attention from external stimuli and minimizing competing physical activity and thought. However, it is not as universally effective as PMR or Yogaform Stretching.

AT requires more skill at focusing/refocusing than either PMR, Yogaform Stretching, Breathing Exercises, or, for some clients, Imagery. The target stimuli, somatic phrases and images such as "warmth and heaviness," are often subtle. The exercise is relatively unchanging, increasing the likelihood of distraction.

R-States

In my clinical experience, AT (at least the beginning exercises), like PMR, may facilitate Sleepiness, Disengagement, and Physical Relaxation. Therefore, I hypothesize that AT may have a pattern of effectiveness similar to PMR and may be useful for clients in psychotherapy for anxiety or depression.

FORMAL CONSIDERATIONS

Placement

I do not recommend using AT at the beginning of an exercise sequence. It works best after PMR or breathing, and may be combined with imagery.

Duration

I recommend that beginners limit their sessions to five minutes. Advanced practitioners may increase the length to fifteen minutes.

Portability

Because of the degree of sustained focus required, AT exercises are less portable than stretching, PMR, or breathing exercises. However, in a quiet environment, they can be practiced with some ease.

APPROPRIATE CLIENTS

Because autogenic exercises require a degree of focusing ability, they are perhaps less appropriate for clients who are easily distracted or need a highly structured and familiar training format. Although proponents claim the approach can be applied to virtually any condition, a conservative strategy is to apply it in situations where autonomic arousal is clearly involved, or to supplement or follow PMR.

Autonomic symptoms such as cold hands (AT suggestion: "hands are warm"), palpitating heart ("evenly beating heart"), dry mouth ("mouth is moist, like tasting a lemon"), watery eyes ("eyes are calm and dry"), digestive problems ("stomach soothed and cool"), migraine headache ("forehead and neck cool and relaxed"), and colitis ("intestines cool and soothed") might respond well to targeted suggestions (see access skills, chapter 4).

One should seek medical approval before attempting autogenic suggestions for organs or processes that are weakened, injured, recovering from surgery, under treatment, or whose functioning is compromised in any way. For example, if a client suffers from abdominal bleeding, it would not be wise to suggest, "My stomach is warm and throbbing." Such a suggestion might conceivably increase blood flow to the abdomen. For a client suffering from cold hands, obviously do not suggest "My hands are cool and relaxed."

OUR VERSION OF AUTOGENIC TRAINING

Our approach to autogenic training targets four groups of sensations: heaviness, warmth in the extremities, evenly beating heart, and warmth in the abdomen (solar plexus). Unlike traditional autogenic training, we do not include exercises focusing on the breath or coolness of the forehead (which overlap with our breathing and meditation/mindfulness sequences).

Both verbal and visual sequences are offered. Verbal exercises resemble traditional AT exercises and present suggestions as words ("warm and heavy"). Visual exercises present suggestions as visual images targeted to the same sensations ("warm sun, breeze, water"). It is appropriate for clients who are adept at visualization, or when combining autogenic and imagery exercises.

TRAINING

Step 1: Select Format, Provide
Overall Orientation, Conduct Assessment

Step 2: Exercise Rationale

When presenting autogenic exercises, explain the key idea of the connection between body and mind. For example, imagining the taste of a lemon can often evoke the somatic response of salivation. Similarly, thoughts can evoke bodily relaxation. When we relax, we feel physical changes, for example, heaviness, warmth, an evenly beating heart, slow breathing, and so on. Autogenic exercises make use of these feelings. The technique is to simply, and passively, repeat phrases or images that suggest these relaxation feelings.

Explain the rationale for each of the four categories of suggestions. Linden (1993) recommends the following:

"Heavy." This suggestion is claimed to increase muscle relaxation. A relaxed muscle will actually feel "heavy," because less effort is exerted keeping the muscle firm. You may notice this when, after an exhausting day, you fall heavily into bed. Or perhaps you become so relaxed in a chair that you can barely get up.

"Warm." This suggestion is claimed to increase blood flow to the fingers, hands, and feet. When relaxed, blood flow increases to the extremities, contributing to feelings of warmth. In contrast, when under stress, blood flows away from the extremities, contributing to "cold, clammy hands."

"Quiet, evenly beating heart." Most people understand that when under stress, the heart starts beating hard, sometimes irregularly. This suggestion fosters a relaxed heartbeat.

"Sun rays streaming, warm and quiet." In this suggestion, one focuses on the solar plexus (enteric nervous system), an important nerve center for internal organs. The solar plexus is halfway between the navel and the lower portion of the sternum ("the pit of the stomach").

Step 3: Demonstration/Warmup

First, demonstrate the importance of passive, as opposed to active, thinking. Here is a demonstration I use (Smith, 1987):

> First, let's demonstrate its opposite, active thinking. Let your right hand drop to your side. Now, actively and effortfully try to make your hand feel warm and heavy. Work at it. Exert as much effort as you can trying to actively and deliberately will your hands to feel warm and heavy. [CONTINUE, WITH A RELATIVELY ELEVATED "COACHING" VOICE.]
>
> Next, simply relax. Let your hand fall limply by your side. Without trying to accomplish anything, simply let the phrase [USE A SLOW, MONOTONOUS TONE OF VOICE] "my hand is warm and heavy" repeat in your mind. Let the words repeat on their own, like an echo. All you have to do is quietly observe the repeating words. Don't try to achieve warmth and heaviness. Just quietly let the words go over and over in your mind. While thinking the words "warm and heavy," you might want to imagine your hand in warm sand, or in the sun, or in a warm bath. Pick an image that feels comfortable, and simple dwell upon it.
>
> We have just tried active and passive thinking. Which one was more effective? (p. 134)

Suggestions should be phrased in a way that is pleasing and simple to recite or think. For example, one might employ simple words, rhymes, and internal rhythms. A useful insomnia suggestion might be "My sleep is deep and peaceful" rather than "I will fall asleep more quickly tonight". Linden (1993) recommends that personalized suggestions be positive ("I feel calmer" vs. "I feel less tense"). Also, they should be consistent with a client's beliefs.

Voice quality for autogenic exercises should be similar to the PMR "let-go" voice (previously discussed). Speak in a slow, boring monotone, adding little color or interest to what you are saying. Match your voice to specific autogenic suggestions. When suggesting "warm," your voice should actually sound warm and soothing. When suggesting "heavy," your voice should sound heavy and relaxed." "Evenly beating heart" involves a voice that is gently rhymical. "Warm glow in abdomen" involves speaking in a way that is "warm" and "glowing," as if you were on the radio promoting a delicious bowl of hot soup or a new brand of hot chocolate.

Step 4: Practice

Practice the entire sequence.

Steps 5 and 6: Review, Revision, and Special Problems

Some clients have a strong dislike for autogenic suggestions. Others may display excessive Disengagement (and report symptoms of depersonalization). For such individuals, perhaps the entire sequence should be avoided.

Clients may complain that they do not experience the suggested effects. At this point it might be useful to remind them that it is important not to seek actual feelings of "heaviness," "warmth," or the like. Significant relaxation may be taking place in the absence of these sensations. To determine if clients are actually relaxed, be sure to note reported R-States, body language, and relaxation aftereffects (see chapter 17). Clients can be "primed" to experience warmth and heaviness by first practicing overt PMR.

ENHANCING AUTOGENIC TRAINING

- This text introduces four autogenic suggestions: warmth, heaviness, evenly-beating heart, and soothed abdomen. This does not exhaust the list of potential autonomic suggestions. For virtually any type of autonomic distress that can be identified and isolated by a client, a corresponding autogenic suggestion can be identified. For example, the physical complaint "My body does not feel well" is too vague for autogenic suggestions. In contrast, cold hands, a throbbing headache, stomach distress, aching eyes, tired feet, palpitating heart, burning sensations in the esophagus are specific and easily targeted. When inventing new autogenic suggestions, I recommend three strategies. First, imagine a corresponding and opposing autogenic suggestion for the targeted symptom ("warm hands," "soothed and cool forehead," "calm and cool stomach," "cool and relaxed eyes," "warm and tingling feet," "evenly beating heart," "and calm and relaxed esophagus)." Second, imagine an autogenic suggestion for a neutral (not in discomfort) body part not associated with a troubled area. For example, for a headache, think "hands and fingers are warm and soothed." For this option, experiment with suggestions that either oppose ("cool hands" for headache) or correspond to the target symptom ("warm hands" for headache). Third, create an autogenic suggestion that does not counter a specific targeted source of discomfort with an opposing sensation, but suggests a new, less aversive meaning for the discomfort. The pain remains, but is reinterpreted. For example, a person experiencing the discomfort of stomach distress might think "warm, healing blood flows to the stomach. Stomach juices soothe away toxins."

- Supplementary autogenic suggestions can be selected from our list of words associated with R-States (chapter 5). For example, words suggestive of Physical Relaxation include "limp, loose, liquid." Words related to Disengagement include "far away, distant, indifferent, safe, isolated." Some words for At Ease/Peace include "relaxed, clam, easy, contented, and soothed." Similarly, a client may have alternative images suggestive of physical relaxation. Encourage clients to think of their own images or words.
- For visual autogenic exercises, creatively incorporate an image agreed to by the client. One might use the image of a "moving spot of light" that "melts tension away" and "brings energy and health". This spot can move from the tip of one's head, down through the torso, and out through the legs and toes. Alternatively, the spot can exit through the fingers. Moving light imagery can be tailored to a client's preferences ("moving glowing hand," "magic flashlight beam," "glowing energy beam," etc.).
- Precede or integrate PMR exercises (which, like AT, tend to evoke the R-States, Physical Relaxation and Disengagement). Letting Go exercises can work especially well.
- Passive breathing exercises may be introduced.
- Avoid yoga stretching or active breathing exercises.
- Avoid active narrative or insight imagery, as these can evoke R-States inconsistent with AT.
- For some clients it may be appropriate to end with a simple meditation, given that this technique can at times cultivate Disengagement.

TABLE 12.1 Autogenic Training Scripts

VERBAL AUTOGENIC EXERCISES

In this exercise we are going to relax by thinking relaxing words about the body. First make sure you are seated upright in a comfort-

---

(continued)

TABLE 12.1 *(continued)*

able position. Place your feet flat on the floor. And close your eyes.

Let yourself sink into a comfortable state of relaxation, far away from the world. This time is just for you. You can forget the problems of the day.
[PAUSE 5 SECONDS]

Heaviness Suggestions

Simply think the words,
"Arms and legs, very heavy."
There is no need for you to achieve any effect.
[PAUSE 3 SECONDS]
Arms and legs are very heavy, as tension goes away.
[PAUSE 3 SECONDS]
Entire body, more and more heavy.
[PAUSE 3 SECONDS]
Let yourself sink into a distant state of pleasant relaxation.
[PAUSE 3 SECONDS]
There is nothing you have to do.
[PAUSE 3 SECONDS]
Let the words go over and over like an echo.
[PAUSE 3 SECONDS]
Arms and legs very heavy. Very heavy. Very heavy.
[PAUSE 3 SECONDS]
There is nothing you have to do.
[PAUSE 3 SECONDS]
Let tension sink away.
[PAUSE 3 SECONDS]
Let your muscles become more relaxed.
[PAUSE 3 SECONDS]
As you sink deeper into relaxation.
[PAUSE 5 SECONDS]
You become more calm and relaxed.
[PAUSE 3 SECONDS]
More quiet.
[PAUSE 5 SECONDS]
Entire body, very heavy. Very heavy. Very heavy.
[PAUSE 5 SECONDS]
Let the words go over and over in your mind.
Your arm becomes more and more loose and limp.
[PAUSE 3 SECONDS]
As tension sinks away.
[PAUSE 3 SECONDS]

TABLE 12.1 *(continued)*

Arms and legs are very heavy.
[PAUSE 3 SECONDS]
Entire body very heavy.
[PAUSE 3 SECONDS]
Arms and legs are very heavy.
[PAUSE 3 SECONDS]

Suggestions of Warmth

Arms and legs are heavy and warm.
[PAUSE 3 SECONDS]
Entire body, nice and warm.
Let the words go over and over in your mind.
[PAUSE 3 SECONDS]
Comfortably relaxed.
[PAUSE 3 SECONDS]
Feelings of tension dissolve.
[PAUSE 3 SECONDS]
Tension melts and flows away.
[PAUSE 3 SECONDS]
Arms and legs are heavy and warm.
[PAUSE 5 SECONDS]
Feelings of tension dissolve.
[PAUSE 3 SECONDS]
Tension melts and flows away.
[PAUSE 3 SECONDS]
Entire body very warm
Let the words go over and over in your mind.
[PAUSE 3 SECONDS]
Warm and relaxed.
[PAUSE 3 SECONDS]
Let yourself sink deeper into a pleasant state of relaxation.
[PAUSE 5 SECONDS]
Relaxed and calm.
[PAUSE 5 SECONDS]
Far away.
[PAUSE 5 SECONDS]
Far away.
[PAUSE 3 SECONDS]
Warm and heavy.
[PAUSE 3 SECONDS]
Sink into deeper relaxation, heavy and warm.
[PAUSE 3 SECONDS]

(continued)

TABLE 12.1 *(continued)*

Heart Suggestions

   [PAUSE 5 SECONDS]
   Think the words, "Heart is beating quietly and strongly, quietly
and evenly."
   [PAUSE 5 SECONDS]
   Heart is beating quietly and evenly.
   [PAUSE 5 SECONDS]
   As your body sinks deeper into comfortable relaxation.
   [PAUSE 3 SECONDS]
   Far away from the world.
   [PAUSE 3 SECONDS]
   Heart is warm, beating quietly and evenly.
   Let the words go over and over in your mind.
   [PAUSE 3 SECONDS]
   Quietly and evenly.
   [PAUSE 3 SECONDS]
   As tension dissolves.
   [PAUSE 5 SECONDS]
   And flows from the body.
   [PAUSE 5 SECONDS]
   You settle into a safe and comfortable relaxation.
   [PAUSE 5 SECONDS]
   Heart is beating, quietly and evenly.
   [PAUSE 5 SECONDS]
   Quietly and evenly.
   [PAUSE 5 SECONDS]
   There is nothing you have to do.

Abdominal Warmth Suggestions.

   And now gently attend to an area above your navel.
   [PAUSE 3 SECONDS]
   An area where you feel warm and good after drinking warm hot
chocolate, or good soup.
   [PAUSE 5 SECONDS]
   As you become more comfortably relaxed.
   [PAUSE 5 SECONDS]
   Feel your abdomen . . . soothed and warm, comfortable and
warm.
   Relaxed and warm inside.
   Let the words go over and over in your mind.
   [PAUSE 3 SECONDS]
   Warmth spreads and relaxes inside.
   [PAUSE 3 SECONDS]

TABLE 12.1 *(continued)*

Let yourself sink deeper into relaxation.
[PAUSE 3 SECONDS]
Far away from the world.
[PAUSE 3 SECONDS]
Your abdomen is comfortably warm and relaxed.
Relaxed and soothed.
[PAUSE 3 SECONDS]
Let yourself become more and more deeply relaxed.
[PAUSE 5 SECONDS]
More and more quiet and calm.
[PAUSE 5 SECONDS]
Soothing away the tensions of the day.
[PAUSE 5 SECONDS]
Let yourself enjoy the pleasant and soothing feelings of relaxation. Warm and heavy. Through your entire body. For the next minute or so.
[PAUSE 30 SECONDS]
Let go of what you are attending to.
Slowly open your eyes all the way.
Take a deep breath and stretch.
This completes our exercise.

VISUAL AUTOGENIC SUGGESTIONS

In this exercise we are going to relax with images that suggest relaxing sensations. First make sure you are seated upright in a comfortable position. Place your feet flat on the floor. And close your eyes.

Let yourself sink into a comfortable state of relaxation, far away from the world. This time is just for you, you can forget the problems of the day.
[PAUSE 5 SECONDS]
Imagine yourself resting on a soft comfortable bed. This bed can be anything, a soft fluffy mattress. A warm sandy beach, a resting spot by the ocean. A soothing and comfortable bed of thick green grass. Imagine yourself resting in a place that is soft and comfortable.

Heaviness Suggestions.

Your arms and legs are getting heavy, very heavy.
There is no need for you to achieve any effect.
[PAUSE 3 SECONDS]

(continued)

TABLE 12.1 *(continued)*

Arms and legs are very heavy, like gravity is pulling them towards the earth. Like a magnet is pulling tension away into your soft comfortable resting spot.
[PAUSE 3 SECONDS]
Entire body, more and more heavy.
You sink deeper into your bed.
[PAUSE 3 SECONDS]
Let yourself sink into a distant state of pleasant relaxation.
[PAUSE 3 SECONDS]
There is nothing you have to do.
[PAUSE 3 SECONDS]
Warm and heavy, like gentle rays of sun are dissolving tension in your body.
[PAUSE 3 SECONDS]
Arms and legs very heavy. Very heavy. Very heavy.
[PAUSE 3 SECONDS]
You feel the gentle pressure and support against your skin.
There is nothing you have to do.
[PAUSE 3 SECONDS]
A soft and soothing breeze touches your skin.
Let tension dissolve and sink away.
[PAUSE 3 SECONDS]
Let gravity pull tension away as you sink into your bed.
[PAUSE 3 SECONDS]
As sink into relaxation.
[PAUSE 5 SECONDS]
You become more calm and relaxed.
[PAUSE 3 SECONDS]
More quiet.
[PAUSE 5 SECONDS]
Entire body, very heavy. Very heavy. Very heavy.
[PAUSE 5 SECONDS]
Your arm becomes more and more loose and limp.
[PAUSE 3 SECONDS]
As tension sinks away.
[PAUSE 3 SECONDS]
Like a magnet pulling tension away.
[PAUSE 5 SECONDS]
Like the warm sun is melting tension.
A gentle breeze touches your skin, dissolving tension.
Arms and legs are very heavy.
You feel the gentle support against your skin.
[PAUSE 3 SECONDS]

TABLE 12.1 *(continued)*

Entire body very heavy.
[PAUSE 3 SECONDS]
Arms and legs are very heavy.
[PAUSE 3 SECONDS]

Warmth Suggestions.

Arms and legs are heavy and warm.
[PAUSE 3 SECONDS]
Entire body, nice and warm.
[PAUSE 3 SECONDS]
Like the warm sun is shining.
[PAUSE 3 SECONDS]
Dissolving feelings of tension.
[PAUSE 3 SECONDS]
A gentle breeze touches your skin.
Tension melts and flows away.
[PAUSE 3 SECONDS]
Arms and legs are heavy and warm.
[PAUSE 5 SECONDS]
A soothing mist carries tension away.
[PAUSE 3 SECONDS]
Dissolving feelings of tension.
[PAUSE 3 SECONDS]
Tension melts and flows away.
[PAUSE 3 SECONDS]
Entire body very warm
[PAUSE 3 SECONDS]
Warm and relaxed.
[PAUSE 3 SECONDS]
Let yourself sink deeper into your pleasant soft bed of relaxation.
[PAUSE 5 SECONDS]
Relaxed and calm.
[PAUSE 5 SECONDS]
Far away.
[PAUSE 5 SECONDS]
Far away.
[PAUSE 3 SECONDS]
Warm and heavy.
[PAUSE 3 SECONDS]
Sink into deeper relaxation, heavy and warm.
[PAUSE 3 SECONDS]

(continued)

TABLE 12.1 *(continued)*

Heart Suggestions

[PAUSE 5 SECONDS]
Your heart is beating quietly and strongly, quietly and evenly.
[PAUSE 5 SECONDS]
The warm sun melts tension from your body.
Heart is beating quietly and evenly.
[PAUSE 5 SECONDS]
As your body sinks deeper into your comfortable bed.
[PAUSE 3 SECONDS]
Far away.
[PAUSE 3 SECONDS]
A gentle breeze touches your body.
Tension flows away.
Heart is warm, beating quietly and evenly.
[PAUSE 3 SECONDS]
Quietly and evenly.
[PAUSE 3 SECONDS]
As gravity pulls tension from your body.
[PAUSE 5 SECONDS]
You settle into a safe and comfortable relaxation.
[PAUSE 5 SECONDS]
Heart is beating, quietly and evenly.
[PAUSE 5 SECONDS]
Quietly and evenly.
A soothing mist carries tension away.
[PAUSE 5 SECONDS]
There is nothing you have to do.
[PAUSE 5 SECONDS]
As you become more comfortably relaxed in your soft and comfortable bed.
[PAUSE 5 SECONDS]

Abdominal Warmth Suggestions.

And now gently attend to an area above your navel.
[PAUSE 3 SECONDS]
An area where you feel warm and good after drinking warm hot chocolate, or good soup.
Imagine sun rays streaming from this area, quiet and warm.
[PAUSE 3 SECONDS]
Warming your abdomen.
[PAUSE 3 SECONDS]
Warming and relaxing your entire inside.
[PAUSE 3 SECONDS]

TABLE 12.1 *(continued)*

Imagine a warm breeze touching you.
Quiet and warm.
Soothing and warm.
[PAUSE 3 SECONDS]
Let yourself sink deeper into relaxation.
[PAUSE 3 SECONDS]
Far away from the world.
[PAUSE 3 SECONDS]
Imagine sun rays streaming quiet and warm.
[PAUSE 3 SECONDS]
Let yourself become more and more deeply relaxed.
[PAUSE 5 SECONDS]
A soothing mist carries tension away.
It flows away.
You feel more and more quiet and calm.
[PAUSE 5 SECONDS]
Soothing away the tensions of the day.
[PAUSE 5 SECONDS]
Sun rays streaming quiet and warm.
[PAUSE 3 SECONDS]
Sun rays streaming quiet and warm.
[PAUSE 5 SECONDS]
A gentle breeze.
The soothing flow of water.
Let yourself enjoy this relaxing place for the next minute or
so, enjoying how your body feels as it relaxes.
[PAUSE 30 SECONDS]
Let go of what you are attending to.
Slowly open your eyes all the way.
Take a deep breath and stretch.
This completes our exercise.

13

Imagery and Relaxing Self-Talk

Imagery involves creating in one's mind a passive relaxing setting or activity, often accompanied by the repetition of relaxing words or self-statements. Imagery exercises are similar to guided fantasy and daydreams about a passive and relaxing theme.

HYPOTHESIZED EFFECTS OF IMAGERY AND RELAXING SELF-TALK

Physical/Autonomic Effects

In general, imagery is not the most effective way of achieving deep muscle relaxation. The topics I suggest for imagery are settings and activities drawn from casual, everyday life (travel, outdoors/nature, water, indoors) that may or may not involve deep muscle relaxation. Indeed, casual everyday relaxation may evoke positive affective states (e.g., the R-State, Joy) that can sustain a degree of muscle tension. The one exception is if a client has already mastered deep muscle relaxation through another technique, perhaps PMR or AT. Then, imagery of this very technique could well evoke the same level of relaxation.

Cognitive and Attentional Effects

All approaches to relaxation can divert attention from self-stressing verbal thought. In imagery this diversion is achieved by shifting the very modality of cognitive activity. One ceases self-stressing verbal activity and engages in nonverbal activity such as thinking about images, sounds and music, touch sensations, and relaxing smells. However, these effects do not occur in settings where one must keep one's eyes open. Imagery requires a moderate level of skill at focusing/refocusing except for those who are already adept at fantasy.

R-States

Of all the families of techniques, imagery has the potential for evoking the widest range of R-States, especially the R-States At Ease/Peace, Energized, Joy, Childlike Innocence, Deep Mystery, Thankful/Loving, and perhaps Disengagement. Indeed, the R-States evoked are limited only by the specific themes selected. In some traditions, for example, Christian prayer of the heart and some forms of Tibetan Buddhism, one focuses more directly on positive affective states, notably the R-State, Thankful/Loving. And in Kundalini yoga one directs attention to presumed body energy centers, the chakras, which are often associated with affective states (the heart and "love").

When imagery is accompanied by self-statements of relaxing words, any R-State may be incorporated or emphasized ("Let yourself feel sleepy . . . limp . . . refreshed . . . energized . . . " etc.)

FORMAL CONSIDERATIONS

Placement

Generally, I recommend placing imagery near the end of an exercise sequence. However, one might begin with imagery in order to set the stage or context for a subsequent sequence of exercises. Imagery may be effectively combined with autogenic visual suggestions, and PMR and imagery can be combined to target muscles.

Duration

I recommend ten-minute sessions for beginners. Advanced practitioners may practice for up to 40 minutes.

Portability

The portability of imagery is severely limited, except for those with highly developed imagery skills. One must practice in a quiet environment, preferably alone.

APPROPRIATE CLIENTS

Imagery should be accessible to a wide range of clients. Children around the age of 12, and females are often particularly good candidates. Clients who are simply not good at, or interested in, generating imagery tend not to like imagery.

Imagery requires a degree of focusing ability and is perhaps less appropriate for clients who are easily distracted or need a highly structured and familiar training format. I hypothesize that imagery is not appropriate for those who use fantasy as a maladaptive avoidance strategy or for individuals with a thought disorder or problems with impulse-control.

OUR APPROACH TO IMAGERY

I find it useful to define imagery as the covert (or mental) generation of any real or imagined passive setting or activity one finds relaxing. For those who are not adept at generating images, they can be described as "verbal descriptions of relaxing settings and situations." This text presents two categories of imagery: sense and insight. In sense imagery, one simply imagines sensations associated with a relaxing setting or activity. Insight imagery has a relaxing theme, typically the cultivation of a deeper appreciation of, or answer to, a topic or question. One important feature of both is that instead of presenting a single standard imagery sequence for everyone, a rich variety of options are demonstrated and the client then selects the one(s) they prefer.

Some clients prefer considerable imagery "talk," whereas others prefer their imagery guide to remain silent while they quietly enjoy their chosen imagery. For this reason, our instructions include both; we begin with relatively extensive trainer guidance, and end with complete silence.

The approach to imagery in this book is not exclusively visual, but involves the senses of sight, sound, touch, and smell. Our reasoning is that actual life relaxation activities or settings involve all the senses; so imagery should involve recreations of such activities or settings. I hypothesize that one does not have to actually experience vivid, lifelike recreations of sense input in order for imagery to be of value. Some clients may prefer to consider imagery as an exercise in which one attends to verbal descriptions of a passive relaxing setting or situation. In a sense, such verbal imagery becomes a type of descriptive prose, song, poetry, or prayer in which the practitioner savors words and their meanings rather than sensory images and experiences.

It is useful to note the close connection between imagery and relaxing self-statements, or words and phrases repeated during an imagery exercise. Such self-statements can be simple suggestions of R-States ("Let yourself feel At Ease and Peaceful"). A slightly more complex approach is to include an affirmation, or internal proclamation of the possibility and value of a specific R-State ("I have the capacity within me to feel Mental Quiet"), or of a philosophical or religious belief that supports relaxation ("I feel Joyful that God loves me").

Sense Imagery is appropriate for most clients who wish to use imagery. The four categories of stimuli I have found most useful include travel (boats, plains, trains, balloons, horses), outdoor/nature settings (mountains, gardens, forests), water (rivers, lakes, ocean, beach, rain), and indoor settings (childhood home, castle, religious institution, cabin). Of these, water imagery tends to be the most preferred. The potential variety of images is nearly infinite (see Table 13.1). For group training, see chapter 21.

Insight Imagery is appropriate for clients who have spiritual interests. The sequence presented in this book guides the relaxer through a peaceful story with a message.

TRAINING

Step 1: Select Format, Provide Overall Orientation, Conduct Assessment

Step 2: Exercise Rationale

It is important to differentiate different types of imagery and to point out that relaxation imagery is different from problem-focused imagery and the mental rehearsal one might employ in preparation for sports or a stressful situation illustrated here:

> Imagine you are going to give a stressful lecture in front of a class. As you walk up to the podium, you feel yourself getting

TABLE 13.1 Menu of Sense Imagery Themes

Travel
Airplane, bird, blimp, bus, car, cruise ship, horse-drawn carriage, floating in air, floating dandelion seed, flying saucer, flying like a bird, hot-air balloon, jet, kite, magic cow, motorcycle, ocean liner, raft, parachute, rocket in space, ship, roller blades, skateboard, submarine, train, wagon, walking

Outdoor/Nature
Church retreat, campgrounds, clouds, desert, forest, garden, island, meadow, monastery, mountain, nature preserve, nudist camp, outer space, park, planet (Mars, etc.) spa, valley, storybook land, zoo

Water
Beach, brook, creek, glacier, hot tub, lake, ocean, pond, rain, rain forest, mist, river, sauna, ski slopes, shower, snow, steam bath, stream, swimming pool, wading pond, waterfall

Indoor
Cabin, castle, cave, cavern, childhood house, church, dream house, meditation room, mosque, palace, prayer room, skyscraper, school room, secret hiding place, synagogue, tavern, temple, tree house, vacation home

© 2005, Springer Publishing Company. Permission granted to use.

> nervous. Your heart beats quickly. You briefly close your eyes, take three deep breaths, and say to yourself, "I can do it." You stand in front of your podium and place your notes in front of you. You feel nervous again, and think "If I forget where I am, I will simply return to my notes. Everyone does that."

Again, this is *not* and example of relaxation imagery. In relaxation imagery one mentally creates or recreates a passive activity or setting where one feels relaxed. Explain that the first steps are to select a topic, fill in the sense details, and check for possible problems that might arise ("booby traps").

Steps 3 and 4: Demonstration/Warmup and Practice

In sense imagery, one first demonstrates four themes: travel, outdoor/nature, water, and indoor. A client then selects the theme of his or her image, and suggests sense details (what is seen, heard, touched, and smelled). The instructor then presents the chosen theme, including the sense details offered by the client. For the remaining ten minutes, the client silently engages in imagery.

There is no demonstration phase for Insight Imagery.

The voice quality appropriate for imagery depends on whether it is disengaging or engaging. Disengaging talk should be quiet and rather monotonous. Talk designed to enhance R-States related to opening up should be a bit more "colorful," with inflections corresponding to key story phrases. Such engaging talk is not unlike the soft and gentle storytelling voice one might use in telling an interesting story to a child.

Steps 5 and 6: Review, Revision, and Special Problems

After completing imagery, ask the client to describe the image they created. Check to make sure it is not a problem-solving or success image ("I imagined planning my vacation," "I imagined winning a football game"). The image should not involve discursive activity (playing games, talking, sports, sex, eating) or have a discrete goal.

The most serious problem with most forms of imagery (especially standardized or taped imagery) is the "booby trap," an unanticipated negative association that emerges after imagery has begun. For example, a client may have chosen beach imagery, only to realize, in the middle of the imagery exercise, that beaches remind him of the time he was seriously sunburned. When a booby trap has been detected, imagery may be replaced or revised so that it is "problem-proof." For example, introduce a cooling palm tree or umbrella on a sunny beach.

Clients may complain of difficulty in producing vivid, lifelike images. Unlike programs such as autogenic training that encourage, and value images that are as vivid as possible, I reassure clients that they can enjoy an image even if visual images are not vivid, or are even absent. One can think of an imagery script as simply a verbal description, akin to descriptive prose, poetry, song, or prayer. After all, one can enjoy a good story, without accompanying illustrations.

Generally, I have clients continue to practice with the full instructions presented in this text even after receiving training in imagery. This permits clients to revise and finetune their imagery each time they listen to instructions. After three or four presentations, clients usually have decided upon the details of their imagery, dispense with full instructions, and practice alone for 10–30 minutes. However, it is acceptable for clients to continue with full instructions, even after they have made their selections. Here, clients find that the tone of voice and occasional choice of words and images support their chosen imagery and they ignore sections of instruction that are unnecessary.

ENHANCING IMAGERY

- Any form of relaxation can precede imagery instructions.
- Simple, unintrusive variations of any exercise can be incorporated into an imagery theme:

> Imagine you are an autumn leaf holding on to a tree. Gently tense up your hands (PMR). As a relaxing breeze flows by, let go (PMR) and float to earth.
> Imagine you are in a warm, relaxing pond of water. Notice how you feel warm and heavy (AT).
> Imagine a relaxing cloud floating overhead. A gentle breeze moves the cloud along. Breathe in the refreshing air and exhale.

- Incorporate self-statement suggestions of desired R-States.
- Incorporate affirmations into imagery, especially verbal imagery. Imagery stories can provide especially appropriate settings for relaxation-enhancing affirmations.
- End imagery with meditation. (If you do this, gradually introduce imagery suggestions that are increasingly passive, simple, and focused. Select a meditation focal stimulus consistent with the image (See "Deepening Imagery" in chapter 19), for example:

> Imagine a wonderful pond. You can see birds and clouds in the air, feel the cool breeze against your skin, and hear the bubbling water. As evening approaches, things grow quiet. The clouds float away. The birds become silent. The air and water are still. And all you see in front of you is the simple pond, like a round mirror reflecting the dark night sky. Meditate on this pond.

TABLE 13.2   **Imagery Scripts**

SENSE IMAGERY

Rationale/Explanation

In this exercise we are going to learn to relax with a special type of daydream or fantasy. It is called imagery. Imagery can give us a relaxing break, a special, safe, and peaceful place removed from outside pressures and distractions. And imagery opens to the wonders of myth and magic, of special places and stories that teach and inspire. And at times imagery can offer a message for living a life of calm and simple focus.

In this exercise, you need to do two things. First, select a special type of theme, one that is especially relaxing to you. Second, pick details for your imagery theme. In today's session, we will first take an imagery journey and explore different types of themes. Next, you will pick the theme you like best. We will close with a ten-minute imagery exercise.

Now, make sure you are seated upright in a comfortable position. Are your feet resting comfortably on the floor? And close your eyes.

Demonstration

In our minds we will take a special journey. Our journey will have four phases. First, we will focus on traveling. Second, we will arrive at a peaceful outdoor nature setting. Third, in this setting we will experience the refreshing and renewing powers of water. And fourth, we will conclude by discovering a special indoor place, our home or final destination at the end of our journey.

We now begin our journey with three travel images.

Travel imagery: the balloon. Imagine yourself floating high in the air in a balloon. Can you see the clouds float by? Far below is the world floating past. The relaxing air touches your skin. You can hear the relaxing sound of wind brushing against the balloon. You can smell the clean air around you.

Travel imagery: the boat. Imagine yourself in a boat floating far out to sea. You can see the distant trees. You can hear the gentle sound of waves lapping against your boat. The water touches your skin. The smell of the water is very peaceful.

Travel imagery: the country train. Imagine yourself moving through a remote countryside in a train. You can see the pastures rushing past. The creaking sound of the train on the tracks has a soothing quality about it. You smell the wood in the train. You can feel the gentle swaying motion.

TABLE 13.2 *(continued)*

And now, for the next minute or so, enjoy the travel imagery of your choosing. Involve all of your senses.

[PAUSE 60 SECONDS]

We are ready to continue with outdoor nature imagery.

Nature imagery: the mountain. Imagine yourself on the top of a mountain. You can see far into the distance. You can hear the songs of birds echoing. You can feel the crisp mountain air. And the mountain pines smell fresh and relaxing.

Nature imagery: the grassy plain. Imagine a faraway grassy plain. Waves of grass extend into the distance. You can hear the wind rushing through the meadow. You can feel the soft grass touching your skin. Its peaceful and refreshing fragrance fills the air.

Nature imagery: the valley. Imagine a peaceful valley. All around are towering mountains. You are next to a giant forest. You can hear the chirping of squirrels. You can feel the warm mountain sun. And you smell the gentle fragrance of flowers.

And now for the next minute or so, enjoy an outdoor/nature image of your choosing. Involve all your senses.

[PAUSE 60 SECONDS]

We are ready to continue with water imagery.

Water imagery: the pond. Imagine yourself floating in a pond. You can see deep into the clear blue water. You can feel the water touching your skin and supporting your body. You can hear the splashing of small fish in the distance. You smell the water's clean scent.

Water imagery: the stream. Imagine sitting next to a stream. Your feet dangle in the cool rush of water. It washes away the concerns of the day. You can see and hear the water splashing against the rocks. You feel its refreshing and renewing mist touching your skin. The fragrance is clean and full of energy.

Water imagery: the mist or rain. Imagine yourself walking through the mist or rain. Far in the distance you can see the soft clouds overhead. Drops gently touch your skin. You can hear the rain as it hits the ground. And you notice how fresh the rain makes the air smell.

And now for the next minute or so enjoy water imagery of your choosing. Involve all of your senses.

[PAUSE 60 SECONDS]

We are ready to continue with indoor imagery.

Indoor imagery: the forest cabin. Imagine yourself in a peaceful forest cabin. You can see the wooden walls and fireplace. You can hear the wind outside and the crackling fire. You can feel the heat

(continued)

TABLE 13.2 *(continued)*

of the fire touching your skin and you can smell the soothing odor of burning logs.

Indoor imagery: the childhood room. Think of your childhood room. What did it look like? Did you have anything special on the walls? Maybe you can smell food cooking in the distance, or hear pets scampering underfoot. What is touching your skin?

Indoor imagery: the holy place. Imagine yourself in a holy place, perhaps church or temple, with its majestic and reassuring arches. You can hear the soft sound of music in the background, or smell flowers or incense. As you sit, you can feel the firm chair holding you.

And now, for a moment, think about the journey we have just taken. What part was most relaxing? What part did you enjoy? Did you like traveling? The outdoor nature setting? The water theme? Or the relaxing indoor setting? Which part of your journey did you enjoy most?

[PAUSE]

And now is the time for you to select a special theme for your imagery. Select the theme that is best for you.

[PAUSE]

Which theme do you want?

Sometimes people pick a theme that runs into problems. It might seem fine at first, but has a hidden booby trap within. For example, you might want to think of the lake you visited as a child, not realizing you nearly drowned in the lake. This painful thought might arise unexpectedly in your daydream and spoil your relaxation. Can you think of any hidden problems in your theme?

[PAUSE]

If there are any problems, simply pick another theme, or revise your theme to remove the problem.

[PAUSE]

Dress Rehearsal

We are now ready to try your daydream.

Let yourself settle into a peaceful state of relaxation.

As you relax, I will begin to count backwards, from five to one. With every count, let yourself sink into a pleasant state of relaxation, far from the concerns of the world.

[PAUSE]

Five.

You begin to settle into a state of relaxation, letting go of the concerns of the day. There is nothing you have to do.

TABLE 13.2 *(continued)*

Four.

The world becomes more and more distant, as you let go and relax. You feel very safe and comfortable.

Three.

Let yourself sink deeper and deeper into relaxation. You notice your breathing become more slow and even. You begin to feel heavy and relaxed.

Two.

You sink farther and farther away from the world. You become more and more relaxed, as if you were sinking into the world of sleep and dreams.

One.

We are now ready to begin our special relaxing daydream. Let's return to the part of our relaxing journey you enjoyed the most. Think of what it was like. Involve all of your senses. [HERE THE TRAINER PRESENTS A SERIES OF SENSE SUGGESTIONS DRAWN FROM CLIENT'S LIST. TRAINER SUGGESTS ONE FROM EACH OF THE FOUR CATEGORIES, UNTIL A TOTAL OF THREE OR FOUR SUGGESTIONS ARE EVENTUALLY PRESENTED FROM EACH CATEGORY. FOR EXAMPLE, TRAINER SAYS: "YOU SEE THE BLUE SKY . . . YOU HEAR THE WIND IN THE TREES . . . YOU FEEL THE WARM SUN ON YOUR SKIN . . . YOU HEAR BIRDS IN THE DISTANCE (NOW ONE SUGGESTION HAS BEEN PRESENTED FROM EACH CATEGORY) . . . YOU SEE THE TREES FAR IN THE DISTANCE . . . HEAR THE BIRDS SINGING QUIET-LY . . . FEEL THE TOUCH OF SPRING MIST . . . AND SMELL THE FRESH SCENT OF FLOWERS . . . CLOUDS FLOAT GENTLY OVERHEAD . . . THE TREES RUSTLE IN THE WIND . . . THE WIND TOUCHES YOUR SKIN . . . THE FRAGRANCE OF FLOWERS IS SO PEACEFUL (NOW THREE SUGGESTIONS HAVE BEEN PRESENTED FROM EACH CATEGORY)."

For the next ten minutes let yourself enjoy your relaxing fantasy. What do you see? What do you hear? What do you feel touching your skin?

[PAUSE 10 MINUTES]

Gently let go of what you are attending to. We have finished our relaxing imagery exercise. Gently open your eyes. And take a deep breath and stretch.

INSIGHT IMAGERY

In this exercise we are going to learn to relax with a special type of daydream or fantasy. It is called insight imagery. First make sure you are seated upright with your feet flat on the floor.

(continued)

TABLE 13.2 *(continued)*

Through the magical powers of imagery we will take a journey, one that is enjoyable and refreshing. In this journey you explore a special question. It is this:

For me, what is the deepest purpose of relaxation? What is the most important reason for mastering a relaxation goal?

We will meet this question again later at a special part of our journey. Now is the time to put this question aside and enjoy our time together.

The setting. Imagine a beautiful outdoor setting, quiet and distant from the concerns of everyday life. This outdoor setting can be any place you choose. A vast garden, extending without end. A beautiful forest, dense with trees and bushes. A river or lake.

Your setting is a world that is full of life and energy. The wind, the sun, trees, grass, water. There is much to experience.

What do you see? The clear blue sky above? Soft, fluffy clouds floating by? Waving leaves and grass that are healthy and green. Rippling water?

[PAUSE 5 SECONDS]

What do you feel touching your skin? The gentle wind. The warm sun? A soothing mist?

[PAUSE 5 SECONDS]

What do you hear? The sound of the wind through grass or leaves. Waves lapping against a beach? The gentle songs of birds in the distance.

[PAUSE 5 SECONDS]

What fragrances are there? The fresh scent of grass, trees, or water? Clean, clear air?

[PAUSE 5 SECONDS]

For the next few minutes, there is nothing you need to do. Simply enjoy your beautiful nature setting. Enjoy all of your senses.

[PAUSE 2 MINUTES]

Release of tension. The world around you becomes more quiet. Wind settles into a gentle breeze. Clouds in the sky move more slowly. The grass and trees are more still.

Now it is the time to let go of excess burdens that weigh you down and keep you from moving deeper, keep you from seeing things clearly.

Attend to your body.

Let any tensions you may feel dissolve and flow away.

Flow away into the gentle breeze, the warm and soothing sun, the cool mist.

For the next minute or so, let tensions flow away.

[PAUSE 1 MINUTE]

TABLE 13.2 *(continued)*

Release your tension and concerns. Let them go. Let them go to the powers that be. Let go of that which you cannot change.

The path. We are ready to move on. Imagine in your beautiful setting is a long path.

It is path that starts at your feet, and extends into the distance out of sight, perhaps hidden by trees, rocks, or water.

The path may be paved with smooth stones.

Or it may be a path of sand or grass.

The path can be anything.

For the next minute or so, simply attend to your path, and when you feel comfortable, begin moving along the path.

[PAUSE 1 MINUTE]

As you move down your path, you move far away from the everyday, deeper into the world of silence.

You are guided by an inner wisdom, the song of a distant bird, or perhaps a glowing light in the distance.

I will begin to count backwards from five to one.

With each count, you find yourself moving deeper and deeper along the path.

5

Breathe in deeply, pause and let go.

Release the tensions and concerns of the day.

4

You are moving deeper along your path.

3

Deeper and deeper, far away from the everyday world.

2

The world grows more quiet and still, the farther you move.

1

And your path ends.

Your Guide and the Place of Wisdom. You have arrived at a special place of wisdom. The air is completely still.

Complete silence.

In this quiet place you can find answers, or deeper questions. In this place you will offer your question to one thing, or one person, we will call your Guide.

The Guide appears different for every person.

It can be a clear, still pond. You can see through the water.

It can be a spiritual or religious symbol, rich with guiding meaning.

It can be a simple flower.

(continued)

TABLE 13.2 *(continued)*

It can be a mysterious box with a guiding message inside.

It can be the night sky, a guiding star.

It can be a person, someone very wise, an old relative or friend, a teacher or religious figure. One who quietly whispers an answer in your ear.

What or who is your Guide?

And now, quietly and simply nod in the direction of your Guide.

There is no need to think about anything or figure anything out. Simply attend. When thoughts or distractions come, simply let them go, and simply attend.

[PAUSE 60 SECONDS]

The question. And now is the time for your question. And ask the question, to your Guide: Why do I need to relax? What is the deepest reason for me?

Do not try to figure out your answer. Simply attend to your Guide.

Simply let ideas come and go. Some will be simple distractions, some will be stirred by your Guide.

Each time a thought comes, any thought, gently take note of it by nodding your head, and let go.

Continue attending, quietly, without effort, without thought. Let thoughts come and go.

[PAUSE 90 SECONDS]

Why do I need to relax? What is the deepest reason for me?

At this time, select for you what seems like the best answer.

[PAUSE 60]

Let go of what you are thinking. We are ready to move on.

Celebration. In these last few moments, let yourself enjoy deep and renewing beauty of your surroundings. Ever changing. Ever new. Full of mystery and wonder.

Freely let your imagery go anywhere it wants. Involve all of your senses. What you see, feel, hear, and smell. Simply enjoy all there is to enjoy in the vast world around you.

[PAUSE 30 SECONDS]

And now we have approached the end of our journey. But we have one final task.

A moment of gratitude. In whatever way feels right for you, express your thanks for wherever your journey has taken you. You may simply nod your head in appreciation, or actually say a few words in your mind. You may do this now.

[PAUSE 30 SECONDS]

Gently let go of what you are attending to. Slowly open your eyes, take a deep breath, and stretch. We have completed our journey and are ready to move on to life's tasks.

14

Meditation and Mindfulness

The instructions for meditation and mindfulness are essentially instructions to sustain passive/effortless simple focus and do nothing else. In concentrative meditation, one attends to one stimulus; in mindfulness, one attends to all stimuli. Put differently, for concentrative meditation, all stimuli other than the target focus are distractions; for mindfulness, all distractions are part of the stream of potential target stimuli. For both, irrelevant discursive analytic and judgmental thoughts are distractions, needless "efforts" to be put aside. One simply attends to one's target stimulus or stimuli, and nothing else. One puts aside all effort, all diversion, and all distraction.

Think of a camera with several lenses. A "micro" lens enables you to move in very close to your subject, for example a single flower in a garden, or little junior at the family reunion. A wide-angle, panoramic (macro) lens enables you to step back and get the broadest perspective, so you can include the entire garden, or the whole family. For both lenses, you of course do not want to include irrelevant distracting stimuli, such as the garbage dump next to the garden, or the irreverent boy next door making obscene faces. Concentrative meditation is like a camera with a micro lens; mindfulness meditation is like the wide-angle, panoramic (macro) lens. Both forms of meditation are like good cameras that enable you to point away and shield your lens from distraction.

HYPOTHESIZED EFFECTS
OF MEDITATION AND MINDFULNESS

Physical/Autonomic/Attentional Effects

For meditation and mindfulness, it is difficult to separate the effects on skeletal muscles, autonomic arousal, and attentional processes. Meditation and mindfulness first require mastery of the access skill of sustained effortless/ passive simple focus. A seasoned meditator can readily detect and release subtle sources of distracting tension or arousal. (See chapter 4 for an extended discussion). One might speculate that during meditation or mindfulness, brain and body processes that support all types of self-stressing become less active or dominant. One learns to be simply aware and not engage in any physical or cognitive activity, including activities that contribute to self-stressing. As a result, well-mastered meditation and mindfulness can be as effective as any other family of relaxation. Finally, concentrative meditation, especially with eyes closed, can be an effective diversion from external stress.

R-States

Relatively little research has explored the R-States associated with meditation and mindfulness. I speculate that Mental Quiet, as well as Aware and Timeless/Boundless/Infinite may be associated with continued and regular practice. Meditation with eyes open (meditation on an external visual image; full mindfulness) may be less effective at evoking Disengagement and Physical Relaxation than meditations that involve closing one's eyes.

FORMAL CONSIDERATIONS

Placement

I recommend placing concentrative meditation near the very end of an exercise sequence. Mindfulness exercises with a bodyfocus ("attend to the sensations of your feet touching the floor") may be placed prior to physical exercises to increase body focus. Stretching may be combined with rocking meditation. Beginning practitioners should precede their practice with at least 15 minutes of physical relaxation.

Duration

Beginning meditators should limit their practice to ten minutes a session. The typical trained practitioner should practice 20–30 minutes. For advanced practitioners, sessions can last up to an hour. Sessions longer than an hour should be broken up into smaller sessions, with intervening periods of non-meditation activity.

Portability

For beginners, meditation and mindfulness are not particularly portable. However, experienced practitioners may find these exercises useful in most situations where one can close one's eyes for a few minutes. Mindfulness, because it can be practiced with eyes open, can be practiced anywhere.

APPROPRIATE CLIENTS

Again, of all techniques, meditation and mindfulness require the highest level of skill at sustaining effortless/passive simple focus. Clients with well-developed relaxation skills (who have tried and found other approaches easy or even "too simple," and do not experience high levels of skeletal muscle tension, autonomic arousal, worry, or negative emotion) may find meditation rewarding. Meditation and mindfulness are also appropriate for those who have spiritual inclinations or are highly motivated to learn these approaches.

Meditation is not appropriate for individuals who have difficulty concentrating, are easily distracted, or need a highly structured and familiar training format. These approaches are not appropriate for those who want to "learn to concentrate or focus better." Other approaches to relaxation, particularly the physical families of techniques, are more useful for those who have difficulties focusing. Caution should be taken when teaching meditation to individuals who may have a strong irrational, religion-based opposition to meditation. Like imagery, eyes-closed meditation may be inappropriate for those who use fantasy as a maladaptive avoidance strategy or for individuals with a thought disorder or problems with impulse control.

OUR APPROACH TO MEDITATION AND MINDFULNESS

Unlike traditional single-technique approaches, this book introduces three meditation sequences: eight meditations, graduated mindfulness, and mindful walking. Because different meditations work for different individuals, we give a choice. The eight-meditations sequence is a global review of concentrative and mindfulness meditation, grouped as meditations of the body, meditations of the mind, meditations of the senses, and finally a simple and highly structured version of mindfulness.

Of the eight meditations, I have found rocking meditation to be the easiest and most readily practiced; the remaining are about equally challenging. Beginners may find meditations of the body easiest when preceded by a 15 minute warmup of physical relaxation exercises. Contrary to the nearly universal preference among Western meditation instructors for mantra meditation, I find this approach no easier than others.

The graduated mindfulness sequence presents a sequence of increasingly challenging mindfulness meditations. The goal is to gradually ease the practitioner into mindfulness and provide practice for attending mindfully to a wide range of stimuli. One begins by imagining the sensations of eating fruit and mindfully attending to the sensations of taste. The subsequent exercises focus on the flow of breath, body sensations, thoughts, sounds, and all other stimuli.

The mindful walking sequence involves taking a slow walk while attending mindfully to each step. In addition, one mindfully gazes at an area directly in front of where one is walking. In a sense this is the most active of mindfulness exercises. However, it is meant to be practiced after attempting the graduated mindfulness sequence. Mindful walking can be considered a strategy for beginning the process of applying mindfulness to active life.

TRAINING

Step 1: Select Format, Provide
Overall Orientation, Conduct Assessment

Step 2: Exercise Rationale

I try to present meditation in a way consistent with the utter simplicity of the technique. For a rationale, I just present the overall instructions, "Attend to a simple stimulus. Return attention after every distraction." Then I give the following rationale:

> The goal of meditation is to learn to silence thinking while remaining effortlessly focused. It is to be very quietly relaxed and wakefully attentive at the same time. This can be a very powerful way of relaxing and overcoming stress. But learning

meditation isn't easy. You can't just tell your mind to stop
thinking. It doesn't work. The more you try to quiet your mind,
the more your mind thinks about getting quiet—and still thinks.
And you can't just force yourself to calmly focus on something.
Forcing anything isn't effortless. The more you think about it,
the skill of meditation seems impossible. How does one silence
thinking without thinking? How does one focus without trying to
focus? This takes a special skill which we shall learn today.

Distraction is perhaps the universal experience of meditation, for beginners
and advanced practitioners alike. All kinds of thoughts may come to mind—
memories, plans for the day, emotions, images, physical sensations, sounds
from the outside, and so on. Many beginners have the mistaken belief that
to practice correctly somehow requires avid unwavering concentration, as if
meditation were akin to playing a video game (where a second's lapse of
attention may cause one to lose millions of points. In fact, distraction is a
normal part of meditation. Indeed, one must be distracted in order to develop
in meditation.

The goal of meditation is not so much to concentrate the mind as it is to
consistently, and calmly, return attention to a focal object after every distraction. This may happen hundreds of times a session. However, one returns
attention as calmly and restfully as possible. It is only through such opportunities to return attention that one gradually trains oneself to focus in meditation.
You might say that meditation is not a concentration exercise; it's a refocus-
ing exercise.

I invite trainees to consider the following two meditators, meditating on
the word "One." Both show exactly the same number of distractions; the
second person is dealing with them properly while the first person is not:

Person #1:

"One . . . One . . . One . . . Hmmm, I want a hamburger.
Darn it! I got distracted. I must concentrate better! DAMMIT!
ONE! . . . ONE! . . . ONE! . . . "

Person #2:

"One . . . One . . . One . . . Hmmm, I want a hamburger.
Oops, One . . . One . . . One . . . "

There are meditative and nonmeditative ways of dealing with distraction.
Some meditative reactions include the following:

"No problem . . . easily return."

"I'm distracted. That's okay, it's a part of meditation. Gently return."

"My mind wandered again. How interesting. Back to meditation."

"Oh, hello, distraction. I can spend time with you later, after my meditation. Goodbye."

Some nonmeditative responses include:

"My mind wandered. I'll never meditate. I feel so frustrated."

"Oh, what an important thought about my work problem. I have to think about it or my problem won't get solved."

"Hmmm, this distraction's fun. I'll just stay with it. This is just as good as meditating."

Several seasoned meditation instructors have some helpful descriptions of this easy, permissive way of dealing with distraction in meditation. LeShan (1974) says:

> Give yourself permission to make constant slips from the directions. You will make them anyway and will be much more comfortable—and get along better with this exercise—if you give yourself permission in advance. Treat yourself as if you were a much-loved child that an adult was trying to keep walking on a narrow sidewalk. The child is full of energy and keeps running off to the fields on each side to pick flowers, feel the grass, climb a tree. Each time you are aware of the child leaving the path, you say in effect, "Oh, that's how children are. Okay, honey, back to the sidewalk," and bring yourself gently but firmly and alertly back to just looking. Again and again you will suddenly notice that you are thinking about something else or translating your perception into words or something of the sort. Each time, you should say the equivalent of "Oh, that's where I am now; back to the work." (p. 54)

Carrington (1978) suggests:

> When meditating never force thoughts out of your mind. All kinds of thoughts may drift through your mind while you are meditating. Treat these thoughts just as you would treat clouds drifting across the sky. You don't

push the clouds away—but you don't hold onto them either. You just watch them come and go. It's the same with thoughts during meditation, you just watch them, and then when it feels comfortable to do so, go back. (p. 25)

Elsewhere, Carrington advises against struggling against intruding thoughts when meditating. Such distractions are a natural part of everyone's meditative experience. Indeed, they can be a sign that meditation is working. She suggests greeting distracting thoughts as you would a friend whom you like, but with whom you do not have time to talk right now. Imagine that you are letting this friend walk alongside you, but you are not becoming involved in conversation with him/her. In other words, flow with the thoughts that turn up during meditation and allow them full play, but do not cling to them. (Carrington, 1978, p. 20)

Some liken distraction to silt at the bottom of a cool and quiet pond. This silt, when stirred, can cloud the waters. The return action of meditation is a way of clearing the mind of potential future distraction. Each meditative return is like a cleaning sweep along the bottom of the pond. Somewhat less poetically, by permitting distractions to come and go we might be releasing or discharging subtle inner tensions that might cloud meditation.

Mindfulness. Mindfulness meditation can be difficult to describe. I find it best to start with very simple and somewhat poetic instructions, and then present elaborations as problems arise. With mindfulness meditation, the object is not to attend to a preselected stimulus. Instead, one quietly attends to, notes, and lets go of every stimulus that enters awareness—every thought, feeling, sensation, sound, idea, and so on. One does not try to figure out, think about, push away, or do anything with the thoughts, feelings, and sensations experienced. Simply let each stimulus come and go and wait for the next stimulus. The mindful meditator is nothing more than a neutral observer, viewing the world as it is, uncolored by reactions, judgments, and evaluations.

Mindfulness meditation can defy verbal description. It can be useful to think of several images, for example, that of sitting beside and gazing at a quietly flowing stream. A variety of unexpected objects slowly and continuously float by. A piece of wood comes into sight and then floats away. Then a patch of leaves. And then a floating seed. In mindfulness meditation, treat every thought, feeling, and sensation as something that drifts into view on its own. The task is utterly simple: acknowledge that it is there ("Oh, a thought . . . this is interesting") and let it drift away after a few seconds. Calmly wait until something else floats into view.

Or one might think of the image of calmly resting in a tent in the evening woods. There is nothing to do or figure out; it is peaceful and secure. Sounds come and go, for example, the rush of the wind. Listen, without thinking or trying to figure things out, and quietly return to listening once again. The trees smell so refreshing. Note this and return to a peacefully quiet and attentive stance. A bird sings far in the distance. One thinks "Oh, the sound of a bird," and returns to quietly listening again. In other words, all the mindful meditator does is note each sensation, let go of what he or she is sensing, and continue attending.

Many people try to do too much with mindfulness meditation. One doesn't have to figure out the connections between each stimulus; often there will be none. The task is not to look for deeper understandings. There is no need to attend to any thought, feeling, or sensation for any length of time. Indeed, one should dwell on any particular "bubble in the stream" or "sound of the night" for only several seconds—about the time it takes a real-life bubble to float in and out of sight on a stream or the time it takes a gentle gust of wind to blow and settle into silence. And in mindfulness meditation one doesn't have to be concerned about distractions. Each time one is distracted, the meditator notes it as yet another passing stimulus ("Ah, a distraction . . . how interesting"), lets go of it, and gently and easily returns to attending to whatever stimuli may drift past awareness.

Steps 3 and 4: Demonstration and Practice

I recommend that clients practice the entire Eight Meditations sequence every day until it becomes clear which meditation they prefer. Usually it takes two or three practice sessions. Then they can practice their preferred meditation.

The meditation/mindful tone of voice should in itself suggest a sense of Mental Quiet. It should be soft and clear, energized, and a bit deliberate. Use short sentences, few words, and many pauses. Imagine your client is savoring each word you say, so it must be said slowly and carefully. Always precede meditation with preparatory relaxation.

Steps 5 and 6: Review, Revision, and Special Problems

- The most frequent "problem" clients report in meditation is inability to concentrate, or difficulty in dealing with distraction. Emphasize that distraction is a normal part of meditation, and that the objective is to gently return to one's meditative task with a minimum of concern, effort, or upset.

- Clients who find it difficult attending to a simple meditative focus may benefit from combined meditations, for example, rocking and breathing, or breathing and mantra meditation.
- First teach concentrative meditation, and practice for a month. Then graduate to mindfulness, using concentrative meditation as a pre-session "warmup."
- Beginners may benefit from brief meditations, 5–10 minutes in length, which can be gradually increased to 20 or 30 minutes over a period of a month.

ENHANCING MEDITATION/MINDFULNESS

Meditation and mindfulness require the highest degree of skill at sustaining effortless/passive simple focus. I hypothesize that meditation and mindfulness are easier when preceded by PMR, AT, yogaform stretching, or breathing. Such techniques may enhance the release of distracting tension. In addition, deepening imagery (which starts discursive and energetic and ends focused and effortless) may be conducive to preparing for the sustained focus required for meditation. Concentrative meditation may be an effective preparation for mindfulness meditation. However, the relative value of different warmups has yet to be subjected to research.

Historically, at least seven preparation strategies have been used to teach meditation: (1) meditation (concentrative or mindfulness) alone, without a presession warmup; (2) meditation (concentrative or mindfulness) with either yoga stretching or breathing or both as warmup; (3) meditation (concentrative or mindfulness) with or without breathing or stretching warmup and gradually increasing in length (over the course of several weeks) from 10 minutes to 25 minutes; (4) graduated mindfulness, beginning with simple physical sensations, progressing to awareness of other sensory input, and ending with awareness of all sense input; (5) mindfulness with concentrative meditation as warmup; (6) mindfulness after several weeks of training in concentrative meditation; and (7) multitechnique concentrative/mindfulness meditation (our approach) in which several techniques are taught and the client selects which works best.

TABLE 14.1 Meditation and Mindfulness Scripts

EIGHT MEDITATIONS

Meditation is a very simple exercise. In fact, the instructions can be said in two sentences: Calmly attend to a simple stimulus. Calmly return your attention after every distraction . . . again and again and again. Begin by making sure you are seated comfortably in an upright position. Your feet should be flat on the floor. And close your eyes.

Meditation of the body: Body sense meditation

For the next minute or so, let go of the concerns of the day. This time is for you alone. There is nothing you have to do or figure out.
  [PAUSE]
Let go of any tensions you might feel. And relax.
  [PAUSE]
Attend to a physical relaxation sensation you can identify in your body. Do you feel warm? Sinking? Heavy? Perhaps you notice a warm glow in your abdomen. Perhaps you feel warmth or tingling in your hands and fingers. For the next minute or so, simply let go of tension, and quietly attend to that one body sensation. Whenever you start thinking about what you are doing, simply let go of these thoughts, and return to attending to how your relaxing body feels.
  [PAUSE 45 SECONDS]

Meditation of the body: Rocking meditation.

Think of all the times in life you have found the gentle movement of rocking very calm and soothing. You might be on a rowboat in a lake, gently bobbing back and forth as waves lap against you. Perhaps you are in a rocking chair on a porch. You are at peace. Nothing is on your mind. There is indeed something very soothing and meditative about simple rocking
At this time let yourself begin to rock back and forth in your chair.
  [PAUSE]
Let each movement become more and more gentle and easy. Let yourself rock effortlessly. Let your body move on its own, in its own way, at its own speed. All you have to do is simply attend.
  [PAUSE]
Let each movement become more and more subtle so that someone watching would barely notice you are rocking. For the next minute or so, quietly attend to gentle and silent rocking.
  [PAUSE 90 SECONDS]

TABLE 14.1 *(continued)*

Gently let go of what you are attending to. Meditation is very simple. If your mind wandered, that's OK. If you got distracted, that's OK.

Meditation of the body: Breathing meditation.

Take in a full breath, and relax. Let your breathing continue on its own in a way that is free and easy. There is nothing you have to so. Simply attend to the flow of breath, in and out. And return your attention whenever your mind wanders or is distracted.
[PAUSE 90 SECONDS]

Meditation of the mind: Mantra meditation.

Let a relaxing word, perhaps the word *peace*, come to you like an echo in the distance. Let the word go over and over and over, at its own pace and volume.

The word doesn't have to go with your breath. Simply attend as the word quietly and easily goes over and over. When your mind wanders or you are distracted, that's OK. Simply return.
[PAUSE 90 SECONDS]

Meditation of the mind: Visual image.

Think of the image of a simple spot of light, a candle flame, or a star.

And calmly attend.

And calmly return after every distraction.
[PAUSE 90 SECONDS]

Meditation of the senses: External image.

Slowly open your eyes halfway. Easily gaze on the candle in front of you. Whenever your mind wanders, gently return.
[PAUSE 90 SECONDS]

Meditation of the senses: A sound.

With your eyes closed, what do you hear? Perhaps there is simply silence. Maybe you can hear the quiet background sound of this recording. For this next meditation, simply pick a sound, one that is continuous, and quietly attend to it. If you wish, you may attend to the background sound. There is no need to think about what you

---

(continued)

TABLE 14.1 *(continued)*

---

are listening to. Whenever your mind wanders, gently return to
simply listening.
  [PAUSE 60 SECONDS]

Mindfulness meditation.

  The world is alive with sounds and sights and sensations. You
are a mirror. Quietly reflect on what passes by. There is no reason
to think about anything.
  [PAUSE]
  With your eyes partly open, and without thinking about anything,
what do you notice about you? What sound or sight or sensation comes
to you?
  [PAUSE]
  Whenever you notice something, fine. Gently name it, put it
aside, and continue attending with an open mind until you notice
something else.
  [PAUSE]
  When you notice something again, just quietly name it, put it
aside, and resume attending.
  You are a neutral observer, waiting very calmly and peacefully
. . . doing nothing but noting what comes to mind.
  Each moment comes and goes.
  The river of time slowly passes by.

GRADUATED MINDFULNESS

  In this exercise we will take a journey through several types of
mindfulness meditation.
  First make sure you are seated upright in a comfortable position.
Place your feet on the floor.
  Mindfulness meditation is very simple. Just attend very calmly
to whatever you are experiencing.
  You put your thinking aside.
  You attend without thought.
  Without analysis. Without effort. Without judgment. Without
trying to hold on to anything or push anything away.
  Just attend and that's all.
  Like a neutral observer, doing nothing to interfere.
  A simple mirror.

Being mindful of taste.

  Imagine a wonderful bowl of pieces of your favorite fruit.
  And now identify your favorite piece.
  [PAUSE 5 SECONDS]

TABLE 14.1 *(continued)*

If you can't make up your mind, select a piece of orange.

Now imagine you have taken a piece of fruit you especially like and have placed it in your mouth.

Feel its cool shape and texture.

Slowly bite down.

You feel the fruit squeezing as it is crushed and releases its juices in your mouth.

You can smell its fresh sweet scent.

You can sense the cool liquid flowing in your mouth.

The fresh fruit flavor spreads over your tongue.

It's cool and delicious.

As you move your tongue, the flavor dissolves.

As you swallow, the juice flows away, leaving a wonderful taste in your mouth.

This was a taste of mindfulness.

You simply attended to a sensation.

Without thought. Without analysis. Without effort.

Being mindful of breathing.

Easily take in a full, deep breath, filling your lungs and abdomen with air.

[PAUSE]

And when you are ready, simply exhale.

And breathe naturally.

Notice the air as it touches and flows into your nose.

Notice the gentle rush of air as it flows in.

Simply attend to the air, as it flows in and out of your nose.

There is no need to control your breathing in any way.

Whenever your mind wanders, or you start thinking about what you are doing, simply let go of your thoughts.

Just attend to the flow of air. That's all. The flow of air.

Attend to the path the air takes as it moves deeper into your nose and throat.

Attend to the flow of air as it fills your lungs.

Being mindful of the body.

Attend to how your body feels.

Can you feel your feet touching the floor? The pressure of your shoes or socks on your feet?

(continued)

TABLE 14.1 *(continued)*

Can you feel your legs and thighs against the chair as you sit firmly and comfortably?

Can you feel your back against the back of your chair?

Simply attend to your body, and notice whatever sensations come and go.

Whenever you notice a sensation, gently note it, let go, and continue attending.

Whenever you find yourself thinking about what you like or dislike, figuring things out, or are distracted in any way, gently let go of the thought or distraction, and attend to your body.

Being mindful of thoughts.

Attend to your mind, as thoughts come and go.

There is no reason to try to do or think anything. No need to try to keep thoughts away. No need to pursue or figure thoughts out. No need to hold onto a thought.

Simply wait and attend.

Whenever a thought or feeling comes to mind, just note it, let go, and continue attending, again and again and again.

Being mindful of sounds.

Attend to the sounds you hear.

Without selecting any particular sound, let sounds come to you.

When you notice a particular sound, do not dwell or cling to it. Do not think about it.

Just gently note it, let it go, and continue waiting.

Sounds come and go, like the wind at night or the songs of birds. Simply attend.

Full mindfulness.

Gently open your eyes and be mindful of the world of the moment.

There is nothing to do, think about, or figure out.

You are simply a mirror, reflecting the river of time as it flows by, minute by minute.

Quietly attend and wait. When you notice something, be it a sight, sound, thought, or sensation, just let it go.

And resume attending. Doing nothing. Waiting for what comes to you. You are the neutral observer, thinking nothing, doing nothing to interfere.

For the next few minutes, continue being mindful of the world around you.

TABLE 14.1 *(continued)*

MINDFUL WALKING

In this type of mindfulness meditation, you will slowly and easily walk for ten minutes.

First, stand upright, look around, and decide your general path. If you are outdoors, you might pick a sidewalk, about a block or so.

Or you might pick an unobstructed nature path.

If you are indoors, in a room, you might choose to walk next to a wall.

Select where you will walk, a path that is not blocked in any way, a path where you won't have to step over anything. A path where you won't have to think about navigating where you are going.

[PAUSE 10 SECONDS]

And begin walking, very slowly and evenly. One foot at a time.

Do not exert much effort to walk.

Easy, slow-motion walking.

Notice the sensation of each foot touching the ground.

Moving.

And then the next foot touching the ground.

[PAUSE 10 SECONDS]

When you feel comfortable walking . . .

When this type of slow walking seems easy to you . . .

Gently gaze at an area of the ground about two or three feet in front of you.

Do not look far ahead at where you are going.

Just gaze at what is immediately in front of you, where you will step next.

Gaze at the area of ground directly in front of you.

Notice what comes in and out of view.

[PAUSE 10 SECONDS]

The ground comes and goes.

[PAUSE 5 SECONDS]

You notice only the patch in front of you as you slowly walk.

You notice it changing as you move ahead.

When your mind wanders, or you start thinking or walking fast, slow down.

Continue walking while gazing slightly ahead for the next ten minutes or so.

[PAUSE 10 MINUTES]

And now, let go of what you are attending to.

You can stop walking.

Take a deep breath and stretch.

We have completed our mindful walking.

Part III

Training Issues

15

Overview of Relaxation Training Formats

One of the first decisions to make when teaching relaxation is to select which of many formats to use. Psychologists used to think that all families of relaxation were more or less interchangeable because all of them were presumed to evoke the relaxation response. From this traditional point of view, training format was not an issue. You would simply present exercises from the family in which you are trained. Because most psychologists are trained in progressive muscle relaxation that is the approach they would teach to all clients. Yoga instructors are trained in yoga, so yoga is what clients would get.

Substantial research (Smith, 1999a, 2001) has shown that the one-technique-fits-all approach does not fit the facts. Different families of relaxation are not interchangeable variations of the same technique, but have quite different effects and work differently for different people and different relaxation goals. Because of this important discovery, I recommend nine training formats: a revised traditional single-technique format and eight combination formats.

REVISED TRADITIONAL
SINGLE-TECHNIQUE FORMAT

I believe one application of the traditional format remains viable. Indeed, it is used in most clinical relaxation recordings available to health professionals.

If, through careful assessment, a relaxation trainer determines that one single family may be best for a client, then selection of exercises primarily from that family alone may be justified. However, I recommend revising this approach by incorporating exercises from other families to augment the desired impact. Such augmentation transforms the traditional format to the revised traditional format.

For example, a therapist may decide to use only progressive muscle relaxation (tense-let go exercises) with a client who suffers from excessive muscle tension. Breathing exercises might be added to augment the main effect of tensing and letting go ("inhale – tense up – exhale and let go"). A visual imagery exercise (from the imagery family of relaxation) may also be inserted to augment PRM ("tense up – let go – imagine muscle tension melting away like candle wax"). The result is an exercise sequence from the PMR family, augmented by occasional selections from the families of breathing and imagery exercises.

If you examine textbook instructions and recordings of seasoned relaxation trainers, you will find that nearly all use the revised traditional format, if unwittingly. Most yoga programs integrate three families of techniques: breathing, yoga stretching, and some form of meditation. Those who teach imagery typically begin with a few breathing and letting go exercises.

I believe there are risks to the revised traditional format. Typically, it is applied, one-for-all, so that all clients receiving relaxation receive the same sequence. As I have already explained, this is a serious mistake, given that different families have different effects and work for different clients. Second, I suspect that no single relaxation family is, in itself, enough and that effective relaxation involves combining several families, not as supplements but as integral components. Relaxation training is like creating a balanced and nutritious meal. Each of the six families of relaxation may well be good for different relaxation access skills, much as different food groups meet different nutritional needs. Just as a balanced diet includes something from many food groups, balanced relaxation should include elements from many families of relaxation.

COMBINATION FORMATS

We consider eight ways of presenting combinations of exercises tailored to client needs and interests:

- Scripting
- Package Programs
- World Tour
- Spot Relaxation
- Mini-Scripts
- Access Zone Scanning
- Workshops
- Group Relaxation

These combination formats start with the core instructions presented in chapters 9–13. Unlike commercially available recordings, each of our instructions presents a relatively pure "unmixed" version of a family of techniques. The yoga stretching instructions include just stretching, with no accompanying breathing. PMR instructions include only PMR, and no "supporting" additional exercises from other families. Thus, clients can more readily identify and explore the unique effects of each family of relaxation. In contrast, when clients receive instructions that premix PMR, breathing, and imagery, they have no way of knowing which type of exercise is most responsible for any obtained effects. Also, sets of unmixed exercises give the trainer maximum freedom to create exercise combinations based on client needs and the latest research. For example, if a headache client needs PMR letting-go exercises and autogenic suggestions of "warmth and heaviness," these two pure sets of exercises can be presented.

Scripting

The most complete way to augment and combine exercises is to create a relaxation script and then transform it to an audio recording. In my opinion, such a scripting exercise is the most effective way for a trainer to master the skills of combining techniques. First, a client receives training for all six families of techniques: full yogaform stretching, full PMR, verbal autogenic training, breathing exercises, sense imagery, and meditation (eight-meditations sequence).

Then, trainer and client select a relaxation goal, preferred exercises, a general theme or "unifying idea" for the entire sequence, and words and phrases suggestive of desired R-States. These basic elements are then artfully combined into a meaningful sequence personally tailored to the client.

Package Programs and the World Tour

The *package program* format goes one step beyond the traditional single-technique format, but is not as comprehensive as scripting. A trainer presents at least three and no more than five exercise sequences. Ideally, one determines through interview or prior relaxation assessment (chapter 17) which approaches are most likely to work for a client. Conversely, one might introduce the six families in an introductory session or workshop.

Once selected, the client practices the selected exercise sequences, with a different sequence for each session. At the end of training, the trainer presents recordings or printed instructions for the sets finally preferred. This is the client's relaxation package.

To illustrate, prior assessment may indicate that a client is not interested in techniques involving imagery or having spiritual overtones. He or she may want simply physical approaches to reduce stress and enhance health. The package program, therefore, might include:

1. Abbreviated Yogaform Stretching
2. Breathing and Stretching.
3. Full PMR
4. Verbal Autogenic Suggestions

The *world tour* is a package program that includes all six families of relaxation, including exercise variations. Put simply, a client starts with yogaform stretching, and proceeds through PMR, autogenic training, breathing, imagery, and meditation, devoting about three days of practice to each. When finished, a set of two to four exercise sequences are selected to be practiced on a rotating basis, one a day. For example, after trying all six families, a client may choose to practice PMR, autogenic training, and sense imagery in rotation over three days. Alternately, one could practice a physical-mental exercise combination every day, PRM plus imagery, for example.

Spot Relaxation and Mini-Script

A *spot relaxation* is a quick exercise created for a targeted problem (for example, taking a deep breath and stretching one's fingers to alleviate fatigue from typing). A *mini-script* is an abbreviated two- to five-minute version of a preferred full relaxation sequence (traditional, scripted, package, or world

tour) that can be practiced once one's full sequence has been mastered. The mini-script can serve as an effective brief substitute for full relaxation.

Access Zone Scanning

Access zone scanning is based on the idea that each family of relaxation initially targets a different relaxation access skill (chapter 4). In this structured exercise, one explores each access skill.

Workshops and Group Relaxation

A *workshop* provides an extended introduction to relaxation, emphasizing general theory as well as goals appropriate to the group. One then presents a 20-minute demonstration of selected exercises from each of the six families. Finally, exercises are processed, and participants are invited to share which R-States they experienced, which sampled exercises they preferred, and which R-States seemed to be associated with specific approaches. A workshop presentation can be an excellent introduction for clients considering relaxation training.

In *group relaxation*, one presents any of the formats discussed in this text, including instruction for specific families of techniques. Whenever selections are called for, group members vote.

SELECTING A FORMAT

When is it appropriate to select one training format over another? Let me conclude with a few simple guidelines.

When to Use the Revised Traditional Format

- A trainer is competent in just one family and, for whatever reason, has no intention of learning or using additional families.
- A client has expressed a clear and strong desire to learn one family of relaxation, even after reviewing the options available.
- There is not enough time to consider more than one family.

When to Use the Scripting Format

- If it is the most desirable and individualized approach to relaxation.
- The client can afford and has sufficient time for full training in all six families and for making an individualized script (generally 10 weeks).

When to Use the Package (or World Tour) Format

- Recommended for most clients.
- Recommended when there is not enough time to consider scripting. Requires about four to five weeks of training.

When to Use Spot Relaxation and Mini-Scripts

- After learning at least three families of techniques.
- When a specific, physical problem has been identified that is clearly related to a specific access skill deficiency.
- As a demonstration in workshops.

When to Use Access Zone Scanning

- In settings where brief relaxation is required.
- Before relaxation training, as an overview.
- After learning several families of techniques, in order to summarize and integrate insights.
- As part of relaxation assessment, to determine which families of techniques a client might need or prefer.
- As a demonstration in workshops.

When to Use the Workshop Format

- To introduce potential clients to relaxation.
- As part of a class or program on stress management or health psychology.

When to Use the Group Format

- Permits simultaneous training of several clients.
- Can be a valuable component of group therapy or counseling and support environments where group interaction and cohesion is desired.

BRIEF RELAXATION TRAINING

Elsewhere I introduce Brief Relaxation Training (BRT; Smith, 1999b), a combination brief format in which a trainer demonstrates six families of relaxation and identifies client preferences during the demonstration. Then, the trainer crafts a combination sequence of exercises based on client preferences.

BRT is an interactive format that requires considerable trainer involvement and ongoing technique modification. Put simply, a trainer demonstrates a family of techniques until it is clear that the trainee wants to abandon that family and move on to the next family. One begins by explaining that a variety of exercises will be presented. A nonintrusive communication system is explained whereby from time to time the trainer asks "Should we include this exercise in your final program?" and the trainee responds by gently nodding "yes," "no," or (with a shrug), "don't know." The standard yogaform stretching sequence of eleven stretches is presented, each stretch followed by the trainer asking if it should be included. When three stretches receive a "no" or "don't know" rating, the trainer smoothly moves on to PMR. When three of the eleven PMR exercises do not receive a "yes" rating, breathing exercises are introduced. Breathing exercises are arranged into three groups: breathing and stretching, diaphragmatic breathing, and passive breathing. When two of any group do not receive a "yes" rating, the next group of breathing exercises is considered. Finally, imagery and meditation are considered. Again, for these final exercises, when two demonstrations do not receive a "yes," one moves on.

At the end of training, the trainer shows the trainee a list of specific exercises that received a "yes" rating (see checklist, p. 266) and asks if these should be included in a final script, given the desired script length. Present the any of the versions of the Smith Relaxation States Inventory (chapter 17) and ask if any of the words on the inventory should be included in the final relaxation script.

Finally, the trainer crafts a relaxation program or recording incorporating client preferences.

16

Orientation

The first phase of relaxation does not involve teaching techniques, but orienting clients to the training they are considering. The orientation phase of training should include six topics:

- A consideration of precautions and risks
- An explanation of the stress, the relaxation engine, and access skills.
- When appropriate, a review of goal-specific relaxation processes
- A review of the mechanics of the selected training format
- A consideration of special training requirements
- An explanation of inventories

EXPLANATION OF PRECAUTIONS AND RISKS

Before you begin with a client, make sure your client does not have special problems or concerns that could significantly impact exercise selection or practice. It is especially important to determine if any exercises may pose a health risk.

- First, avoid any movement exercise (PMR, yoga stretching, breathing stretching) that could conceivably aggravate any physical pain, discomfort, injury, infection, illness, weakness, wound, or lesion. These involve problems concerning skin, muscles, ligaments, bone, lungs, and nerves. Simply inform all clients of this concern and ask if they have any conditions that fit. A client may be advised to seek the advice of his or her physician or nurse before beginning a series of exercises.

- Evoking the relaxation response is associated with reductions in metabolic rate. This in turn may lower blood pressure and alter blood chemistry levels in such a way as to change required dosage levels of prescription medications. Ask clients if they are on any prescription medications and inform them of this risk. Again a client may be advised to consult with his or her physician or nurse.
- Clients should stop practicing and consult a physician if they experience any of the following possible cardiac symptoms:

  - Pain or tightness in the chest
  - Irregular heartbeat
  - Extreme shortness of breath
  - Feeling lightheaded, nauseated, or dizzy (these can be normal effects associated with breathing exercises)

- Any seriously adverse experience with previous relaxation training should be addressed. This includes relaxation taught ineptly, or as part of a religious group a client has rejected (church, temple, synagogue, mosque, cult). Emphasize that the exercises to be taught are based on psychological science, not religious dogma, and have a record of safety and effectiveness. If a client continues to have negative associations with previous experiences, the problematic approach may be avoided.
- Conversely, a client may have strong attachments to a certain specific exercise. A meditator may like his version of Zen or transcendental meditation. A religious client may have a favorite quieting prayer. A student of a particular family of yoga may feel strong allegiance to this family of techniques. A graduate of therapy may have strong emotional connections to the version of progressive muscle relaxation the therapist taught. Often clients who have such strong attachments view alternatives as inferior and respond to training with hostility. In such situations, invite the client to explore alternatives to supplement what they already know.

In sum, these precautions are most important when relaxation is taught as a part of psychotherapy, counseling, or rehabilitation. It is assumed that those receiving professional treatment are under appropriate medical supervision, and that any relaxation techniques to be taught have received appropriate medical approval as a part of normal supervisory review. When relaxation is taught not as a part of therapy or treatment (in schools, workplaces, religious institutions, etc.) I recommend distributing the Relaxation Precautions Fact Sheet (see Table 16.1).

EXPLANATION OF STRESS, THE RELAXATION ENGINE, AND ACCESS SKILLS

Your explanation of the stress and relaxation engines should be viewed as an essential part of relaxation training. Indeed this introduction can reassure client and evoke enthusiasm for practice. It is here that a client is motivated to practice and learns in general why a technique has an effect. A client who understands an exercise, believes that it works, and is enthusiastic about its promise, is more likely to practice it and benefit from it.

Make your explanation brief, in as few as five minutes. If you wish to elaborate, you may assign homework reading or present a general orientation lecture for potential clients. (For an extended example of client-oriented introductions, see Smith, 2004.) A minimal introduction might include the material in Table 16.2.

TABLE 16.1 Relaxation Precautions Fact Sheet

Relaxation Precautions Fact Sheet
You are about to receive training in professional deep relaxation. Although relaxation exercises are generally safe for most people, some groups should display simple common-sense precautions. Generally, consider relaxation training to involve a modest level of exertion, perhaps a little more than climbing a flight of stairs. You, and possibly your physician or nurse, should be aware of the following two precautions:

1. You may be taught exercises that involve bending, stretching, moving, tensing up muscles, or breathing deeply. Avoid any such exercise that could conceivably aggravate any physical pain, discomfort, injury, infection, illness, weakness, wound, or lesion. These include problems concerning skin, muscles, ligaments, bone, lungs, and nerves.
2. The relaxation techniques you will learn can evoke reductions in metabolic rate. This in turn may lower blood pressure and alter blood chemistry in such a way as to change the required dosage levels of prescription medications.

TABLE 16.2   Brief Introduction to Stress and Relaxation

Some stress is good and can help you cope. However, under excessive stress, your body and brain are subjected to levels of tension that can contribute to considerable wear and tear, illness, and poor performance at work and school, and in sports and relationships. Eventually, your body and brain become "set" or "tuned" to more readily experience harmful tension in the future.

With relaxation training, the body and brain are relieved of harmful levels of tension and can recover from impairments in physical and mental functioning. Eventually, they are "reset" or "retuned" to a more healthy and relaxed state.

See Smith (2004).

If clients are to be taught all six families of relaxation, or Access Zone Scanning, it is important to provide a rationale as in Table 16.3.

EXPLANATION OF GOAL-SPECIFIC RELAXATION PROCESSES

If a client or group has expressed a specific relaxation goal, this can be addressed in the general introduction to the program. Counselors in a hospital setting or stress management clinic might be presumed to have an interest in the goal of stress management. Recovering heart surgery patients may want relaxation to enhance healing. Business executives may be interested in health and energy. Those in a substance abuse or weight reduction program may want relaxation for calm directed action. Students may want help with work or school. Individuals confronting issues that require creative problem-solving (jobseekers, singles exploring dating prospects) may want relaxation as a tool for creativity and insight. Vacationers may want to supplement relaxing beach activities with relaxation targeted to spontaneous enjoyment. A church group may want a focus on God-based spirituality or meditation and mindfulness. If you are meeting a client for the first time, with little prior background information, simply ask what their relaxation goal is (after giving and explaining the list).

TABLE 16.3   Self-Stressing and the Six Families of Relaxation

We psych ourselves up for stress by our thoughts and feelings. This is called "self-stressing." Once we have encountered a stressor, appraised it as a threat, and decided that perhaps our coping resources are not sufficient, we experience heightened stress energy. We stress our bodies and minds in six ways. Stress shows in our posture, muscle tension, and breathing. In our minds, we experience stressed body focus, stressed emotions, and stressed attention. This self-stressing is natural and often very valuable for coping with very difficult situations. Let's first explore the six types of self-stressing. The first three involve things we do with our bodies.

Stressed Posture. We develop tense, stress-maintaining postural habits, like slouching, bending over our desks to examine the computer, clenching our jaws, holding our hands in a "carpal tunnel position," and so on. Our stressed postures get us ready for vigorous coping—to fight or flee, for example.

Stressed Muscles. We tighten the muscles of our shoulders, arms, face, neck, and legs, to get ready for vigorous action.

Stressed Breathing. We tighten up our stomachs and chests, often like boxers in a fight. We force ourselves to breathe deeply, or to hold our breaths. Our breathing becomes stressed and inefficient.

The remaining types of self-stressing involve the mind:

Stressed Body Focus. Under stress, we may direct attention to parts of our bodies and think about what is happening there ("Gosh, am I really sweating that much!" "I think my stomach is getting queasy." "Wow, my heart is pounding!") This type of body focus and thinking about the body can create additional bodily upset and stress.

Stressed Emotion. We feel stressed emotions, anxiety, depression, irritation, frustration, and so on. These feelings fuel vigorous action.

Stressed Attention. We concentrate hard on the stressful challenge at hand, divide our attention in multitasking, and sometimes become preoccupied with worry about what we are doing. Worn out, our minds wander and we become less aware. These are the signs of stressed attention.

Through each of these we stress ourselves up to get ready for vigorous fight or flight action. So, self-stressing can be good—up to a point. But too much self-stressing can hurt your health, your well-being, and your ability to be and do your best at work, school, home, and sports.

(continued)

TABLE 16.3 *(continued)*

Summary of How We Self-Stress

1. Stressed Posture
2. Stressed Muscles
3. Stressed Breathing
4. Stressed Body Focus
5. Stressed Emotion
6. Stressed Attention

Relaxation Techniques to Reduce Stress

Relaxation techniques help us recover from self-stressing. For thousands of years, people have been inventing and testing out ways of relaxing. The many techniques that have evolved can be sorted into six groups or "families." Remarkably, each family of relaxation techniques goes with a given type of self-stressing, as indicated below:

Types of Self-Stressing	*Relaxation Families*
Stressed Posture	Yoga
Stressed Muscles	Progressive muscle relaxation
Stressed Breathing	Breathing exercises
Stressed Body Focus	Autogenic training
Stressed Emotion	Imagery
Stressed Attention	Meditation/Mindfulness

However, it is perhaps better not to think of any technique as a generic pill just for one type of stress. Yoga isn't good for just stretching out the kinks. Instead, each family of relaxation is a gateway to a different type of peace and calm. The first step on the path of relaxation may be reduced self-stressing. But those who practice relaxation regularly go far beyond this initial goal.

The best way to learn relaxation is to explore all six families. It's like a balanced meal. Each family of relaxation is like a different food group—fruits and vegetables, proteins, carbohydratees, and so on. A complete and balanced meal would include something from each group, perhaps emphasizing the groups in which you have nutritional deficiencies. Relaxation training is like creating a balanced meal in which you explore all basic food groups (i.e., families of relaxation techniques). Then you pick which meal is most nutritious for you.

> **Note to Practitioners and Trainers**
>
> **For all client goals, never say, "research proves this effect" or "it is a scientific fact that relaxation does this." Instead, present goals as reasonable hypotheses, supported by anecdotal reports, relaxation theory, and some research. No matter how passionate a trainer may believe in a specific technique, no matter how sure or speculative a goal may seem, it is up to practitioners to experiment and find what works for the client. This applies to specific goals that may be "strongly supported" by research. It is important to keep in mind that even for technique effects found to be highly significant statistically, there are often a sizable number of exceptions.**

Below are examples of introductions to goal-specific processes.

Sleep and napping. Relaxation can be a good way of enhancing sleep, and giving a boost to a ten-minute power nap. It can reduce everyday tensions that interfere with the natural flow of sleep and napping processes, resulting in a more satisfying and refreshing sleep or nap.

Managing stress. Relaxation is a powerful tool in managing stress. When we experience too much stress for too long a time, potentially harmful changes occur in the body and brain. The body's stress alarm is reset so that one is increasingly likely to react with stress. Relaxation addresses each of these effects of stress.

Healing. Relaxation can help strengthen healing processes. The body's immune system is enhanced. Even basic healing from physical injury or illness may be facilitated.

Health and energy. You want to stay healthy and have enough energy and stamina for daily challenges. Relaxation is more than a "power nap" and can give you that edge, important for work, school, sports, and just having fun.

Calm direction. Learning a special type of calm direction is an important part of relaxation training. One learns to keep one's mind on what one wants to do and be less distracted by worry, fatigue, or urges to do something else or give in to an addictive or compulsive urge.

Productivity and effectiveness. Relaxation has been used to enhance performance at sports and effectiveness at work and

school. All of the previous goals we have listed can contribute
to this overall goal.

Spontaneous enjoyment. We're here to have fun. Before beginning (our nature walk, dance, trip to the concert) let's warm up
with some relaxation exercises. This can help us put aside some
of the unnecessary leftover concerns of the day so we can more
freely and fully enjoy ourselves.

Creativity and insight. Relaxation can give you a tool for
enhancing creativity and insight. It can give you renewing energy when you are in a rut. It can stir the creative juices when
you need new ideas for work, school, or fun.

God-based spirituality. People often use relaxation in con-
junction with God-based spirituality. If your life of prayer has
grown stale, relaxation techniques can add new life and meaning.
And relaxation can deepen worship and contemplation of religious texts, music, and art.

Meditation/mindfulness. Meditation involves simply focusing on a single thing, like a candle flame, religious symbol, or
even nature. Beginners often find meditation deeply frustrat-
ing and filled with distraction. Practicing a preliminary relaxation exercise can speed the mastery of meditation. In
addition, when one becomes "stuck" and bored with meditation,
accompanying relaxation can add life. Mindfulness is a special
type of meditation in which one approaches all of life with simple, easy, efficient focus. All approaches to relaxation can
contribute to mindfulness.

EXPLANATION OF SELECTED TRAINING FORMAT

Explain to the client how training will proceed and the format to be used
(revised traditional, packages, scripting, or group). Which specific exercises
will be included (and why)? How many sessions will be required and how
long will each session run? What are the expectations for home practice?

SPECIAL TRAINING REQUIREMENTS

Finally, review the following special requirements.

Clothing and Attire

Whenever possible, clients should wear comfortable, casual, loose-fitting
clothing. Remove glasses or contact lenses. Remove or loosen shoes or ties.
Handbags should be put aside.

Practice Time

Explain to clients that the most difficult problem beginners have with relaxation training is learning to set aside a specific daily time for relaxation. This might seem like an easy thing to do, but it is important not to underestimate the difficulties. There are many hidden forces that can get in the way. First, our society has a deep and often hidden prejudice against inactivity and rest. Relaxation is associated with laziness and wasting time. Society tells us it is alright to take it easy, *after* we have completed our work. *In fact, rest can be just as important and meaningful as work.* Second, we often have the mistaken belief that success must always be preceded by strain and toil. It can take time to see that rest-related skills are also important.

There is a third, more insidious, resistance as well. People with a high-stress pattern of living may actually become accustomed to and perhaps even crave a chronic, high level of stress arousal. Just as the alcoholic craves alcohol when sober, the "stressoholic" craves stressful activity even when at rest.

When clients begin practicing a relaxation technique, they may well experience the combined effects of society's pressures and their own stress addiction. They may feel impatient, bored, and restless. They may want things to happen immediately.

There are several ways to approach the problem of establishing a practice time. First, do not pick a time that you already know, may cause problems, for example:

- Do not practice after eating; once blood is diverted to the stomach for digestion, less blood is left for practicing. One might feel tired, or worse, experience a cramp.
- Do not practice at times typically associated with high levels of stress. Relaxation is a young and delicate skill that should be developed in a safe, low-stress environment. New relaxation skills are less likely to take hold and have an effect in times of high stress. Apply relaxation to stress management after the appropriate skills have been mastered.
- Some trainers argue that certain special times are ideal for relaxation, for example the evening or morning. I am a realist. Few clients have the luxury of such selection. Any time that does not stir up special problems will work.
- At least five sessions a week should be scheduled. Our research suggests that one of the most important variables influencing success at relaxation is daily practice.

- Do not select a time in which the possibility of interruption is high. For example, if a client talks with friends in the early evening, it would not be a good idea to select this time for practicing relaxation. Finally, clients should not select a time when there is urgent unfinished business to complete. It is difficult to relax when thinking about other things to do. Remind your client that time off is a special time, just for them.

The Relaxation Place

- Pick a chair that is comfortable and permits you to sit up with back support. A sofa that causes you to slouch is not a good idea. I do not recommend practicing on the floor or in bed. Because reclining is associated with sleep, such a position may evoke undesired sleepiness. Relaxation texts are full of special standing or seating recommendations. Some may or may not be of value for advanced practitioners. For our purposes, a comfortable chair is good enough. First, the chair is often our "stress position." Often we need to relax most when seated—in a car, bus, office, classroom, church pew, etc. So, we should learn relaxation in the seated position we will use when practicing relaxation.
- Select a practice place that is quiet, isolated, and free from interruption. If you are in a room, close the door, unplug the phone, and turn off the television. If you are living with others, ask them to leave you alone. If you are at school or work, find some quiet unused room.
- Avoid extras like incense and music until you have mastered training. When you are learning a basic approach to relaxation, you want to experience the effects of just the exercise, and not accompanying music or fragrance. After you have mastered basic techniques, you can creatively augment your practice.

Special Problems With Finding a Time or Place

For clients who have particular difficulty in finding time to practice, I recommend teaching a preparatory time-off activity. A time-off activity is a 10–30 minute quiet and pleasant activity designed to counter some of the many sources of resistance to relaxation. Through the behavioral procedure of shaping, a client is taught to tolerate regular periods of inactivity by incorporating a pleasurable and simple relaxing activity he or she already knows. Such an activity also has the effect of reinforcing the healthy habit of taking time off.

First, a client selects a practice time and place, then a quiet pleasant activity. Many find the following guidelines helpful:

- Select an activity that involves a minimum of physical movement and effort. Thus, avoid jogging, sports, dancing, or similar pastimes.
- Choose an activity that can be done alone without outside distraction. Avoid talking over the phone, chatting with friends, playing games, engaging in sexual activity, and the like.
- Make sure your activity is not especially goal-directed or analytic. Avoid activities that have a serious purpose, such as doing homework, practicing a musical instrument (for a class or professional purposes), solving highly complex puzzles, doing difficult reading, planning the day's activities, or working on personal problems.
- Pick an activity that is different from what you usually do. Try to think of something you find restful and enjoyable that you just haven't had time to do recently. Avoid activities you already do. For example, if you already spend time each day listening to pleasant music, do not choose this as your time-off activity.
- Choose something that is indeed fun and easy. Don't make it a chore or burden. You should like doing it.
- Take care to select an activity that will last no less than 20 minutes and no more than 30 minutes. It is important that you stick to this time period very carefully. If you are restless after 10 minutes, continue until you have finished 20 minutes (don't let your stress addiction get to you). If after 30 minutes you aren't finished and want to continue, stop anyway. It is important that you condition your mind and body to understand that a certain period of time is for time off and nothing else. Consistency and discipline are very important when teaching small children, and stress-addicted minds and bodies often act like cantankerous children. Be firm.
- Finally, avoid the following: eating, drinking, smoking, taking drugs, and sleeping.

Often clients will have great difficulty thinking of pleasant, quiet things do. This itself may be a sign of stress addiction. I "prime the pump" by inviting clients to brainstorm with me. Try to think of as many activities as possible, for example:

- Crafts (simple)
- Daydreaming

- Doing one's nails
- Doodling
- Knitting
- Listening to quiet music
- Looking at collected postcards or stamps
- Looking out the window
- Magazine reading
- Novel reading
- Playing a simple musical instrument just for fun
- Sewing

EXPLANATION OF INVENTORIES

Many clinicians chose to introduce various inventories (chapter 17) as a part of training in order to assess training needs, select relaxation techniques, or evaluate progress. The purpose of these inventories needs to be explained. This is particularly important for tests based on the R-State pyramid (chapter 5) that assess R-States (Smith Relaxation States Inventory-Revised [SRSIr]; Smith Relaxation States Inventory Brief Version [SRSIbv]; Smith Relaxation States Inventory Alternative Brief Version [SRSIabv]).

The R-State pyramid is a formidable and challenging construction. The complete model can be presented to health professionals as well as ambitious and interested clients. However, let me suggest three simplified versions that may be more appropriate for some clients.

Simplified Two-Category Version

This two-category simplification divides R-States into those directly associated with relaxation and those reflecting positive emotional states associated with relaxation. The two-category version is the basis of the Smith Relaxation States Inventory Brief Version (SRSIbv, Table 17.7)

> People experience two groups of psychological states of mind when practicing: relaxation/meditative states and positive relaxation emotional states. Relaxation/meditative states include:
>
> - Sleepiness
> - Disengagement

- Rested/Refreshed
- Energized, Strengthened
- Physical Relaxation
- At Ease/Peace
- Mental Quiet
- Aware, Focused, Clear

Positive relaxation emotional states include:

- Joyful
- Childlike Innocence
- Thankful/Loving
- Deep Mystery
- Awe and Wonder
- Prayerful
- Timeless/Boundless/Infinite

Simplified Three-Category Version

Elsewhere (Smith, 2004) I have found it useful to divide the R-State pyramid into three levels, without differentiating columns. Level 1 is "Stress Relief and Feeling Good" (Disengagement, Rested/Refreshed, Energized, Physical Relaxation, At Ease/Peace, Joyful). Level 2 is "Selflessness." Level 3 is "Spiritual and Transcendent Feelings," which combines both Spirituality and Transcendence (Levels 4 and 5 in the original pyramid). Sleepiness and Aware are described as basic types of relaxation and wakefulness. These are illustrated in Figure 17.1 and can be assessed with the Smith Relaxation States Inventory Revised (SRSIr, Table 17.5) or the Smith Relaxation States Inventory—Alternative Brief Version (SRSIabv; Table 17.9).

Brief Professional Explanation

In this final, brief explanation, ignore distinctions between columns of states, and simply present five levels, with three R-States grouped per level.

In all these versions we emphasize that the R-States near the base of the pyramid (Sleepiness, Disengagement, Rested/Refreshed, Energized, Physical Relaxation, At Ease/Peace) are "basic R-States" which most people experience when practicing. The R-States near the middle of the pyramid (Mental Quiet, Childlike Innocence, Joy, and Thankful/Loving) are less frequently experienced, and are some of the special "rewards" of continued regular practice. R-States near the peak of the pyramid (Deep Mystery, Awe and Wonder, Prayerful, Timeless/Boundless/Infinite, and perhaps Aware) are somewhat rare.

Emphasize that relaxation can be working very well when R-States near the base are experienced. The fact that one does not experience R-States closer to the peak does not mean that relaxation is not having an effect.

17

Assessment Tools

A client can select among many relaxation families of exercises. This book offers a variety of assessment tools that can be used throughout training. We will consider four types of assessment: symptom, behavioral, psychological, and relaxation sampling. All clinically useful tools are printed in this book for client and trainer use. Relaxation researchers are strongly advised to consult Smith (2001) for further assessment suggestions.

PHYSICAL SYMPTOM REVIEW

Occasionally clients desire relaxation to treat highly specific and localized target symptoms. A relaxation trainer should first determine if this is an appropriate goal, and consider forgoing extensive training in lieu of a specific exercise. Typically, treatable symptoms correspond very closely to one of the first four types of self-stressing (stressed posture and position, stressed skeletal muscle tension, stressed breathing, stressed body focus. One simply applies corresponding exercises. It is important to note that some physical symptoms such as headaches, hot flashes, or diarrhea may appear to be localized but, in fact, may have complex causes. Here, simple technique-symptom matching may not be appropriate. Also, I do not recommend directly applying meditation/mindfulness for problems of "stressed attention." Table 17.1 lists symptoms that often respond well to targeted relaxation training.

TABLE 17.1 Target Symptom Fact Sheet

Target Symptom Fact Sheet

Do you want to learn relaxation in order to treat any of the following?

Postural problems
Joint stiffness
Tension and fatigue from standing, sitting, maintaining a specific posture
Breathing difficulties
Foot pain
Eye fatigue
Lower back pain
Neck tension
Shoulder tension
Stomach distress
Wrist pain (from typing, writing, etc.)
Muscle pain in general

BEHAVIORAL ASSESSMENT

Behavioral observation is the least intrusive way to measure relaxation. (For an excellent review of behavioral assessment of relaxation, see Poppen, 1988). Behavioral observation is valuable for assessing overall level of physiological arousal. The Behavioral Signs of Relaxation Rating Scale (Table 17.2) focuses on three types of readily observable behavior indicative of relaxation: breathing, posture, and movement.

Breathing

A variety of breathing behaviors can indicate deepened relaxation. Most generally, breathing that is rapid and jerky (with gasping or holding breath) and involves movement of the chest suggests arousal. When breathing becomes slower and more even, with greater use of the diaphragm (indicated by a slowly rising and falling stomach), one can infer deepened relaxation.

Posture

It is fairly easy to observe a client's posture during relaxation. Generally, in a relaxed posture, limbs are partially open, not stretched out or tightly closed.

TABLE 17.2   Behavioral Signs of Relaxation Rating Scale

Below are a number of behavioral signs of relaxation. Indicate how well each fits or describes the person you are rating. Do this by putting a number in the space to the left of each statement. Please use the following scale:

HOW WELL DOES THE ITEM YOU ARE READING FIT
THE PERSON YOU ARE RATING?

① NOT AT ALL   ② SLIGHTLY/   ③ MODERATELY   ④ VERY WELL
                                    SOMEWHAT   WELL

Breathing

1. ① ② ③ ④   Slow breathing pace
2. ① ② ③ ④   Even breathing rhythm
3. ① ② ③ ④   Greater use of diaphragm (stomach rising and falling)
4. ① ② ③ ④   Reduced chest extension

Posture

5. ① ② ③ ④   Shoulders sloped
6. ① ② ③ ④   Head slightly tilted
7. ① ② ③ ④   Limbs and other body parts are in open, relaxed position
   a. Jaws slightly parted
   b. Palms open
   c. Fingers curled and not straight or clenched
   d. Knees and feet pointing apart

Muscle Activity

8. ① ② ③ ④   Little restless movement
   a. Eyes closed; no blinking, looking around, staring
   b. Palms open
   c. No chewing, biting lips, swallowing
9. ① ② ③ ④   Little clenching and bracing
10. ① ② ③ ④   Face, neck, arms and hands are smooth and unwrinkled with no sign of twitching or extended veins or muscles.

Look for slightly sloped shoulders, slightly tilted head, and a general openness of jaws, palms, fingers, knees, and feet. Jaws may be slightly parted, palms open, fingers curled, and not straight or clenched, and knees and feet pointing apart. In exercises emphasizing opening up (yoga, breathing, and some forms of meditation), the neck and back are more likely to be calmly, not rigidly, erect. It is as if each vertebra were precisely stacked so that no effort is needed to keep the back and neck erect.

Movement

A tense muscle is moving, a relaxed muscle is still. Movement can be voluntary (blinking, open eyes, looking around, chewing, biting lips, swallowing, clenching, bracing) or involuntary (twitching, ticks). Often, the degree of skin smoothness can indicate a certain level of muscle tension (furrowed brow, bulging muscles). A yoga practitioner is engaged and relaxed when he or she can execute and maintain a stretch or posture smoothly (without jerks) and slowly.

A variety of subtle nonverbal cues may suggest various R-States. Some are relatively direct. Most people can recognize the behavioral signs of Sleepiness (nodding, deep breathing, etc.). The R-State, Physical Relaxation, may be reflected by the behavioral signs just outlined. Obviously, a smile suggests Joy. Considerable empathic skill may be required to detect the R-States, Disengagement, Mental Quiet, Aware, Thankful/Loving, and Timeless/Boundless/Infinite. For these, a trainer may have to resort to verbal communication.

FINGER/HEAD-NOD SIGNAL SYSTEM

At times it can be important to ask clients how well an exercise is working before the end of a practice session. Interrupting a session with a question can be too intrusive. Instead, I have found it useful to use a simple behavioral signal system. Before training begins, inform the client that you will ask if he or she is relaxed or likes an exercise. Generally, a client is to indicate "Yes," "No," or "Unsure" with the eyes closed. The finger system involves raising the right index finger about an inch to indicate "Yes," the left finger for "No," and both fingers simultaneously for "Unsure." Alternatively, with a head-nod system, a client nods "Yes," "No," or simply and gently shrugs his or her shoulders for "Unsure." The head nod system is preferable for group training and enables a trainer to see responses of many participants.

SMITH RELAXATION INVENTORY SERIES

The *Smith Relaxation Inventory Series* offers a rich catalog of assessment tools useful in a wide range of training contexts. All are presented at the end of this chapter.

Smith Relaxation Preferences Inventory (SRPI)

Clients are given a description of the six families of relaxation and indicate which they prefer. Give the SRPI after presenting the Relaxation Sampler sequence (preferably at least three times). (See Table 17.3.)

Smith Relaxation Goals Inventory (SRGI)

This inventory describes and asks one to select a relaxation goal from 10 possibilities (sleep/naps, stress management, healing, health and energy, calm directed action, productivity and effectiveness, spontaneous enjoyment, creativity and insight, God-based spirituality, and meditation/mindfulness). It gives a trainer or workshop leader an idea of what to consider in the orientation and how to target exercises. (See Table 17.4.)

The Smith Relaxation States Inventories

The Smith Relaxation States Inventories assess all 15 R-States as well as the states of physical stress, worry, and negative emotion. Three versions are available: the Smith Relaxation States Inventory Revised (SRSIr; Table 17.5), the Smith Relaxation States Inventory Brief Version (SRSIbv; Table 17.7), and the Smith Relaxation States Inventory Alternative Brief Version (SRSIabv; Table 17.9).

The Smith Relaxation States Inventory Revised is a full version that is appropriate for clinical and research settings. The brief and alternative brief abbreviated versions are for training purposes. At this time I have no particular preference for one brief version over the other, and offer both to practitioners to try. The brief versions differ in item layout. Finally, instead of the SRSIr, SRSIbv, or SRSIabv, one can use the Simplified R-State Pyramid Map. This map presents the 15 R-States organized into a pyramid. One simply puts a check mark by the R-States that are experienced. When giving the Relaxation Sampler sequence (see Appendix), the effects of each of six families demonstrated is noted on the map by a few letters (P = progressive muscle relaxation).

VERBAL REPORT

Another relatively simple approach to relaxation assessment is to listen to spontaneous client reports. In addition to providing overall appraisals of their

TABLE 17.3 Smith Relaxation Preferences Inventory (SRPI)

Please complete this inventory only after you have tried some relaxation exercises. Below are a number of relaxation exercises you may have tried. How well did each work for you? Please indicate the extent to which you preferred each, using this key. SKIP THOSE EXERCISES YOU HAVE NOT TRIED.

HOW WELL DID THIS EXERCISE WORK?

① NOT AT ALL   ② A LITTLE   ③ MODERATELY WELL   ④ VERY WELL

1. ① ② ③ ④   YOGA STRETCHING. (Not breathing or meditation; see below for these choices)
2. ① ② ③ ④   PROGRESSIVE MUSCLE RELAXATION. ("Tense up . . . let go.")
3. ① ② ③ ④   AUTOGENIC EXERCISES. (Suggestions like "your arms are feeling warm and heavy.")
4. ① ② ③ ④   BREATHING EXERCISES. If you selected this, please check one or more of the below:
   - ❏ Breathing exercises combined with stretching exercises; for example, reaching reach up to the sky while taking in a deep breath.
   - ❏ Breathing exercises in which you squeeze or touch your abdomen/stomach with your hands while breathing out.
   - ❏ Breathing exercises in which you do nothing but breathe in and out, perhaps slowly through your lips, or slowly through your nose.
5. ① ② ③ ④   IMAGERY/VISUALIZATION. If you checked this, please specify type:
   - ❏ Imagery in which you enjoy a pleasant place or setting.
   - ❏ Imagery in which you seek deeper insight or an answer to a question
6. ① ② ③ ④   MEDITATION. If you checked this, please specify type. If you aren't sure, please skip
   - ❏ Meditating on physical sensations or feelings in your body
   - ❏ Meditating while rocking
   - ❏ Meditating on your breath
   - ❏ Meditating on a mantra
   - ❏ Meditating with eyes closed on a simple image in your mind
   - ❏ Meditating on an external sound, like a bell
   - ❏ Meditating with eyes open on some simple object, like a candle
7. ① ② ③ ④   MINDFULNESS MEDITATION. If you aren't sure, please skip.
   - ❏ Meditating on whatever comes in or out of awareness. (Do not check this if you meditated on your breath. Check "I meditate on my breath" in question 6).

TABLE 17.4   Smith Relaxation Goals Inventory (SRGI)

People practice relaxation for many reasons. What are your reasons for wanting to learn a relaxation technique? What relaxation goals interest you?

TO WHAT EXTENT DOES THIS RELAXATION GOAL INTEREST YOU?

① NOT AT ALL   ② A LITTLE   ③ MODERATELY   ④ VERY MUCH

1. ① ② ③ ④   To prepare for sleep; combat insomnia.
2. ① ② ③ ④   To have more effective "catnaps" or "powernaps."
3. ① ② ③ ④   Reduce or manage stress, tension, negative emotion, or worry.
4. ① ② ③ ④   To manage physical pain, discomfort, or other negative symptoms.
5. ① ② ③ ④   To recover from maintaining a fatiguing posture or position for an expended time (standing, sitting, bending over, crouching)
6. ① ② ③ ④   To help recover from illness, injury, or surgery.
7. ① ② ③ ④   To use relaxation as a "healthy behavior" to maintain health and resistance to disease, and increase energy resources, strength, and stamina for work, sports, and life and its activities.
8. ① ② ③ ④   To increase my ability to calmly sustain focus on a desired task, ignore external distraction, and cope with diverting impulses and desires to do something else. To finish what I want to do and resist various distracting or destructive impulses and urges (to smoke a cigarette, drink, eat, take drugs, give in to boredom)
9. ① ② ③ ④   To enhance my effectiveness at work, school, or sports.
10. ① ② ③ ④   To have fun and enjoy myself; to contribute the enjoyment of other activities.
11. ① ② ③ ④   To increase my creativity, overcome "creative blocks," and nurture an expressive source of ideas and insight.
12. ① ② ③ ④   To enhance personal spirituality, to celebrate and relate to God or my Higher Power. To deepen my relationship to God or my Higher Power.
13. ① ② ③ ④   To develop a meditative or mindful state of awareness in which I am calmly aware and focused, both during times of quiet and times of action.

techniques ("this technique worked very well," "the second technique did not work"), the client's choice of words can reveal underlying relaxation processes. For example, clients who report feeling "limp" or "loose" are obviously describing R-State Physical Relaxation. Those who feel "indiffer-

TABLE 17.5   Smith Relaxation States Inventory Revised (SRSIr)

HOW DO YOU FEEL RIGHT NOW?
PLEASE CHECK ALL THE ITEMS USING THIS KEY.

I AM EXPERIENCING THIS . . .

① NOT AT ALL	② A LITTLE/ SOMEWHAT	③ MODERATELY	④ VERY MUCH

① ② ③ ④	1.	My mind is SILENT and calm (I am not thinking about anything).
① ② ③ ④	2.	My muscles feel TIGHT and TENSE (clenched fist or jaws; furrowed brow).
① ② ③ ④	3.	I feel AT PEACE.
① ② ③ ④	4.	I feel DROWSY and SLEEPY.
① ② ③ ④	5.	Things seem AMAZING, AWESOME, and EXTRAORDINARY.
① ② ③ ④	6.	My muscles are SO RELAXED that they feel LIMP.
① ② ③ ④	7.	I am HAPPY.
① ② ③ ④	8.	I am WORRYING
① ② ③ ④	9.	I feel AT EASE.
① ② ③ ④	10.	I feel DISTANT and FAR AWAY from my cares and concerns.
① ② ③ ④	11.	I feel ENERGIZED, CONFIDENT, and STRENGTHENED.
① ② ③ ④	12.	I am DOZING OFF or NAPPING.
① ② ③ ④	13.	I feel THANKFUL.
① ② ③ ④	14.	Things seem TIMELESS, BOUNDLESS, or INFINITE.
① ② ③ ④	15.	I feel IRRITATED or ANGRY.
① ② ③ ④	16.	I feel JOYFUL.
① ② ③ ④	17.	I feel SAD, DEPRESSED, or BLUE.
① ② ③ ④	18.	I feel AWARE, FOCUSED, and CLEAR.
① ② ③ ④	19.	My hands, arms, or legs are SO RELAXED that they feel WARM and HEAVY.
① ② ③ ④	20.	I feel INNOCENT and CHILDLIKE.
① ② ③ ④	21.	My BREATHING is NERVOUS and UNEVEN (or shallow and hurried).
① ② ③ ④	22.	I feel LOVING.
① ② ③ ④	23.	I feel INDIFFERENT and DETACHED from my cares and concerns.
① ② ③ ④	24.	I feel PRAYERFUL or REVERENT.
① ② ③ ④	25.	I feel PHYSICAL DISCOMFORT or PAIN (backaches, headaches, fatigue).
① ② ③ ④	26.	My mind is QUIET and STILL.
① ② ③ ④	27.	I feel ANXIOUS.
① ② ③ ④	28.	I sense the DEEP MYSTERY of things beyond my understanding.
① ② ③ ④	29.	I feel RESTED and REFRESHED.
① ② ③ ④	30.	I feel CAREFREE.
① ② ③ ④	31.	TROUBLESOME THOUGHTS are going through my mind.

TABLE 17.6 Smith Relaxation States Inventory Revised (SRSIr) Scoring Key

SCALE	SCORING INSTRUCTIONS	SCORE
R-STATE SCALES		
Basic Stress Relief		
Sleepiness	(Add item 4 + item 12) Divide this sum by 2	
Disengagement	(10 + 23) Divide by 2	
Rested/Refreshed	29	
Energized	11	
Pleasure and Joy		
Physical Relaxation	(6 + 19) Divided by 2	
At Ease/Peace	(3 + 9 + 30) Divided by 3	
Joy	(7 + 16) Divided by 2	
Selflessness		
Mental Quiet	(1 + 26) Divided by 2	
Childlike Innocence	20	
Thankfulness and Love	(13 + 22) Divided by 2	
Spirituality and Transcendence		
Mystery	28	
Awe and Wonder	5	
Prayerfulness	24	
Timeless/Boundless/Infinite/At One	14	
Aware		
Aware	18	
STRESS SCALES		
Somatic Stress	(2 + 21 + 25) Divided by 3	
Worry	(8 + 31) Divided by 2	
Negative Emotion	(15 + 17 + 27) Divided by 3	

TABLE 17.7 Smith Relaxation States Inventory Brief Version (SRSIbv)

HOW DO YOU FEEL RIGHT NOW?
PLEASE CHECK EACH ITEM BELOW USING THIS KEY

RIGHT NOW, I'm feeling this way . . .

① NOT AT ALL   ② A LITTLE/SOMEWHAT   ③ MODERATELY   ④ VERY MUCH

STRESS	RELAXATION/MEDITATIVE R-STATES	POSITIVE R-STATES
① ② ③ ④ **PHYSICAL STRESS, DISCOMFORT** Muscles feel TIGHT, TENSE (Clenched fist jaws; furrowed brow) PHYSICAL DISCOMFORT or PAIN (back/headaches, fatigue)	① ② ③ ④ **SLEEPY, DROWSY, DOZING OFF**	① ② ③ ④ **HAPPY or JOYFUL**
	① ② ③ ④ **DISTANT OR DETACHED** I feel DISTANT and FAR AWAY from my cares and concerns	① ② ③ ④ **CHILDLIKE INNOCENCE**
① ② ③ ④ My BREATHING is NERVOUS and UNEVEN (or shallow, hurried)	① ② ③ ④ I feel INDIFFERENT and DETACHED from my cares and concerns	① ② ③ ④ **THANKFUL or LOVING**
	① ② ③ ④ **PHYSICAL RELAXATION**	① ② ③ ④ **FEELING the DEEP MYS-TERY of things beyond my understanding**
① ② ③ ④ **CONCENTRATION** (Problems with concentration; feeling distracted, confused)	My muscles are SO RELAXED they feel LIMP Hands, arms, or legs are SO RELAXED they're WARM and HEAVY	① ② ③ ④ **THINGS SEEM AMAZ-ING, AWESOME, EXTRAORDINARY**
① ② ③ ④ **WORRY** I am WORRYING and TROUBLE-SOME, NEGATIVE THOUGHTS go through my mind	① ② ③ ④ **RESTED OR REFRESHED**	① ② ③ ④ **PRAYERFUL or REVERENT**
	① ② ③ ④ **AT EASE, CAREFREE, AT PEACE**	
	① ② ③ ④ **ENERGIZED, STRENGTHENED**	① ② ③ ④ **THINGS SEEM TIMELESS, BOUNDLESS, or IN-FINITE**
① ② ③ ④ **ANXIETY**	① ② ③ ④ **MENTAL QUIET** My mind is SILENT and calm (I'm not thinking about anything)	
① ② ③ ④ **IRRITATION/ANGER**	My mind is QUIET and STILL	
① ② ③ ④ **DEPRESSION, SADNESS, BLUE**	① ② ③ ④ **AWARE, FOCUSED, CLEAR**	

TABLE 17.8   Smith Relaxation States Inventory Brief Version (SRSIbv) Summary Sheet

NAME YOUR TECHNIQUES →										

STRESS STATES

PHYSICAL STRESS, DISCOMFORT
④ ④ ④ ④ ④ ④ ④ ④ ④ ④
③ ③ ③ ③ ③ ③ ③ ③ ③ ③
② ② ② ② ② ② ② ② ② ②
① ① ① ① ① ① ① ① ① ①

CONCENTRATION
④ ④ ④ ④ ④ ④ ④ ④ ④ ④
③ ③ ③ ③ ③ ③ ③ ③ ③ ③
② ② ② ② ② ② ② ② ② ②
① ① ① ① ① ① ① ① ① ①

WORRY
④ ④ ④ ④ ④ ④ ④ ④ ④ ④
③ ③ ③ ③ ③ ③ ③ ③ ③ ③
② ② ② ② ② ② ② ② ② ②
① ① ① ① ① ① ① ① ① ①

ANXIETY
④ ④ ④ ④ ④ ④ ④ ④ ④ ④
③ ③ ③ ③ ③ ③ ③ ③ ③ ③
② ② ② ② ② ② ② ② ② ②
① ① ① ① ① ① ① ① ① ①

IRRITATION, ANGER
④ ④ ④ ④ ④ ④ ④ ④ ④ ④
③ ③ ③ ③ ③ ③ ③ ③ ③ ③
② ② ② ② ② ② ② ② ② ②
① ① ① ① ① ① ① ① ① ①

DEPRESSION
④ ④ ④ ④ ④ ④ ④ ④ ④ ④
③ ③ ③ ③ ③ ③ ③ ③ ③ ③
② ② ② ② ② ② ② ② ② ②
① ① ① ① ① ① ① ① ① ①

RELAXATION AND MEDITATIVE STATES

SLEEPY
④ ④ ④ ④ ④ ④ ④ ④ ④ ④
③ ③ ③ ③ ③ ③ ③ ③ ③ ③
② ② ② ② ② ② ② ② ② ②
① ① ① ① ① ① ① ① ① ①

DISTANT, DETACHED
④ ④ ④ ④ ④ ④ ④ ④ ④ ④
③ ③ ③ ③ ③ ③ ③ ③ ③ ③
② ② ② ② ② ② ② ② ② ②
① ① ① ① ① ① ① ① ① ①

PHYSICAL RELAXATION
④ ④ ④ ④ ④ ④ ④ ④ ④ ④
③ ③ ③ ③ ③ ③ ③ ③ ③ ③
② ② ② ② ② ② ② ② ② ②
① ① ① ① ① ① ① ① ① ①

RESTED, REFRESHED
④ ④ ④ ④ ④ ④ ④ ④ ④ ④
③ ③ ③ ③ ③ ③ ③ ③ ③ ③
② ② ② ② ② ② ② ② ② ②
① ① ① ① ① ① ① ① ① ①

(continued)

TABLE 17.8 *(continued)*

NAME YOUR TECHNIQUES →										

AT EASE, AT PEACE	④③②①	④③②①	④③②①	④③②①	④③②①	④③②①	④③②①	④③②①	④③②①	④③②①
ENERGIZED	④③②①	④③②①	④③②①	④③②①	④③②①	④③②①	④③②①	④③②①	④③②①	④③②①
MENTAL QUIET	④③②①	④③②①	④③②①	④③②①	④③②①	④③②①	④③②①	④③②①	④③②①	④③②①
AWARE	④③②①	④③②①	④③②①	④③②①	④③②①	④③②①	④③②①	④③②①	④③②①	④③②①

POSITIVE MENTAL STATES

HAPPY, JOYFUL	④③②①	④③②①	④③②①	④③②①	④③②①	④③②①	④③②①	④③②①	④③②①	④③②①
CHILDLIKE INNOCENCE	④③②①	④③②①	④③②①	④③②①	④③②①	④③②①	④③②①	④③②①	④③②①	④③②①
THANKFUL, LOVING	④③②①	④③②①	④③②①	④③②①	④③②①	④③②①	④③②①	④③②①	④③②①	④③②①
MYSTERY	④③②①	④③②①	④③②①	④③②①	④③②①	④③②①	④③②①	④③②①	④③②①	④③②①

TABLE 17.8 *(continued)*

NAME YOUR TECHNIQUES →										
AWE AND WONDER	④③②①	④③②①	④③②①	④③②①	④③②①	④③②①	④③②①	④③②①	④③②①	④③②①
PRAYERFUL	④③②①	④③②①	④③②①	④③②①	④③②①	④③②①	④③②①	④③②①	④③②①	④③②①
TIMELESS, BOUNDLESS, INFINITE	④③②①	④③②①	④③②①	④③②①	④③②①	④③②①	④③②①	④③②①	④③②①	④③②①

© 2005 Springer Publishing Company. Permission granted for use.

ent" or "forgetting" are describing Disengagement. If a client uses words that do not appear on our word lists, look for similarities. For example, feeling "limber" most resembles words listed for Physical relaxation; "in my own space" resembles distancing/letting go, "unburdened" resembles mental Relaxation, and so on. See chapter 5 for an extended listing of words associated with various R-States.

RELAXATION SAMPLING

The most direct way of quickly determining which families a client likes or dislikes is to provide demonstration samples of exercises from six families of relaxation. Simply use the Relaxation Sampler sequence (see Appendix). The sampler provides five-minute demonstrations of yogaform stretching, PMR, breathing exercises, AT, imagery, and meditation/mindfulness. One first plays a recording of, or presents, the sampler demonstration, and asks a client to indicate which exercises were preferred or disliked, perhaps using the Smith Relaxation Preferences Inventory (Table 17.3). In addition, as

TABLE 17.9 Smith Relaxation States Inventory–Alternative Brief Version (SRSIabv)

HOW DO YOU FEEL RIGHT NOW?
PLEASE CHECK ITEM BELOW USING THIS KEY:
RIGHT NOW, I'm feeling this way . . .

① Not at all ② A Little, Somewhat ③ Moderately ④ Very Much

THE QUICK STRESS TEST

1. ① ② ③ ④ Physical Stress, Discomfort
   Muscles feel tight, tense (Clenched fist, jaws, furrowed brow)
2. ① ② ③ ④ Problems with concentration; feeling distracted, confused
3. ① ② ③ ④ Worry
   I am worrying
   Troublesome, negative thoughts go through my mind
4. ① ② ③ ④ Anxiety, feeling fearful
5. ① ② ③ ④ Irritation/Anger
6. ① ② ③ ④ Depression, sadness, feeling blue

R-STATE QUESTIONNAIRE

Basic R-States

1. ① ② ③ ④ Sleepy, Drowsy, Dozing off
2. ① ② ③ ④ Aware, Focused, Clear

Level 1: Stress Relief, Feeling Good

3. ① ② ③ ④ Distant or detached
   I feel distant and far away from my cares and concerns
   I feel indifferent and detached from my cares and concerns
4. ① ② ③ ④ Rested or Refreshed
5. ① ② ③ ④ Energized, Strengthened
6. ① ② ③ ④ Physical Relaxation
   I feel physically relaxed, warm and heavy.
   I feel physically relaxed, loose and limp.
7. ① ② ③ ④ At ease, Carefree, At Peace
8. ① ② ③ ④ Happy or Joyful

Level 2: Selflessness

9. ① ② ③ ④ Mental Quiet
   My mind is quiet, without thought
   My mind is still
10. ① ② ③ ④ Childlike innocence
11. ① ② ③ ④ Thankful or Loving

Level 3: Spirituality and Transcendence

12. ① ② ③ ④ Feeling the Deep Mystery of things beyond my understanding
13. ① ② ③ ④ Things seem amazing, awesome, extraordinary
14. ① ② ③ ④ I feel prayerful or reverent
15. ① ② ③ ④ Things seem timeless, boundless, or infinite

TABLE 17.10 Smith Relaxation States Inventory Alternative Brief Version (SRSIabv) Summary Sheet

NAME YOUR TECHNIQUES →									

QUICK STRESS TEST

1. Physical stress, Discomfort
   ④ ④ ④ ④ ④ ④ ④ ④ ④ ④
   ③ ③ ③ ③ ③ ③ ③ ③ ③ ③
   ② ② ② ② ② ② ② ② ② ②
   ① ① ① ① ① ① ① ① ① ①

2. Problems with concentration . . .
   ④ ④ ④ ④ ④ ④ ④ ④ ④ ④
   ③ ③ ③ ③ ③ ③ ③ ③ ③ ③
   ② ② ② ② ② ② ② ② ② ②
   ① ① ① ① ① ① ① ① ① ①

3. Worry
   ④ ④ ④ ④ ④ ④ ④ ④ ④ ④
   ③ ③ ③ ③ ③ ③ ③ ③ ③ ③
   ② ② ② ② ② ② ② ② ② ②
   ① ① ① ① ① ① ① ① ① ①

4. Anxious, Fearful
   ④ ④ ④ ④ ④ ④ ④ ④ ④ ④
   ③ ③ ③ ③ ③ ③ ③ ③ ③ ③
   ② ② ② ② ② ② ② ② ② ②
   ① ① ① ① ① ① ① ① ① ①

5. Irritation, Anger
   ④ ④ ④ ④ ④ ④ ④ ④ ④ ④
   ③ ③ ③ ③ ③ ③ ③ ③ ③ ③
   ② ② ② ② ② ② ② ② ② ②
   ① ① ① ① ① ① ① ① ① ①

6. Depression
   ④ ④ ④ ④ ④ ④ ④ ④ ④ ④
   ③ ③ ③ ③ ③ ③ ③ ③ ③ ③
   ② ② ② ② ② ② ② ② ② ②
   ① ① ① ① ① ① ① ① ① ①

R-STATE QUESTIONNAIRE

BASIC R-STATES

1. Sleepy
   ④ ④ ④ ④ ④ ④ ④ ④ ④ ④
   ③ ③ ③ ③ ③ ③ ③ ③ ③ ③
   ② ② ② ② ② ② ② ② ② ②
   ① ① ① ① ① ① ① ① ① ①

2. Aware, Focused, Clear
   ④ ④ ④ ④ ④ ④ ④ ④ ④ ④
   ③ ③ ③ ③ ③ ③ ③ ③ ③ ③
   ② ② ② ② ② ② ② ② ② ②
   ① ① ① ① ① ① ① ① ① ①

STRESS RELIEF, FEELING GOOD

3. Distant, Detached
   ④ ④ ④ ④ ④ ④ ④ ④ ④ ④
   ③ ③ ③ ③ ③ ③ ③ ③ ③ ③
   ② ② ② ② ② ② ② ② ② ②
   ① ① ① ① ① ① ① ① ① ①

4. Rested, Refreshed
   ④ ④ ④ ④ ④ ④ ④ ④ ④ ④
   ③ ③ ③ ③ ③ ③ ③ ③ ③ ③
   ② ② ② ② ② ② ② ② ② ②
   ① ① ① ① ① ① ① ① ① ①

(continued)

TABLE 17.10 *(continued)*

NAME YOUR TECHNIQUES →										

5. Energized, Strengthened

④ ④ ④ ④ ④ ④ ④ ④ ④ ④
③ ③ ③ ③ ③ ③ ③ ③ ③ ③
② ② ② ② ② ② ② ② ② ②
① ① ① ① ① ① ① ① ① ①

6. Physical Relaxation

④ ④ ④ ④ ④ ④ ④ ④ ④ ④
③ ③ ③ ③ ③ ③ ③ ③ ③ ③
② ② ② ② ② ② ② ② ② ②
① ① ① ① ① ① ① ① ① ①

7. At Ease, Peace

④ ④ ④ ④ ④ ④ ④ ④ ④ ④
③ ③ ③ ③ ③ ③ ③ ③ ③ ③
② ② ② ② ② ② ② ② ② ②
① ① ① ① ① ① ① ① ① ①

8. Happy or Joyful

④ ④ ④ ④ ④ ④ ④ ④ ④ ④
③ ③ ③ ③ ③ ③ ③ ③ ③ ③
② ② ② ② ② ② ② ② ② ②
① ① ① ① ① ① ① ① ① ①

SELFLESSNESS

9. Mental quiet

④ ④ ④ ④ ④ ④ ④ ④ ④ ④
③ ③ ③ ③ ③ ③ ③ ③ ③ ③
② ② ② ② ② ② ② ② ② ②
① ① ① ① ① ① ① ① ① ①

10. Childlike innocence

④ ④ ④ ④ ④ ④ ④ ④ ④ ④
③ ③ ③ ③ ③ ③ ③ ③ ③ ③
② ② ② ② ② ② ② ② ② ②
① ① ① ① ① ① ① ① ① ①

11. Thankful, Loving

④ ④ ④ ④ ④ ④ ④ ④ ④ ④
③ ③ ③ ③ ③ ③ ③ ③ ③ ③
② ② ② ② ② ② ② ② ② ②
① ① ① ① ① ① ① ① ① ①

TABLE 17.10 *(continued)*

NAME YOUR TECHNIQUES →									

SPIRITUAL/TRANSCENDENT

12. Deep mystery

④ ④ ④ ④ ④ ④ ④ ④ ④ ④
③ ③ ③ ③ ③ ③ ③ ③ ③ ③
② ② ② ② ② ② ② ② ② ②
① ① ① ① ① ① ① ① ① ①

13. Awe and Wonder

④ ④ ④ ④ ④ ④ ④ ④ ④ ④
③ ③ ③ ③ ③ ③ ③ ③ ③ ③
② ② ② ② ② ② ② ② ② ②
① ① ① ① ① ① ① ① ① ①

14. Prayerful

④ ④ ④ ④ ④ ④ ④ ④ ④ ④
③ ③ ③ ③ ③ ③ ③ ③ ③ ③
② ② ② ② ② ② ② ② ② ②
① ① ① ① ① ① ① ① ① ①

15. Timeless, Boundless, Infinite

④ ④ ④ ④ ④ ④ ④ ④ ④ ④
③ ③ ③ ③ ③ ③ ③ ③ ③ ③
② ② ② ② ② ② ② ② ② ②
① ① ① ① ① ① ① ① ① ①

indicated in the script (see Appendix), one notes specific R-State evoked by different exercises on the Simplified R-State Pyramid Map (Figure 17.1).

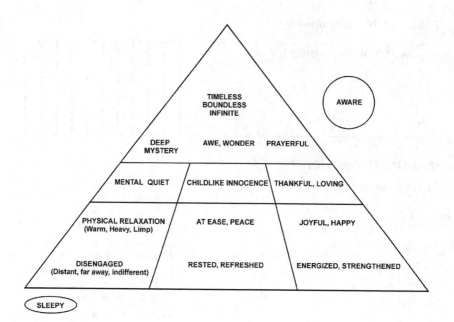

FIGURE 17.1   Simplified R-State Pyramid map.

© 2005 Springer Publishing Company. Permission granted for use.

18

Troubleshooting and Enhancing Relaxation

Once a client has completed a relaxation program, training is not complete. A conscientious trainer will address any problems that could interfere with progress in practice and introduce strategies for enhancing skills a client has already learned. Troubleshooting and enhancing relaxation can help ensure that a client maintains practice and derives maximum benefit from what has been taught. Here are some ideas based on my experience as a trainer.

TROUBLESHOOTING

N-States and Relaxation-Induced Anxiety

Any form of relaxation can evoke unwanted or aversive states of mind. Such paradoxical effects have been termed relaxation-induced anxiety (Heide & Borkovec, 1984). I prefer the term negative states, or simply N-States. N-States can include physical sensations, negative emotions, images, and worry. Their sources are many. Some N-States reflect how one appraises relaxation:
   Previous aversive experiences with relaxation. Perhaps one of the most frequent sources of discomfort with relaxation is previous adverse experience. Clients have been sexually harassed by hypnotists, manipulated and threatened by yoga instructors, lied to by meditation gurus, proselytized by preachers, taught ineptly by coercive PMR trainers, or simply taught that relaxation is

"weird and/or occult." Past negative experiences with relaxation can limit a client's willingness to attempt relaxation and stir distress in the course of relaxation training.

Negative appraisal of letting go. In everyday life we accomplish our tasks through planning and effort; in relaxation, we must let go of planning and effort. A beginning relaxer can find this basic shift difficult, feeling that the task of "letting go" in order to achieve the possible benefits of relaxation is impossible. A client may even fear the task of "letting go," and mistakenly think it means "going crazy," "becoming sick," and so on. Or, reduced control may simply suggest reduced personal efficacy, "laziness," reduced ability to perform at one's peak, and so on.

Negative appraisal of R-States. Clients may not be familiar with many of the R-States we have previously identified, including physiological signs of reduced arousal (for example, increased blood flow to the extremities, reduced breathing and heart rate), symptom reduction, feelings of somatic and cognitive tension relief, as well as Disengagement, and Mental Quiet. Not knowing such experiences are a normal part of relaxation, clients may find them threatening and fear becoming ill, "going crazy," etc.

Negative associations with relaxation techniques. A relaxation technique may remind a client of a negative experience that has nothing to do with the technique itself. For example, a client may relax with imagery that involves an ocean or beach, only to remember a painful childhood sunburn. Such relaxation "booby traps" are most common when techniques are mechanically imposed on clients with little attempt to individualize.

Other forms of N-States reflect secondary processes set in motion through the act of sustaining relaxation.

Increased sensitivity. One consequence of all relaxation training is the reduction of potentially distracting internal and external stimuli. In the quiet of a practice session, a relaxer may simply notice subtle sources of stimuli that ordinarily go undetected. He or she may be aware of breathing, heart rate, underlying emotional state, and so on. Unprepared, a client may perceive such experiences as threats.

Disengagement, disorientation and depersonalization. Through Disengagement the relaxer pulls away from and becomes less aware of the outside world. In relaxation this contributes to a singular focus on a restricted stimulus by minimizing distraction. However, if a relaxer resumes everyday activities while remaining disengaged, he or she may experience disruptive depersonalization or disorientation.

Reduction of defensive barriers. Relaxation can reduce defensive efforts to deny or ignore threatening thoughts and feelings. For a skilled psychotherapist, the resulting emergence of threatening material can provide a basis for treatment. However, such uncovered material can interfere with the course of relaxation if not properly managed.

Reductions in critical thinking and reality testing. As one relaxes, one reduces deliberate efforts at analysis and control, including critical and analytic thinking. In some contexts this can contribute to spontaneous enjoyment, as when one temporarily suspends disbelief and becomes absorbed in a movie or novel. However, lessened critical thinking and reality testing may make one more susceptible to troublesome thoughts and fantasies that might arise in relaxation. For example, in the course of a day's events a client may casually wonder, "Sometimes I feel like I am floating in relaxation. Do I really float?" He or she may ordinarily appraise such a feeling reasonably, "Of course, I am not really floating; I'm just experiencing a relaxation effect." However, if such a thought were to arise in deep relaxation, rational and reality-based assessment has decreased. Our client may well "suspend disbelief" and actually believe he or she is levitating, thus experiencing distress.

Hyperventilation/Hypoventilation. We have seen that changes in breathing during relaxation can result in decreased or increased blood levels of CO_2. Such hyper- or hypoventilation can lead to aversive subjective states, including dizziness, anxiety, and so on.

Presumed shifts in brain functioning. As relaxation deepens, parts of the brain, perhaps the cerebral cortex, may become relatively less active. Other parts, perhaps those less active in normal daily life, become relatively more active. This could result in increased spontaneous wakeful dream-like activity, including vivid imagery, novel or intense emotional states, changes in body image (sensations of floating, changing size), and even felt paranormal phenomena.

N-States: A Sign That Relaxation Is Working

Students of relaxation, like students of any other discipline such as sports, dance, and so on, experience "ups and downs." Such cycles are a natural part of growth and movement in relaxation. The very process of "going deeper" in a relaxation session can unearth distractions and problems. In the relaxation session itself, the proper response to such nonspecific distractions is generally to let go of the distraction and resume practice. This, indeed, is how one develops many of the access skills of relaxation. Put differently, the emergence of N-States in relaxation can be a sign that relaxation is indeed working.

If problems persist, or are disruptive beyond the practice session, a trainer might experiment with the following modifications:

- Shorten the exercise
- Practice the exercise with less vigor (especially important for physical approaches)
- Precede the exercise (especially mental) with five to ten minutes of preferred physical relaxation exercises as a "warmup"
- Select less focused or passive exercises within a family of exercises (for example, instead of meditating on a mantra, a client might attempt rocking meditation). Note that for all the families of relaxation presented in this book, exercises are presented in order of increased focus and passivity.
- Attempt exercises from a different family.
- Provide greater structure, perhaps by shortening pauses and periods of silence and continuing instructional "patter"
- Increase exercise complexity by introducing elements of several exercises
- Revise an exercise, deleting any elements that trigger distressing associations
- Introduce phrases of encouragement and support
- Supplement exercises with music or recordings of nature sounds
- Increase extraneous stimulation (turn up lights, open the windows, select a familiar and somewhat complex relaxation environment, practice in an upright seated position, practice standing up)
- Practice in a group
- Take a break or vacation from professional relaxation, and emphasize familiar casual approaches that are not likely to cause problems
- In the instructions, remove phrases suggestive of Disengagement
- In the instructions, emphasize phrases suggestive of specific effects (symptom reduction, tension relief, positive feelings)

If relaxation-induced distress persists, professional counseling or psychotherapy may be advised.

Unwanted Sleepiness

Nearly everyone who has learned a relaxation technique has fallen asleep from time to time. Clients often wonder if drowsiness and sleep are normal and what can be done if they become a problem. The R-State, Sleepiness, is a normal part of most relaxation. When sleepiness interferes with instruction or practice, it needs to be addressed.

Sleepiness can be a needless distraction if it is caused by factors unrelated to relaxation. Some of these are associated with low levels of skill acquisition, or the misapplication of skills.

Lack of relaxation skill. A client who lacks the access skills required for an approach may simply fall asleep during relaxation training.

Inability to differentiate relaxation from sleep. The beginning practitioner often has a vague, undifferentiated perspective of the nature of relaxation. Just as a beginning chef may see all oriental cuisines as the same, a novice relaxer may find it difficult to differentiate R-States and see all in terms of the one relaxation experience he or she may know well, falling asleep.

Inability to differentiate R-State Disengagement from sleep. Because feelings of Disengagement often precede normal sleep, clients may often think they are falling asleep when disengaging from distracting stimuli in relaxation. In relaxation, unlike sleep, Disengagement is accompanied by maintained attention on a simple stimulus. As relaxation skills develop, clients learn to differentiate Disengagement from sleep.

Excessive relaxation. Clients differ in the length of practice they can tolerate. For some 15 minutes is enough, for others, one hour is quite comfortable. But clients who practice too long run the risk of falling asleep.

Misapplication of the relaxation technique or level. A client may practice a technique that is too advanced or simply inappropriate. Unable to effectively deploy skills related to passive attention, he or she may fall asleep.

Sometimes sleepiness can be traced to problems in the environment in which one practices.

Relaxing in a position or at a time and place associated with sleep. Clients often chose to practice relaxation in a reclining position, at bedtime, in bed, or in their bedrooms. Unfortunately such practices are likely to evoke associations of sleep and suggest it is time to fall asleep rather than relax.

Relaxing in a poorly ventilated setting. Reduced oxygen and increased carbon dioxide contribute to feelings of drowsiness.

Relaxing in a distracting setting. A setting may be too noisy, uncomfortable, warm, or unpleasant. A client may then respond by tuning out such aversive stimuli by falling asleep.

Clients may also experience difficulties with relaxation because of a variety of simple physiological reasons.

Relaxing after eating or consuming alcohol. After a meal, one often feels sleepy. Blood is diverted from the brain for digestion. Consumption of alcohol, although relaxing, contributes to reductions in awareness.

Consuming medications that can contribute to drowsiness. Many medications, for example, some common antihistamines and pain relievers, have drowsiness as a side effect. Such medications, if taken immediately before a practice session, can increase the likelihood of falling asleep.

Lack of sleep. A client who is tired or sleep deprived will likely fall asleep during a relaxation session. This is a normal physiological response to a normal physiological need.

Illness. If a client is recovering from illness or surgery, the body may need recuperative sleep.

At times, more complex psychological reasons underlie difficulties with sleepiness.

A wish to avoid a relaxation technique, instructor, or setting. A client who simply does not like a technique, an instructor, or a setting, may respond by becoming drowsy and falling asleep.

Avoidance of negative relaxation effects. Clients may become drowsy or fall asleep to avoid the threatening negative effects we have considered earlier.

Avoiding external stress through relaxation. At times, clients employ relaxation as a strategy for passively avoiding coping with the demands of living. For example, a client may have the unpleasant task of scheduling an income tax audit. He or she may quite innocently cope with such emotional distress by practicing a relaxation technique. However, if no action is taken or planned, relaxation may become a tool for avoiding responsibility. The relaxer may be more likely to fall asleep.

If a sleep response is temporary and occasional, it can be ignored. If it becomes a persistent problem, the instructor may consider a number of interventions:

- Precede training with stretching or breathing stretches
- Precede exercises with walking
- Recommend a 10 minute nap prior to relaxation
- Do not eat prior to relaxation
- If possible, do not take prescription meditations before relaxation
- Do not drink alcoholic beverages before relaxation
- Practice in a well-ventilated room
- Lower the temperature of the setting
- Do not practice in a room associated with sleep (bedroom, lounge)

- Do not practice at bedtime, naptime, or any other time associated with sleep
- Practice at a time when you are ordinarily most alert and awake
- Do not practice in a position associated with sleep (lying down, reclining)
- Practice sitting up or in a less comfortable chair
- Practice sitting on the floor or kneeling with legs crossed in a yoga "lotus" position
- Precede preferred relaxation exercise with exercises designed to increase arousal and blood flow, or the R-State Strength and Awareness (walking, singing, yoga, breathing)
- Try a different approach to relaxation
- Practice with eyes open
- Make the relaxation exercise shorter
- Make the relaxation exercise more physical
- Make a relaxation exercise more complex
- Introduce suggestions of "wakefulness" in the relaxation exercise
- Speak louder
- Practice in a group
- Practice with the lights on
- Include music or background nature sounds

Negative, Anti-Relaxation Beliefs

Clients may harbor a variety of negative beliefs about relaxation. A clinician may view these as forms of "resistance" to training. At the least, negative, anti-relaxation beliefs can prevent potential clients from considering or continuing techniques that may offer substantial benefit. Our research has identified six categories of N-Beliefs (R-Attitudes; Smith, 2001):

Concerns over relaxation-induced anxiety (increased sensitivity to problems, emergence of anxiety symptoms). Previous negative experiences with relaxation may lead a client to associate practice with any of the N-States we have considered. If such apprehensions are uncovered, a trainer might:

- Explain the extent to which the fears are unfounded and how they usually emerge
- Discuss the possibility of augmenting training using any of the strategies we have previously considered for reducing N-States in relaxation

Concerns over disengagement (concerns that relaxation will cause one to slow down, withdraw from the world, become less effective, not solve one's problems, waste time. Here it can be useful to:

- Focus on which relaxation goals a client desires and to select a goal that is least troublesome
- Emphasize that some families of relaxation are much less likely to contribute to Disengagement and more likely to evoke Energy and Awareness

Trainer concerns (having a trainer who does not individualize techniques). I sympathize with clients who are cautious about selecting a relaxation trainer. Indeed, concerns about trainer qualifications are well founded. In this case, it is crucial to:

- Emphasize the importance of professionalism and proper trainer credentialing. A client should ask where and how a trainer was educated. If a client is receiving training for clinical purposes, then the trainer should be part of a professional team, supervised by a licensed psychologist, psychiatrist, counselor, social worker, or psychiatric nurse.

Fantasy concerns (fear of getting lost in fantasy or daydreaming in relaxation). These concerns can be realistic if a client has a history of avoiding challenges through fantasy, or has a clinical history suggesting that withdrawal into imagery may not be advised.

- Suggest highly structured physical techniques or introduce the precautions suggested for minimizing N-States

Practical concerns (not slowing down enough for relaxation, being distracted, finding it hard to put relaxation to use, finding time to practice).

- Reassure clients that such concerns are extremely common among relaxation trainees. There are numerous strategies for countering such practical concerns, ranging from proper selection of techniques to relaxation time-management
- Proper preparation (chapter 16) is essential to motivate clients to find time to practice

Concerns over being subjected to unwanted religious indoctrination or hypnotic control.

- Explain that at all times the client is in complete control during every exercise presented in this book. In fact, a client learns a higher level of "calm control" requiring less effort and planning.
- Hypnosis is a highly specific procedure in which suggestions are made by a hypnotist and a client feels he or she "automatically" responds. For example, a hypnotist may suggest that a client lose the sense of smell or act like a chicken, and the client automatically complies. At no point are such suggestions used here. At every moment training is a collaborative effort between trainee and "guide." The trainee can stop at any time, and indeed the trainee is ultimately responsible for the course and length of training.
- Even though some of the families used here, yoga and meditation, may have roots in Hindu and Buddhist religion, and other techniques are used in many religions, including Christianity, Judaism, and Islam, the approaches here are strictly nonreligious. The techniques are no more intrinsically religious than a book or piano, both of which are at times used in and out of a religious setting. Of course, religious clients may choose to incorporate relaxation techniques into their own religious practice. However, that is entirely the client's choice. Here the trainer is available to help if called upon (see chapter 24).

Initial Resistance, Discomfort, Embarrassment

Beginners may find the mechanics of a relaxation technique (especially a physical technique) unexpected and awkward. They may respond with feelings of self-consciousness and embarrassment. Reactions may range from amusement and giggling to refusal to practice a specific technique because it "has sexual connotations," "is too intimate," or "makes me feel open and vulnerable to others."

Here are some strategies to use. A good initial rationale should allay many of these concerns. Blending a demonstration of an exercise with a rationale can divert attention from disruptive thoughts to the task at hand. Change any phrases that can even remotely have sexual connotations ("go limp," "tighten muscles," "tension flows out"). Include references to images that are familiar and somewhat serious and competitive. Also, initial brief demonstrations and group practice of very safe sample exercises should help beginners get used to the types of movements and actions involved.

ENHANCING EXERCISES

Two variables are most likely to determine if a relaxation exercise works. First, daily practice. Relaxation is like nutrition—a complete meal every other week isn't enough. You need to do it just about every day. The second is belief. Clients who are able to integrate relaxation with deeply held philosophical and religious beliefs are more likely to practice with regularity and benefit.

R-Beliefs

We have identified eight beliefs that seem to make the greatest difference (Smith, 1999a). The first three are a bit more abstract and nonspecific and generally do not apply to a specific external situation. These beliefs support regular practice of a relaxation technique, but they are somewhat less likely to change as a result of practice.

Deeper perspective. Life has a purpose greater than one's personal wants and desires. There's more to life than personal concerns and worries.

God. One can trust that God guides, loves, and provides comfort. One can put oneself in God's hands.

Inner wisdom. One can trust the healing and wisdom of the body. There are sources of strength and healing deep within.

The remaining R-Beliefs are situational and refer to one's relationship to some aspect of the outside world. They, too, support relaxation but are more likely to change as a result of practice.

Optimism. One can be optimistic about how well one will do with current hassles. One believes in being optimistic.

Love. It is important to love and respect others, and to treat others with compassion and understanding.

Honesty. It is important to be direct and clear in what one says, thinks, and does; one should be honest and open with one's feelings.

Acceptance. It is important to be able to accept things as they are. There's no need to try to change what can't be changed.

Taking it easy. It is important to know when to let go and simply take it easy. It is important to know when to stop trying, let go, and relax.

It is important to recognize that R-Beliefs reflect ways of coping with the task of relaxation, not necessarily with external stressors. The R-Belief "forget your problems for now" may well facilitate the relaxation skills of letting go of thought and activity, diverting attention, and sustaining attention. But it may prove disastrous when applied to external stressors (and, for example, prompt one not to get out of the way of an approaching train).

We see how R-Beliefs can function in the following hypothetical internal dialogues of relaxers.

A practitioner of yoga stretching: "I want my yoga to produce immediate effects. I am impatient with how slow it seems to be working. However, I realize it takes time. Everyone grows at his own pace. I'll just have to accept things as they are and continue practicing." *R-Belief: Accept things as they are.* Articulation of this belief enabled the practitioner to put his frustration aside and continue.

A practitioner of imagery: "I chose as my relaxation image a peaceful vacation with my two small children. I forget my everyday hassles and pains, and attend, filled with feelings of love and gratitude." *R-Belief: Love and respect others.* This belief provides the motivation to continue attending to the object of attention. The R-State Thankful/Loving facilitates sustained attention.

A skin cancer patient and practitioner of autogenic training: "I think the phrase, 'warmth and healing are flowing to my tumor, I feel warm and healing blood flowing to my tumor. Let the healing powers do their work." *R-Belief: Trust the healing powers of the body.* This provides the rationale for proceeding with relaxation exercise.

A client receiving a massage: "It makes no sense to think about work during my massage session. Sometimes it is important just to take time for relaxation, and enjoy myself." *R-Belief: Know when to let go and take it easy.* This enables the client to put aside distracting thoughts, and let go of muscle tension.

A client practicing a series of breathing exercises before an interview: "I can't keep my mind on breathing slowly and deeply. I keep thinking about my upcoming interview. I have prepared for this interview, and will do the best I can. I'm optimistic about how I will deal with this challenge. I can now put this thought aside and relax." *R-Belief: View the world with optimism.* An optimistic appraisal of a distracting concern about a future challenge facilitates putting the distracting thought aside and focusing on the relaxation exercise.

The same client above, not so sure about readiness for upcoming interview: "I want to prepare for my interview, but I need to relax. So I confront myself and do some honest soul-searching. Frankly, which is more important at this moment, preparing more for my interview or relaxing? To be honest, there is nothing I can do about the interview now; I must relax." *R-Belief: Honesty.* Here the client openly and honestly confronted her conflicting motivations.

A client engaged in prayer. "I am very worried about my life situation, I do my nightly prayer. At first, I find myself hoping for an instant solution to my problems. When I decide to put myself in God's hands and trust His wisdom, I relax." *R-Belief: Trust God's love and guidance.* Belief in God enables client to put distracting concern aside.

A student of meditation. "My daily routine is ultimately less important when seen in deeper perspective. I feel deeply at peace when I attend to the night sky above and realize that I am part of a larger universe." *R-Belief: Put your concerns in deeper perspective.* This provides a rationale for putting distractions aside (distractions are less important) and meditating on the night sky. It also cultivates an R-State (Timeless) that supports sustained focus.

For a receptive client, a skillful relaxation trainer can introduce relaxation in the context of a client's R-Beliefs. However, the client must approve of this strategy, otherwise the trainer risks taking on the role of a preacher imposing a belief.

At risk of appearing sexist, our research (Smith, 2001) has found that females are much more likely to profess R-Beliefs and report R-States higher on the R-State Pyramid. Generally, I feel more comfortable integrating such beliefs and R-States into training for females. Males display more pragmatic beliefs, and concrete level R-States, which can be readily incorporated into training.

Pauses

The simplest way of fostering skill development is to increase pause time between exercise elements and reduce instructional "patter" (the number of words used in instruction). So, when teaching PMR, increase the pause at the end of each release cycle (to 10 or 20 seconds). For AT, increase the pause time when shifting to a different target suggestion (pause 60 seconds between the end of the "heaviness" and the beginning of "warmth" exercises, etc.).

Immediate and Gradual Enhancements of Milieu

Relaxation training can be facilitated when practiced in a milieu conducive to skill development. Here one makes full use of the practice environment and stylistic elements of a practice session to support the metaskill of sustained effortless/passive simple focus. To elaborate, imagine a relaxation sequence that begins with a half hour of yoga stretching and ends with 15 minutes of imagery. One could prepare the practice room by dimming the lights before training and keeping them dim throughout training. Immediately, this may create a "calm environment." Such reduced stimulus facilitates the task of diverting attention from external stimuli, makes it easier to focus and refocus attention by introducing fewer external distractions, and enhances efforts to evoke reinforcing R-States such as Mental Quiet and Disengagement.

The effect may be different if the trainer begins training with lights on bright and gradually diminishes lighting throughout training, so that by the time meditation begins, lights are low. The slowly dimming light contributes to the process of slowly increasing the level of skill deployment.

Immediate enhancements are perhaps relatively easy to understand. Turn down the lights. Put on relaxing clothing. Close the doors. Light the incense. Play quiet music. In other words, establish a milieu that is from the beginning conducive to sustained, effortless, simple focus, and begin. Gradual enhancements are a bit more difficult. Instead of selecting a variable that can be switched on or off, or removed or placed, one selects something that can be introduced in increments, with each increment suggesting greater relaxation, specifically increased levels of the access skill sustained effortless/passive simple focus. Here are some examples:

> When teaching meditation, try introducing candlelight. One might begin a mindfulness walking exercise by lighting 10 candles. After every five steps, candles are extinguished, one by one.
>
> Yoga might be practiced with a background of recorded nature sounds. At the beginning, a variety of peaceful sounds might fill the air—wind, birds, rustling of leaves, splashing of waves. As training progresses, gently decrease the volume so that the sound of the wind becomes more quiet, the birds seem farther away, fewer leaves rustle, or waves in a lake become gentle ripples. And later in the same recording, some sounds simply cease, so that the "sound landscape" is even more focused and simple.
>
> When guiding an imagery exercise, gradually lower the intensity and variety of one's voice. At first, one's voice might be filled with energy and enthusiasm. As the story progresses, ones voice becomes more quiet, slow, and gentle, enhancing the deepening effects of the guided imagery.

To summarize, immediately establishing a relaxation milieu helps a trainee note and articulate variables that contribute to relaxation, especially the skill of sustained effortless/simple focus. In contrast, a gradual shift is more likely to condition a trainee to actually experience changes in skill level. The trainee may not even articulate or recognize the gradual environmental changes that are occurring, but may still experience deeper relaxation.

Part IV

Combination Training Formats

19

Scripting

Relaxation scripting is both an instructional tool that can help trainers consolidate and integrate their skills and an application for making individualized relaxation audio recordings for clients. As a tool for trainers, scripting provides a unique opportunity to compare families of techniques and master a wide range of deepened and enhanced skills. For the client, the advantages are substantial.

Over the last two decades, I have introduced relaxation to thousands of individuals. They have taught me one very unexpected lesson. I used to think that most clients have very specific relaxation preferences and respond best to just one general strategy, whether it be PMR, stretching, meditation, or the like. I spent many years of research attempting to identify the "PMR," "yoga," or "meditation" type of person. So far I have found few patterns. All this time, my clients were teaching me something very different; virtually all of them preferred combined exercises, typically highly individualized mixtures of many approaches. Very few people prefer just one or two strategies alone. This discovery has led me to develop a new approach to teaching relaxation, scripting.

Scripting is based on the following ideas:

1. Different approaches to relaxation have different effects and work differently for different people.
2. The best way to teach relaxation is not to impose one or two approaches on everyone, but to introduce a variety of approaches.
3. I try to present a relatively "pure" version of each approach, so that clients can discover its unique effects independently of other ap-

proaches. For example, I present PMR tense-let go cycles, minimizing breathing and imagery, so clients can clearly note the relaxation effect of tensing up and letting go.

4. Once one is trained in a variety of approaches, select those that work best and construct an individualized script and tape.
5. The goal of relaxation training goes beyond the relaxation response of lowered arousal. Additional objectives are cultivating appropriate R-States and acquiring beliefs and personal philosophies conducive to deepening relaxation and extending its rewards to all of life.

Many instructors present trainees with relaxation recordings of technique combinations, often standardized versions available from various mental health catalogues. However, giving everyone the same recording can pose a variety of problems. Not only does such a strategy ignore client preferences, but it also risks exposing trainees to exercises that may evoke negative associations. My approach is to craft an individualized relaxation recording based on a mutually developed verbatim script of exercise instructions. There are several advantages to such script writing:

*   The client includes only what works best. (Different exercises work for different people.)
*   Different exercises may be selected for a targeted relaxation goal. (Different exercises can be better for different goals.)
*   Since the client is inventing his or her own relaxation exercise, he or she is more likely to take it seriously and practice it regularly. Indeed a client may well treasure his or her script as a truly personal possession, and practice it very seriously.
*   Given that training is varied and changing, interest and motivation is maintained, reducing premature quitting.
*   Special suggestions and exercises can be included to deepen relaxation.
*   Finally, relaxation can be used as a reminder of personal philosophies conducive to living a life of peace and calm.

OVERVIEW OF THE SCRIPTING PROCESS

Relaxation scripting takes at least 10 sessions. (For group training, see chapter 21.) It is noteworthy that the first seven sessions (Part 1: Preparation) are devoted to training each of the six families of relaxation. In sessions 8–10

(Part 2: Making a Script) you create a script based on the exercise elements that worked best. The schedule in Table 19.1 summarizes the scripting process.

Session 1

First explain the stress and relaxation engines.
Next, describe the scripting approach.

> In this approach to relaxation we will first learn the six families of relaxation most popular among experts. Why all six? Because research has shown that each approach has a different effect and works for different problems. Complete relaxation is like a balanced meal in which you make selections from several basic food groups. The six families of relaxation are like basic food groups and we will construct a "balanced meal" of relaxation tailored just for you.
>
> Here's how we will accomplish this goal. After learning the basics, you and I will select exercises from the menu of six families and construct a special, individualized relaxation recording tailored to your needs and interests. Because we will include the exercises that work best for you, we will do our best to create a recording that is most powerful and effective for you. Training will take 10 sessions (*more or less, depending on available time*). The first six sessions will be devoted to training in the basic six families, and the last sessions will be devoted to making your personalized recording.

You may wish to present clients with a training schedule. Here is a minimal sequence I suggest (Table 19.2).

End by giving the Relaxation Precautions Fact Sheet (Table 16.1) and the Target Symptoms Fact Sheet (Table 17.1). Discuss any potential problems.

Sessions 2–7: Training in Six Families of Relaxation

Teach one complete exercise sequence for each of the six families of relaxation. Devote at least one week to each of the six approaches. Home practice is recommended, but not absolutely required. Follow the instructions provided for each family. Be sure the client completes the Smith Relaxation States Inventory Brief Version or Smith Relaxation States Inventory Alternate Brief Version (SRSIbv, SRSIabv; Tables 17.7–17.10) after every presentation.

TABLE 19.1   Scripting Schedule

Part 1: Preparation

Session 1

- Orientation. Explain general relaxation processes. If a client has already stated a desired relaxation goal, describe goal-specific relaxation processes
- Explain program and 10 sessions
- Give Relaxation Precautions Fact Sheet (Table 16.1)
- Give Target Symptoms Fact Sheet (Table 17.1)

Session 2

- Introduce and teach Yogaform Stretching (Full script)
- Give SRSIbv or SRSIabv (Tables 17.7, 17.9), and record results on Summary Chart (Tables 17.8, 17.10)

Session 3

- Introduce and teach Progressive Muscle Relaxation (Full script)
- Give SRSIbv or SRSIabv, record results on Summary Chart

Session 4

- Introduce and teach Breathing Exercises
- Give SRSIbv or SRSIabv, record results on Summary Chart

Session 5

- Introduce and teach Autogenic Training (verbal)
- Give SRSIbv or SRSIabv, record results on Summary Chart

Session 6

- Introduce and teach Sense Imagery
- Give SRSIbv or SRSIabv, record results on Summary Chart

Session 7

- Introduce and teach Meditation (eight meditations)
- Give SRSIbv or SRSIabv, record results on summary chart

Part 2: Making a Script

Session 8

- Complete Relaxation Scripting Workbook (Table 19.4) with client

Session 9

- Present first draft of relaxation recording
- Review and suggest improvements

Session 10

- Present final version of relaxation training

TABLE 19.2 Scripting Schedule for Clients

SESSION 1:	Orientation
SESSION 2:	Full Yogaform Stretching
SESSION 3:	Full Progressive Muscle Relaxation
SESSION 4:	Breathing Exercises
SESSION 5:	Verbal Autogenic Training
SESSION 6:	Imagery
SESSION 7:	Eight Meditations
SESSION 8:	Selecting what to put in personalized relaxation recording.
SESSION 9:	Presentation of first draft of relaxation recording; review and suggest improvements.
SESSION 10:	Presentation of final version of relaxation recording.

Record results on Summary Chart. This inventory assesses the specific impact of each approach and provides essential information for comparing and combining exercises. After all six families have been taught, the client is ready for a personalized script.

If resources permit, suggest a more open-ended schedule. Additional sessions may be scheduled to explore further sequences in those families of relaxation a client may prefer. For example, if a client has strong preferences for the presented instructions of full progressive muscle relaxation, consider adding one or two additional sessions for abbreviated PRM and letting go. Similarly, if a client enjoys the eight meditations consider presenting graduated mindfulness in the following session.

Session 8: Scripting-Writing Specifics and the Relaxation Scripting Workbook

In general, this process involves filling out with the client the Relaxation Scripting Workbook (see the following section, "How to Use the Relaxation Scripting Workbook" Table 19.4). Generally, writing a script takes 10 steps.

1. Select relaxation goal or goals
2. Identify R-States consistent with relaxation goal(s)
3. Select specific exercises that work best at evoking desired R-States
4. Arrange exercises and add detailed instructions
5. Incorporate unifying idea

6. Add imagery and mediation details (when relevant)
7. Add deepening R-State words and affirmations
8. Incorporate deepening imagery
9. Add concluding segment
10. Evaluate script

Session 9: Presentation of First Draft of Client's Relaxation Recording

Present your first version of your client's relaxation recording. Play and practice the exercises on the recording. Invite client feedback.

Session 10: Final Presentation of Client's Relaxation Recording

Give client final revised recording.

ELABORATION OF SESSION 8: HOW TO USE THE RELAXATION SCRIPTING WORKBOOK

Of the 10 sessions we have reviewed, Session 8 (Scripting) is the most elaborate. We now consider the scripting process and how to use the Relaxation Scripting Workbook (Table 19.4).

Step 1: Select Relaxation Goal

The client first needs to determine why he or she wants to relax. Present the nine goals of relaxation (chapter 6) and ask the client what their relaxation goal is. Explain the goal-specific processes that may be associated with each technique (chapter 16). Record your client's selected goal on the Scripting Workbook (Step 1).

Step 2: Identify R-States Consistent with Relaxation Goal

At this time, the client will have tried six basic approaches to relaxation, and assessed R-States for each. Enter client responses to the SRSIbv (or SRSIabv) for each technique on the R-States Summary Sheet. Identify which R-States seem consistent with the client's goal and are desired by client. For example, if one wants a relaxation script to prepare for going to sleep, the R-States, Sleepiness, Disengagement (distant/indifferent), and Physical Relaxation might be appropriate. For those desiring to use relaxation as a quick pick-me-up before work, the R-States At Ease/Peace and Energized might be more appropriate.

Step 3: Select Specific Exercises

First, the client determines how long he or she wants the relaxation script to be (5–10 minutes, 15–20 minutes, 30 minutes).

A client looks at a list of all exercises tried and selects which to include in his or her script. If a client needs and prefers PMR, yoga stretching, or breathing, I recommend selecting no fewer than five for each family. Note that an exercise and its repetition on both sides of the body count as one exercise, not two; the right-hand stretch and left-arm stretch count as one exercise.

Select exercises consistent with desired R-States. For example, a client might want to experience the R-States, Disengagement, Mental Relaxation, and Aware. Furthermore, he or she may discover that some progressive muscle relaxation, breathing exercises, and imagery evoke these very states. If so, the preferred PMR, breathing, and imagery exercises should be selected. If the R-State, Sleepiness, is evoked by autogenic training, and Sleepiness is not desired, then autogenic training should not be selected. Finally one should avoid exercises that evoke the highest levels of stress. Note that when selecting specific exercises, one does not select an entire sequence, for example, all 11 PRM exercises; instead, one picks those parts of the sequence that work best.

If a client has noted symptoms (Table 17.1) consider suggesting specific targeted exercises. For example, a client with a stiff neck might consider using yogaform neck stretches.

Note that the estimated time for each exercise is listed on the exercise selection sheet and make sure the times for the selected exercises add up to the desired sequence length.

Step 4: Arrange Exercises and Add Detailed Instructions

Both clinician and client then decide how to sequence exercises. The default order is that in which exercises are presented in this book. Generally, for purposes of stress management, it is a good idea to begin with exercises that foster the R-States, Disengagement and Physical Relaxation, then proceed to exercises the enhance the R-State, Mental Relaxation, and end with the R-States, Energized, Aware, Joy, Mental Quiet, and Thankful/Loving. Spiritual R-States (and those higher on the R-State Pyramid) should be presented later. Again, use the SRSIbv (or SRSIabv)Summary Sheet as a guide for selecting which techniques to place first, last, and in the middle of a script. Your script should be recorded on the Relaxation Scripting Worksheet. On a word processor or computer, include the complete instructions for each exercise component selected.

Step 5: Incorporate Unifying Idea

The most important and difficult part of script writing is selecting a unifying idea. This should be selected and placed on the Relaxation Scripting Worksheet. Then, the unifying idea is mentioned and incorporated throughout the entire sequence of exercises, at least once for every family of techniques a client has chosen.

One way to appreciate the value of the unifying idea is to consider what a relaxation sequence is like that has no unifying idea. Traditionally, relaxation exercises are presented in a disconnected fashion, much like workout routines at a health club. In a workout one might do a few pushups, ride the exercycle, complete some situps, lift weights, and so on. Similarly, a relaxation sequence might involve a yoga standing stretch, stretching one's arms, bowing and stretching, and taking a few deep breaths.

In scripting, exercises are woven together so they form a coherent whole, an integrated and meaningful sequence with a beginning, middle, and end. In other words, exercise sequences become something of a work of art. One tool for achieving this is the unifying idea, a statement of a sequence's justification, what it is all about. A unifying idea is an exercise's "title," which explains the gist of an exercise sequence. An exercise sequence with meaning and structure is more likely to be remembered and valued.

Clients often have difficulty understanding a unifying idea. Several analogies can help. If a relaxation sequence can be seen as a necklace, the beads are specific exercises whereas the thread that brings them together is the unify idea. A television drama consists of various characters doing various things; these elements are all unified by means of a plot. The plot is the unifying idea.

Here is an exercise sequence without a unifying idea (instructions are severely abbreviated):

YOGA
Slowly, smoothly, and gently raise your arms high in the air.
Higher and higher, until they are stretching all the way.
Hold the stretch.
Then slowly, smoothly, and gently unstretch.

BREATHING
Slowly take in a deep breath, filling your abdomen with air.
And gently exhale through your lips, very smoothly and gently.

IMAGERY
Imagine a beautiful tree.
You can hear a breeze flow through the leaves, feel the wind touch your skin, and smell the gentle fragrance of leaves.

MEDITATION
Very gently rock back and forth. Attend only to your rocking motion.

Notice how these exercises are disconnected. Here is the same sequence pulled together with a unifying idea, in this case the image of a tree swaying in the wind.

UNIFYING IDEA: THE TREE IN THE WIND
YOGA
Imagine you are a tree gently swaying in the wind. Your arms are like branches. The wind begins to blow against your branches and they begin to move.
Slowly, smoothly, and gently raise your arms high in the air.
Higher and higher, until they are stretching all the way.
Hold the stretch.
Then slowly, smoothly, and gently unstretch.

BREATHING
The wind begins to subside into a gentle breeze. The flow of air is a gentle as your breath. As you easily breathe in, a gentle breeze touches your nose. As you breathe out, air flows out into the breeze.
Slowly take in a deep breath, filling your abdomen with air.
Pause.
And gently exhale through your lips, very smoothly and gently.
The breeze has become even more quiet.

IMAGERY
   You can hear a breeze flow through the leaves, feel the wind touch your skin, and smell the gentle fragrance of the leaves.

MEDITATION
   Very gently rock back and forth. Attend only to your rocking motion.
   And now the air is almost completely silent. And the tree very slowly rocks back and forth as the air gently touches its branches.

In the following segment the unifying idea is "breathing out tension and settling into calm." Notice how this idea is woven into each exercise:

UNIFYING IDEA: BREATHING OUT TENSION AND SETTLING INTO CALM
   Take in a deep breath. Slowly bow over, let go, and **breathe out tension.**
   Let tension begin to melt and **flow out** with your breath.
   Now we become **more calm.** While sitting upright, breathe in deeply and slowly and exhale. As you begin to **settle into calm**, let more and more tension dissolve and float away.
   Now, let yourself become even **more calm.** Let your breathing be effortless and unforced. Simply attend to each incoming and outgoing breath. Let yourself settle into a deeper and deeper state of relaxation as any remaining tension begins to **flow away.**

A unifying idea can be the goal selected for an exercise sequence:

UNIFYING IDEA: COMBATING INSOMNIA AND PREPARING FOR SLEEP
   Let tension flow from your arms and hands.
   Tension flows away, as you let go of the cares that **keep you awake.**
   You release your cares and sink deeper into **sleepy relaxation.**
   Your arms and hands feel heavy and warm.
   You are melting into your **bed of relaxation**
   You are melting into comfortable **slumber.**
   Deeper and deeper.
   With every outgoing breath, let yourself sink into **sleepiness.**
   Deeper
   Deeper.
   Let your slow and easy breathing **cradle you into sleep.**
   And in your mind, imagine **cradling a sleeping child.**

Slowly back and forth with every breath.
Very sleepy.

There are many types of unifying ideas. One may use a very simple story, for example, "a leaf floating down the river," "a bubble rising to the surface of the pond," or "the sun dissolving a block of ice into a puddle of water." Here is an example in which such story changes are woven into a sequence of exercises:

UNIFYING IDEA: THE BUBBLE RISING IN A POND
Tense and let go. Imagine a **bubble is released from the floor of a pond**.
Quietly attend to your breathing. Let tension flow with every outgoing breath. As breath flows, **the bubble slowly rises**.
In your mind's eye simply attend to the **bubble as it reaches the surface. It touches the air and bursts, releasing its tension**. Let go of remaining feelings of tension.

Here are some more examples unifying ideas and how they can weave exercise components together:

UNIFYING IDEA: A PERSONAL RELAXATION PHILOSOPHY, "LET GO OF NEEDLESS CONTROL"
Tense up your shoulders. Notice how this is like trying to control your life. Now relax and **let go. Let go** of the needless tension you have created.
Take in a deep breath. Hold it in, like you hold in needless tension through the day. Then relax and breathing out, **let go** of needless tension.
Imagine in your mind a flowing stream. The stream is peaceful, flowing through life without needless control.

UNIFYING IDEA: THE IMAGE OF A BALL OF STRING UNWINDING
Tense up your shoulder muscles. Imagine tension as a **tight ball of string**.
Then relax and let go.
Imagine the **ball of string slowly unwinding**.
Take in a deep breath. Hold it in. Then relax and breathe out. The **ball of string unwinds even more**.

UNIFYING IDEA: A MODIFIED FRAGMENT OF REINHOLD NEIBUHR'S "SERENITY PRAYER": "GRANT ME THE SERENITY TO ACCEPT THINGS I CANNOT CHANGE, THE COURAGE TO CHANGE THINGS I CAN, AND THE WISDOM TO KNOW

THE DIFFERENCE. LIVING ONE DAY AT A TIME, ENJOYING ONE MOMENT AT
A TIME, ACCEPTING HARDSHIP AS THE PATHWAY TO PEACE. "
 Calmly meditate on the word **"peace."** Let it float through your
mind. **"Peace . . . Peace."** Tend to that which truly matters.
 Gently tense up. Let go, and release the tension. **Let go of**
that which does not matter.
 Accept the easy flow of breath, in and out. Attend to the flow
of breath. **Accept that which cannot change**.
 It is peace that truly matters.
 Breathe gently and easily.
 With each breath, think: **"Peace . . . peace . . . peace."**

In incorporating a unifying idea, it is important to make sure that each
exercise element flows easily and logically into the next. Pay attention to
the transitions between exercises. For example, the following elements, the
shoulder squeeze and deep breathing, are not logically connected and do not
flow from one to the next:

 Squeeze and release the tension in your shoulders. Let the
tension go. Let the tension flow out.
 Take a deep breath, filling your lungs and abdomen with air.
Then exhale, letting the air out.

Here, the same exercises are not only linked by a unifying idea, "let go of
tension," but have a transition so that one exercise flows to the next:

 Squeeze and release the tension in your shoulders. Let go of
tension. Let the tension melt and flow out of your muscles as
you let go. With every easy breath let tension flow out. [NOTE:
THIS IS A TRANSITION TO THE NEXT SEGMENT, WHICH EMPHASIZES
BREATHING]
 Take in a deep breath. Hold the air, then let go, let go of
tension, let the air flow out. Let the tensions of the day flow
out with the air.

The preceding three steps (Steps 3, 4, and 5) are central to the process of
writing a script, and should be completed together. Briefly, one selects specific
exercises, decides on their sequence, and what theme or unifying idea can
integrate the exercises. Roughly at this time, begin to enter concrete verbatim
instructions of your client's beginning script either on paper or on a word
processor or computer.

Steps 3, 4, and 5 are rarely completed in strict sequence. For example, the process of selecting exercises may suggest a theme or unifying idea. The selected unifying idea may in turn suggest additional exercises to include, and which should come first and last. Focusing on the sequence of chosen exercises may reveal that some are missing, for example, an appropriate beginning warm-up exercise. In other words, when completing Steps 3, 4, and 5, go back and forth from step to step.

Step 6: Add Imagery and Meditation Details

If imagery has been selected to be part of a relaxation, this is the time to elaborate and add details. The same is true if meditation has been selected. Imagery should include all the senses (what one sees, hears, feels, and smells) and should be tied in with a unifying idea. Everything you have selected should be recorded on the Relaxation Scripting Worksheet.

Step 7: Add Deepening R-State Words and Affirmations

A relaxation script can be enhanced and "spiced up" with words associated with the R-States experienced for each relaxation technique. First, examine the SRSIbv or SRSIabv Summary Sheet and determine any R-States associated with each technique. Then weave selected words into the script. Additional words may be obtained from the extended discussion of R-States in chapter 5.

To illustrate the single-word approach, imagine the R-State word "Energized" has been selected. This can be introduced in a breathing exercise, like this:

```
As you take in a deep breath, let yourself feel relaxed and
energized.
```

Supportive R-State affirmations are phrases that indicate that one accepts the possibility of experiencing an indicated R-State ("I acknowledge I have the potential for experiencing deep inner peace"), and that the R-State has a value ("It is important to accept feelings of Joy"). In addition, the identified R-State can be presented in the context of an underlying philosophical or religious R-Belief ("I am thankful for God, the inner guide for my relaxation, the source of love and joy").

It takes a bit of judgment to place R-State words and supportive affirmations appropriately. First, consider which R-States are typically associated with a technique (See instructions in chapters 9–14). Then, examine scores on the SRSIbv or SRSIabv and determine which R-States are actually associated with each technique practiced. For example, imagine a practitioner wants to insert the words "feeling far away" somewhere in a script. First, "feeling far away" appears to suggest R-State Disengagement. Disengagement is associated with progressive muscle relaxation, suggesting that this is where the words should appear. In addition, perhaps one's Relaxation Summary Sheet reveals that breathing exercises are associated with the lowest levels of Disengagement, and indeed tend to evoke the opposite R-State, Strengthened and Aware. If so, one would definitely not place the words "feeling far away" in instructions for breathing.

In addition to adding R-State words and supportive affirmations, a relaxation script can be deepened and enhanced if linked with a relaxing philosophy or belief not explicitly linked to R-States. The beliefs most frequently chosen by relaxation practitioners include:

Deeper perspective
God
Inner wisdom
Love
Honesty
Acceptance
Taking it easy
Optimism

Generally it is best to incorporate a relaxation affirmation near the end of a script, unless the affirmation itself is the unifying idea.

Step 8: Add Deepening Imagery

Deepening imagery begins relatively active, complex, and discursive (moving to and fro), and then becomes increasingly passive, simple, and focused. This enhances the relaxation metaskill of sustained effortless/passive simple focus. We can see this in the following example:

> You are relaxing on a beach. As you sit up and look around, you
> notice the blue water and sky. [STARTS WITH AN ACTIVITY, NOT A

PASSIVE POSTURE] The sun is directly overhead, its warm rays dissolve tension in your body. You can feel the wind and hear the soothing waves splash against the shore. Birds are everywhere. The sky is full of clouds. [DETAILS ARE COMPLEX AND ENERGIZED] As you become more relaxed, you recline on the beach. The wind dies down to a gentle breeze. Your attention narrows to the sky above and the peaceful clouds slowly floating by. [DETAILS BECOME MORE SIMPLE AND PASSIVE, LESS ENERGIZED] There is nothing you have to think about or do. The air is now completely still. The sky is pure blue and empty. There are no clouds. The sea is silent. Simply attend to the sea and nothing else. [MOST SIMPLY FOCUSED AND PASSIVE; LEAST ENERGIZED]

Step 9: Concluding Segment

When finished with a script, conclude with a "coming out" segment which gently guides a relaxer to let go of what he or she is attending to and return to the everyday "waking world."

Step 10: Evaluating a Script

Once a script has been written, it is useful to check for possible problems.

Be concrete. Are the instructions concrete and specific? Include every detail and leave very little to the imagination. The client should not be concerned with filling in missing details or figuring out what ambiguous instructions mean. So instead of saying "Do some yoga stretching with your arm," say "Slowly, smoothly, and gently stretch and reach with your right arm." This instruction is far too vague: "Imagine a cool pond and relax." This one is better: "Picture yourself next to a clear, cool pond. There is barely a ripple. The water is blue. The sky is clear without a cloud. You can feel a calm wind."

Avoid overstated and absolutistic claims. One should examine a script for overstated claims that might be questioned. Avoid phrases like:

You will immediately recover from your cold.
You will find the answer to your problem.

Frankly, one may not immediately recover from a cold, find an answer to a problem, or become more relaxed than ever. So avoid making promises that might not be kept.

Similarly, a scriptwriter should be cautious with absolute statements, such as "become completely relaxed," "sink more deeply into relaxation than you have ever sunk before," "you will experience the deepest peace you can imagine at this moment." For some people, such statements can indeed enhance and deepen relaxation. However, others find absolute statements worrisome ("What if I'm very relaxed, but not 'completely' relaxed?" "Just how far is 'sinking deeper than I have ever sunk before'?" If problems arise, change absolute statements into relative statements that cannot be questioned, "Become more relaxed," "Sink deeper," "Experience deep peace."

Avoid arbitrary insertions. One should avoid abruptly introducing exercise elements or images without a previously established context. For example, in the following exercise, the image of a candle flame seems to be arbitrarily introduced:

```
Your hands feel warm and heavy, warm and heavy.
With every outgoing breath, feel warm and heavy, warm and
heavy.
Let your breathing be slow and easy, as your hands become warm
and heavy.
Your breathing is slow and easy and relaxed.
Attend to the candle flame in front of you.
```

Here, the image of a candle flame is given a context.

```
You are seated by a candle, relaxing in the glowing light it
provides.
On your hands, you can feel its warmth.
Your hands feel warm and heavy, warm and heavy.
Let your breathing be slow and easy, so gentle you barely cause
the candle flame to flicker.
And your hands feel warm and heavy.
Your breathing is slow and easy and relaxed.
As you attend to the flame in front of you, it burns and flick-
ers freely and effortlessly.
```

Select an appropriate level of verbal description. The client should be comfortable with the quantity and quality of verbal description you have included. Some want to be left alone with relatively little verbal patter. Others prefer to have their exercise filled with patter. Similarly, some are uncomfortable with too much visual and poetic imagery, whereas others prefer it.

ADVANCED SCRIPTING

Once a trainer has mastered the basics of writing a relaxation script, a rich assortment of options can be considered for enhancing the effectiveness of a script. Generally, these enhancements have two effects: (1) they increase the coherence or internal integrity of a script, making it more of a unified and meaningful work of art, and (2) they subtly and gradually call for increased skill deployment through the course of the exercise sequence.

Combining and Sequencing Exercises

Exercises that have similar or overlapping features can be combined or taught in sequence. Traditional package programs and audio recordings present exercises already mixed and combined. Our strategy is to first teach relatively pure families of techniques, sensitize clients to the unique effects and access skills associated with each, and combine and sequence exercises at the end of training. Combining and sequencing strategies can be used to enhance the impact of an exercise, shorten training, and contribute the overall coherence of a relaxation script. See Table 19.3 for suggestions.

Deepening Techniques

Deepening suggestions. Perhaps the simplest deepening strategy is to incorporate R-State words as suggestions of movement and change. For example, the simple suggestion "you are relaxed" can be made into a deepening suggestion "you are becoming more and more relaxed." Similarly, one can say "you are becoming more distant," "more strengthened and aware," "more joyful," and so on.

　　Cascading deepening imagery. A cascading deepening image is a sequence of linked deepening images. Each image begins active, complex, and discursive, and ends passive, simple, and focused. However, the ending of one image serves as the beginning of another image, and in the context of what follows, is relatively active, complex, and discursive. Notice how the two images below, one of a rainstorm, and one of a waterfall, have been linked. The beginning rainstorm is active, complex, and discursive. Much is going on in the image: thunder, lightning, and a rapidly flowing stream. This image then becomes more passive, simple, and focused as the storm subsides and the stream settles to a ripple. The end of this image is a quiet, simple waterfall.

TABLE 19.3   Suggestions for Combining and Sequencing Exercises

- Yogaform stretching and active breathing stretches are often most effective at the very beginning of a sequence (to reduce residual tension from the day) or the very end (to warm up for the rest of the day's activities).
- PMR and autogenic warmth/heaviness exercises evoke somatic sensations and can be combined and sequenced: "Tense up . . . let go . . . feel warm and heavy as the tension flows away."
- I do not recommend placing AT at the beginning or end of an exercise. It works best after PMR or breathing, and may be combined with imagery.
- PMR and imagery can be designed to both target muscles.
- PMR and breathing exercises both directly instruct one to "let go" or "release." Combination/sequencing option: "Breathe in . . . tense up . . . and as you let go, exhale, letting the air easily flow through your lips."
- PMR and stretching both involve movement of muscles. Combination option: "Tense up your fingers and make a fist. Release the tension. Then slowly stretch open your fingers all the way, and slowly release the stretch."
- Passive breathing exercises can be combined with any other family of techniques.
- PMR and imagery can both target muscles. Combination/sequencing option. "Tense up your muscles, as if you were squeezing a wad of paper. Let go, and let the wad of paper slowly relax and open."
- Yoga stretching and rocking meditation can involve movement of the torso. Combination/sequencing option: "Bow over and stretch your back . . . reach up to the sky . . . and now sit and gently rock back and forth, attending to your rocking movement."
- Imagery and autogenic visual suggestions are both visual. Combination/sequencing option: "Imagine relaxing on a beach. You can see the soft clouds, hear waves splashing, and smell the clean water. As the sun touches your skin, you feel warm and heavy, warm and heavy." I recommend placing imagery near the end of an exercise sequence. Imagery may be effectively combined with autogenic visual suggestions.
- I recommend meditation at the end of a sequence, with other exercises serving as preparation. Mindfulness exercises with a body-focus may be placed prior to physical exercises to increase body focus.

The waterfall then becomes the beginning of another deepening image. It now is relatively active, complex, and discursive. We see water splashing on many rocks and hear the sounds of water flowing and bubbling. We follow the flow of water to a passive, simple, quiet pond. And our attention is again focused.

> You are safe and sound in a forest cabin. It is raining outside.
> You hear the wind blowing hard, and the thunder in the distance.

A torrent of rain pours against the roof and windows. But you are safe inside, beside a warm fireplace. The outside turbulence seems a far and distant concern.

Gradually the rain begins to subside, the wind grows quiet, and the thunderclouds float away. Looking outside, you can see the weather clearing. The air is calm and still. And in the distance, you can see a waterfall. The water is quietly rushing over the rocks.

As you settle into quiet relaxation, your attention dwells on the waterfall. You notice it splashing over rocks, catching an occasional twig or leaf as it flows into hundreds of tiny eddies. You notice the soothing sound of bubbling water, the rushing of water against the rocks and shore, and in the distance, the waterfall itself. As you become more relaxed and calm, your attention centers on a small swirl of water in the pond below the waterfall. You notice the water slowly circling, again and again. You attend to this simple motion.

Zoom imagery. Zoom imagery is a variant of deepening imagery. Here, the inclusiveness of an image broadens or narrows, resulting in a reduction of activity, complexity, and discursiveness and an increase in passive simple focus. With open-focus zoom imagery (or zoom-out imagery) one's stance regarding a focal stimulus recedes, including more and more surrounding stimuli. As a result, the target stimulus is seen with increased perspective and detachment. Details, which once may have contributed to activity, complexity, and discursiveness, become less prominent. Here is an example:

Attend to a small flower in the field. Notice the detail in its red petals, drops of dew, and a buzzing insect busily gathering pollen. The flower shimmers in as the breeze flows by. This is a small world alive with activity and energy. Slowly we move above the flower and notice it is in a cluster of flowers, each swaying in the wind. We no longer notice the occasional bee as we move farther away. As we continue to step back, the flowers merge into a colorful garden, filled with soft pastel colors. Seen as a whole, the garden is still, at peace, a rainbow of stillness.

Another image, almost a cliché in this day of space exploration, dramatically illustrates the effect of open-focus zoom imagery.

You are resting on the grass in a busy park. Children play. Dogs and cats run about. A small band plays in the distance. Much

```
is going on. Imagine yourself slowly, and safely, rising into
the air. At first only a few feet, and you see the ground directly
below. Then a few more feet, and you can see the tops of bushes,
then of trees. As you rise farther and farther, you see more of
the park below, then the lake near the park. Soon, you see an
entire landscape begin to unfold below, rivers, lakes, cities.
Eventually, you are far in space, looking at the serene blue orb
of earth. Everything is so peaceful and quiet seen in this
perspective.
```

Centered-focus zoom imagery (or zoom-in imagery) moves in the opposite direction. One moves closer to the object of attention, excluding stimuli that are extraneous, active, complex, and discursive.

```
Imagine you are seated next to a waterfall and a pond. You
notice the spray of water as it cascades across the rocks and
splashes onto surrounding trees, and into the water. You notice
the foaming water below, as floating leaves and twigs rise and
fall. Your attention is drawn to one shiny rock, the size of a
closed hand. The rock is smooth from ages of flowing water. As
your attention focuses on the rock, slowly you forget the spray
of water around, the bubbling pond, and all the surrounding
sounds. The shiny rock, in its peaceful simplicity, becomes the
focus of your attention.
```

Deepening metaphors. The use of metaphors can enhance relaxation by symbolizing both concrete exercise procedures and R-Beliefs. A swaying tree can signify a yoga stretch or the philosophical statement "Flow with the here and now." Crashing ocean waves can signify the exhalation of breath, or a commitment to "let go of that which cannot be changed." Such metaphors are, in a sense, more abstract than exercises and more concrete than R-Beliefs. Because they exist at an intermediate level of abstraction, they can be used to foster transitions from concrete exercises to affirmations of R-Beliefs, as illustrated here:

```
Stretch and unstretch your arms.
Stretch and unstretch your legs.
With each stretch, you are like a tree swaying in the wind.
Stretch, unstretch, and sway in the wind.
A tree sways in the wind, firmly rooted in the earth, yet flow-
ing with the moment.
Remember how, firmly supported by the ground of life, you can
flow with the moment.
Simply think the words, "Flow with the moment."
```

Deepening transitions. If more than one exercise is selected for a script, deepening transitions can be introduced between each. Such transitions reinforce the expectation that exercises are not an arbitrary assortment, but lead into further relaxation. A transition phrase can be as simple as this:

> We have now completed one exercise and will move on to an exercise that is even more passive and calm.

Such transitions can incorporate any R-State as in: "As we proceed, you feel more Strengthened and Aware." One might also cultivate a more general expectation of change: "Something wonderful is about to happen," "You will discover something very interesting," "You will discover a message of peace of serenity."

Deepening countdowns. Another way to deepen relaxation is to introduce a relaxation countdown. Start with any number, usually 5 or 10, and slowly count back to 1. Each count is associated with increased experience of an access skill or R-State Introduce the countdown with an explanation of the countdown, for example:

> We will now count from 5 to 1. With each number, let yourself become more relaxed.

Then slowly proceed with the count, introducing a transitional suggestion between each number:

> 5
> Let yourself become more relaxed.
> 4
> Let feelings of tension flow away.
> 3
> Notice how you feel as you become increasingly calm.
> 2
> Your entire body becomes calm and relaxed.
> And 1.
> Enjoy the feelings of relaxation you have created.

Countdowns can be woven into any approach to relaxation. For example, PMR "let-go patter" can include a countdown. In stretching and breathing sequences, countdowns can be incorporated into unstretching and exhaling. Imagery provides the richest opportunity for the countdown strategy. Here the actual content of an image can change or reflect increased tension relief, disengagement, or engagement, as illustrated below.

> In this exercise you will imagine yourself beginning to float into the air. I will count from 5 to 1. With each count you will feel more relaxed, calm, and peaceful.
>   5
> You begin to float. As you let go of your tensions, you become lighter and lighter.
>   4
> Your mind centers on the peaceful sensations of floating and relaxation.
>   3
> You float higher and higher. The houses and trees below become smaller and smaller. Your everyday pressures and concerns seem so distant.
>   2
> As you approach the peaceful soft clouds, your mind feels more and more free, more and more open to the possibilities of relaxation.
>   1
> You float into the clouds, completely without effort and concern. You feel free and peaceful.

Deepening markers. Deepening markers are very similar to countdowns. A relaxation word or exercise element can acquire meaning from the context of surrounding exercises. For example, the phrase "let go" has a concrete meaning in PMR ("**let go** of the tension in your hands"). The same phrase can be an affirmation of an R-Belief in a different context ("Remember that you can trust in God. It is okay to **let go** of your personal hassles and concerns.") A deepening marker is a relaxation word or exercise strategically repeated through an exercise sequence. Each time the marker appears, it is in a different context of surrounding exercises, and acquires new, deeper meaning. Such repetition and shifts in meaning reinforce the suggestion of movement in relaxation. In the following example, the simple act of exhalation is a marker:

> Let yourself become more relaxed with every **breath**.
> Let tension begin to dissolve and flow away.
> You sink deeper and deeper into relaxation.
> **Take a deep breath, and slowly exhale.**
> Let muscle tension flow away as you **exhale**.

You sink into deeper relaxation.
Far away from the world.
There is nothing to do or think about.
Let your thoughts flow away with every **breath you exhale**.
You feel as light as the **breath** you breathe.
Sink even more deeply into relaxation.
Far away.
Into a private world of inner calm.
Let yourself inhale and exhale freely and easily, without
effort.
Live one day at a time.
Do not try to change that which cannot be changed.
The **flow of breath** is free and easy, like the coming and going
of each moment.

The following example incorporates PMR, breathing, imagery, and mantra
meditation. The marking phrase "let it be" is introduced in each part of the
sequence; however, it acquires subtle new meanings depending on its context.
Here are excerpts of the sequence:

You are about to take a walk in a forest. To get ready, you
squeeze out the tension of the day.
[PMR]
Tighten up and shrug the shoulder muscles.
Let the tension grow.
Create a nice complete squeeze in your shoulders.
And let go.
Let it be.
Let the tension begin to flow from your shoulders.
Let your shoulders become more and more relaxed and limp.
There is nothing you have to do but **let it be**.
You are now ready to begin your walk in the forest.

[BREATHING]
Slowly take in a complete breath.
Fill your lungs with air.
[PAUSE]
And relax, letting the air flow.
Easily exhale.
And now let yourself breathe at a natural pace, without trying
to make yourself breathe in any particular way.
Simply let yourself breathe. **Let it be**.
Let the air flow in and out on its own.
[INSIGHT IMAGERY]

You begin your journey through the forest and discover a flat and shiny rock on the ground.

Your first urge is to lift the rock and see what secrets are underneath.

You **let it be**, and simply attend to the rock's shimmering surface.

The rock has a message of peace for you, which will appear if you simply and calmly attend. You **let it be**, and attend to what the rock has to say.

[MEDITATION]

Calmly, the words "**let it be**" slowly float through your mind like an echo.

There is nothing you have to do. Quietly attend to the words, as they go over and over in your mind. Whenever your mind wanders, that's okay. Simply return to attending to the words "**let it be**". You are in God's hands.

Deepening cycles. A deepening cycle is a sequence of exercises and images that repeats again and again. With each repetition, suggestions are incorporated that suggest movement into a desired R-State. For example, the following deepening cycle incorporates passive breathing, PMR letting go, autogenic heaviness exercises, and the image of a pebble sinking deeper into a pond. The entire exercise has as its goal fostering sleepiness and combating insomnia.

Take in an easy breath, and slowly exhale.
Let yourself breathe slowly and easily.
Let tensions flow out with every breath. Let tensions flow out of your hands.
You are feeling heavy.
Let yourself sink deeper and deeper.
A pebble is tossed into a pond and begins to sink.
[NEW CYCLE]
Take in another easy breath, and slowly exhale.
Let yourself breathe slowly and easily.
Let tensions flow out with every breath.
Let tensions flow out of your arms and sides.
Let yourself sink deeper and deeper.
As the pebble sinks deeper.
And you sink into sleepiness.
[NEW CYCLE]
Breathe in and out very slowly.
Let yourself breathe slowly and easily.

```
Let tensions flow out with every breath.
Let tensions flow out of your shoulders and face.
Feeling heavy, you sink deeper and deeper.
The pebble sinks into the pond.
You sink deeper into sleepiness.
[NEW CYCLE]
Take in an easy breath, and slowly exhale.
Let yourself breathe slowly and easily.
Let tensions flow out with every breath. Let tensions flow
out of body and legs.
Let yourself sink deeper and deeper.
You become heavy and sleepy.
The pebble sinks deeper and deeper.
You become more and more sleepy.
```

HOW TO MAKE AN AUDIO RECORDING

One does not have to be an accomplished actor to record a relaxation script. Simply read script instructions into a tape recorder. However, here are a few guidelines:

- Speak slowly. Most beginning relaxation trainers (and a few clinicians who should know better) speak too quickly.
- Speak softly. Use the voice appropriate for each type of exercise. Reading a script is not the same as giving a lecture in a hall without a loudspeaker to a group of elderly who have left their hearing aids at home.
- Most beginners are stingy with pauses and silences. Pauses and silences are essential to relaxation and provide the client with time to complete instructions and enjoy their effects. If one is going to make a mistake, it is better to make pauses and silences too long rather than too short. Few things are more annoying than a rushed relaxation script.

In making an individualized relaxation script, the trainer examines scripts presented in this book for each exercise (at the end of each instruction chapter). These scripts are then selected and inserted on a blank page, forming the basic skeleton of a client's script. Then the skeleton instructions are repeatedly revised, combined, and expanded. One "cuts and pastes," inserting the unifying idea, R-State words, and so on.

TABLE 19.4   Scripting Workbook

The following workbook will guide you through the process of developing a relaxation script for your client. The items marked ✎ must be completed in consultation with the client. The other steps can be completed before a preliminary version of a relaxation tape is shared with the client.

1.   ✎   What is your client's relaxation goal?

☐   1.   To prepare for sleep; combat insomnia.

☐   2.   To have more effective "catnaps" or "powernaps."

☐   3.   Reduce or manage stress, tension, negative emotion, or worry.

☐   4.   To manage physical pain, discomfort, or other negative symptoms.

☐   5.   To recover from maintaining a fatiguing posture or position for an ex-pended time (standing, sitting, bending over, crouching).

☐   6.   To help recover from illness, injury, or surgery.

☐   7.   To use relaxation as a "healthy behavior" to maintain health and resis-tance to disease, and increase energy resources, strength, and stamina for work, sports, and life and its activities.

☐   8.   To increase my ability to calmly sustain focus on a desired task, ignore external distraction, and cope with diverting impulses and desires to do something else. To finish what I want to do and resist various distracting or destructive impulses and urges (to smoke a cigarette, drink, eat, take drugs, give in to boredom).

☐   9.   To enhance my effectiveness at work, school, or sports.

☐   10.   To have fun and enjoy myself; to contribute the enjoyment of other activities.

☐   11.   To increase my creativity, overcome "creative blocks," and nurture an expressive source of ideas and insight.

☐   12.   To enhance personal spirituality, to celebrate and relate to God or my Higher Power. To deepen my relationship to God or Higher Power.

☐   13.   To develop a meditative or mindful state of awareness in which I am calmly aware and focused, both during times of quiet and times of action.

(continued)

TABLE 19.4 *(continued)*

If there is more than one goal, circle the one that is most important and indicate in the box below how other selected goal(s) may help achieve the circled goal.

My most important goal is:

My other relaxation goal or goals are:

Here is how my other relaxation goals are related to my most important relaxation goal.

2. ✎ Enter client responses on the SRSIbv on the R-States Summary Sheet on the following page. Identify which R-States seem consistent with the client's goal and are desired by client. (NOTE: If you are using the Smith Relaxation States Alternate Brief Version, or SRSIabv, use the inventory and summary Sheet I Tables 17.9 and 17.10.

The R-State Summary Sheet is a tool for summarizing responses on the Smith Relaxation States Inventory Brief Version (SRSIbv). At the very top of the Summary Sheet is a boldface instruction. To the right of this instruction are boxes. In each box, simply put the name of each technique practiced. For example, if a client practiced "Full PMR," "Breathing," or "Mindfulness," these techniques would be entered like this:

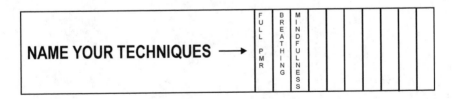

Now, note that each item on the SRSIbv corresponds to a row on the Summary Sheet. For example, the first item, "PHYSICAL STRESS, DISCOMFORT," is also the first row on the Sheet. You are ready to enter your client's scores. Here is an example: if a client filled in the ③ mark for FULL PMR, the illustration below shows how you would enter this score. And if you filled in the ① mark for BREATHING, you would enter the score like this. And if your MINDFULNESS SCORE on PHYSICAL STRESS, DISCOMFORT was "④," you would enter the score like this:

NAME YOUR TECHNIQUES →	F U L L P M R	B R E A T H I N G	M I N D F U L N E S S							
PHYSICAL STRESS, DISCOMFORT	④ ✗ ② ①	④ ③ ② ✗	✗ ③ ② ①	④ ③ ② ①	④ ③ ② ①	④ ③ ② ①	④ ③ ② ①	④ ③ ② ①	④ ③ ② ①	④ ③ ② ①

How to use the Summary Sheet: Look for patterns. Which techniques get the highest scores on which stress state, relaxation/meditative states, and positive relaxation states? Note this on the Sheet. Then Circle the R-States consistent with the selected relaxation goal.

(continued)

TABLE 19.4 *(continued)*

NAME YOUR TECHNIQUES →										

STRESS STATES

PHYSICAL STRESS, DISCOMFORT
④ ④ ④ ④ ④ ④ ④ ④ ④ ④
③ ③ ③ ③ ③ ③ ③ ③ ③ ③
② ② ② ② ② ② ② ② ② ②
① ① ① ① ① ① ① ① ① ①

CONCENTRATION
④ ④ ④ ④ ④ ④ ④ ④ ④ ④
③ ③ ③ ③ ③ ③ ③ ③ ③ ③
② ② ② ② ② ② ② ② ② ②
① ① ① ① ① ① ① ① ① ①

WORRY
④ ④ ④ ④ ④ ④ ④ ④ ④ ④
③ ③ ③ ③ ③ ③ ③ ③ ③ ③
② ② ② ② ② ② ② ② ② ②
① ① ① ① ① ① ① ① ① ①

ANXIETY
④ ④ ④ ④ ④ ④ ④ ④ ④ ④
③ ③ ③ ③ ③ ③ ③ ③ ③ ③
② ② ② ② ② ② ② ② ② ②
① ① ① ① ① ① ① ① ① ①

IRRITATION, ANGER
④ ④ ④ ④ ④ ④ ④ ④ ④ ④
③ ③ ③ ③ ③ ③ ③ ③ ③ ③
② ② ② ② ② ② ② ② ② ②
① ① ① ① ① ① ① ① ① ①

DEPRESSION
④ ④ ④ ④ ④ ④ ④ ④ ④ ④
③ ③ ③ ③ ③ ③ ③ ③ ③ ③
② ② ② ② ② ② ② ② ② ②
① ① ① ① ① ① ① ① ① ①

RELAXATION AND MEDITATIVE STATES

SLEEPY
④ ④ ④ ④ ④ ④ ④ ④ ④ ④
③ ③ ③ ③ ③ ③ ③ ③ ③ ③
② ② ② ② ② ② ② ② ② ②
① ① ① ① ① ① ① ① ① ①

DISTANT, DETACHED
④ ④ ④ ④ ④ ④ ④ ④ ④ ④
③ ③ ③ ③ ③ ③ ③ ③ ③ ③
② ② ② ② ② ② ② ② ② ②
① ① ① ① ① ① ① ① ① ①

PHYSICAL RELAXATION
④ ④ ④ ④ ④ ④ ④ ④ ④ ④
③ ③ ③ ③ ③ ③ ③ ③ ③ ③
② ② ② ② ② ② ② ② ② ②
① ① ① ① ① ① ① ① ① ①

RESTED, REFRESHED
④ ④ ④ ④ ④ ④ ④ ④ ④ ④
③ ③ ③ ③ ③ ③ ③ ③ ③ ③
② ② ② ② ② ② ② ② ② ②
① ① ① ① ① ① ① ① ① ①

(continued)

TABLE 19.4 *(continued)*

NAME YOUR TECHNIQUES →										

AT EASE, AT PEACE

④ ④ ④ ④ ④ ④ ④ ④ ④ ④
③ ③ ③ ③ ③ ③ ③ ③ ③ ③
② ② ② ② ② ② ② ② ② ②
① ① ① ① ① ① ① ① ① ①

ENERGIZED

④ ④ ④ ④ ④ ④ ④ ④ ④ ④
③ ③ ③ ③ ③ ③ ③ ③ ③ ③
② ② ② ② ② ② ② ② ② ②
① ① ① ① ① ① ① ① ① ①

MENTAL QUIET

④ ④ ④ ④ ④ ④ ④ ④ ④ ④
③ ③ ③ ③ ③ ③ ③ ③ ③ ③
② ② ② ② ② ② ② ② ② ②
① ① ① ① ① ① ① ① ① ①

AWARE, FOCUSED, CLEAR

④ ④ ④ ④ ④ ④ ④ ④ ④ ④
③ ③ ③ ③ ③ ③ ③ ③ ③ ③
② ② ② ② ② ② ② ② ② ②
① ① ① ① ① ① ① ① ① ①

POSITIVE MENTAL STATES

HAPPY, JOYFUL

④ ④ ④ ④ ④ ④ ④ ④ ④ ④
③ ③ ③ ③ ③ ③ ③ ③ ③ ③
② ② ② ② ② ② ② ② ② ②
① ① ① ① ① ① ① ① ① ①

CHILDLIKE INNOCENCE

④ ④ ④ ④ ④ ④ ④ ④ ④ ④
③ ③ ③ ③ ③ ③ ③ ③ ③ ③
② ② ② ② ② ② ② ② ② ②
① ① ① ① ① ① ① ① ① ①

THANKFUL, LOVING

④ ④ ④ ④ ④ ④ ④ ④ ④ ④
③ ③ ③ ③ ③ ③ ③ ③ ③ ③
② ② ② ② ② ② ② ② ② ②
① ① ① ① ① ① ① ① ① ①

MYSTERY

④ ④ ④ ④ ④ ④ ④ ④ ④ ④
③ ③ ③ ③ ③ ③ ③ ③ ③ ③
② ② ② ② ② ② ② ② ② ②
① ① ① ① ① ① ① ① ① ①

TABLE 19.4 *(continued)*

NAME YOUR TECHNIQUES →										

AWE AND WONDER

④ ④ ④ ④ ④ ④ ④ ④ ④ ④
③ ③ ③ ③ ③ ③ ③ ③ ③ ③
② ② ② ② ② ② ② ② ② ②
① ① ① ① ① ① ① ① ① ①

PRAYERFUL

④ ④ ④ ④ ④ ④ ④ ④ ④ ④
③ ③ ③ ③ ③ ③ ③ ③ ③ ③
② ② ② ② ② ② ② ② ② ②
① ① ① ① ① ① ① ① ① ①

TIMELESS, BOUNDLESS, INFINITE

④ ④ ④ ④ ④ ④ ④ ④ ④ ④
③ ③ ③ ③ ③ ③ ③ ③ ③ ③
② ② ② ② ② ② ② ② ② ②
① ① ① ① ① ① ① ① ① ①

Circle the above states consistent with desired relaxation goal.

3. ✎ From the list on the following page, select exercises to include in a script. Ask client about how long the exercise should be:

❐ 5–10 minutes ❐ 10–20 minutes ❐ About 30 minutes

Select from 4 or 5 schools. Note the times for each exercise.

4. ✎ Arrange selected exercise instructions and add details. Ask the client if they have any suggestions about the sequence of exercises, i.e., which should be first, last, etc.

At this point you actually begin to write the client's relaxation script, which will eventually be recorded. It is essential that you include *complete concrete details of every instruction component.* Leave nothing to the imagination. What you put on paper, or your word processor, is the skeleton of your client's actual script. From this point on, you will be adding to and revising this script.

(continued)

CHECKLIST OF EXERCISES (CHECK PREFERENCES, NOTE TIMES SO THEY ADD UP TO DESIRED LENGTH).

YOGAFORM STRETCHING

FULL YOGAFORM STRETCHING

❑ HAND STRETCH (4 min)
❑ ARM STRETCH (4 min)
❑ ARM AND SIDE STRETCH (4 min)
❑ BACK STRETCH (2 min)
❑ SHOULDER STRETCH (2 min)
❑ BACK OF NECK STRETCH (2 min)
❑ FACE STRETCH (2 min)
❑ FRONT OF NECK STRETCH (2 min)
❑ STOMACH AND CHEST STRETCH (2 min)
❑ LEG STRETCH (4 min)
❑ FOOT STRETCH (4 min)

BRIEF STRETCHING

❑ BOTH HAND STRETCH (2 min)
❑ BOTH ARM STRETCH (2 m in)
❑ BOTH ARM AND SIDE STRETCH (2 min)
❑ BACK STRETCH (2 min)
❑ SHOULDER STRETCH (2 min)
❑ BACK OF NECK STRETCH (2 min)
❑ FACE STRETCH (2 min)
❑ FRONT OF NECK STRETCH (2 min)
❑ STOMACH AND CHEST STRETCH (2 min)
❑ BOTH LEG STRETCH (2 min)

PROGRESSIVE MUSCLE RELAXATION

FULL PROGRESSIVE MUSCLE RELAXATION

❑ HANDS (4 min)
❑ ARMS (4 min)
❑ ARMS AND SIDES (4 min)
❑ BACK (2 min)
❑ SHOULDERS (2 min)
❑ BACK OF NECK (2 min)
❑ FACE (2 min)
❑ FRONT OF NECK (2 min)
❑ STOMACH AND CHEST (2 min)
❑ LEGS (4 min)
❑ FEET (4 min)

ABBREVIATED PMR

❑ BOTH HANDS (2 min)
❑ BOTH ARMS (2 min)
❑ ARMS AND SIDES (2 min)
❑ BACK (2 min)
❑ SHOULDERS (2 min)
❑ BACK OF NECK (2 min)
❑ FACE (2 min)
❑ FRONT OF NECK (2 min)
❑ STOMACH AND CHEST (2 min)
❑ BOTH LEGS (2 min)
❑ BOTH FEET (2 min)

LETTING GO

❑ ALL MUSCLE GROUPS (10 min)

BREATHING

❑ SLIGHT BOWING AND BREATH-ING (3 min)
❑ LEANING BREATHING (2 min)
❑ BOWING BREATHING (2 min)
❑ STRETCHING BREATHING (2 min)
❑ SLOW BOWING BREATHING (3 min)
❑ STOMACH SQUEEZE BREATH-ING (3 min)
❑ STOMACH TOUCH BREATH-ING (2 min)
❑ BOOK BREATHING (2 min)
❑ SNIFFING (2 min)
❑ BLOWING (2 min)
❑ OCCASIONAL DEEP BREATHS (2 min)
❑ FOCUSED BREATHING (3 min)

AUTOGENIC TRAINING

❑ AUTOGENIC TRAINING VER-BAL SUGGESTIONS
    HEAVY, WARM, HEART, ABDOMEN (2–5 min)
❑ AUTOGENIC TRAINING VISUAL SUGGESTIONS (2–5 min)

IMAGERY

❑ SENSE IMAGERY (2–20 min)
    TRAVEL IMAGERY—BALLOON, BOAT, COUNTRY TRAIN
    NATURE IMAGERY—MOUNTAIN, GRASSY PLAIN, VALLEY
    WATER IMAGERY—POND, STREAM, MIST OR RAIN
    INDOOR IMAGERY—FOREST CABIN, CHILDHOOD ROOM, HOLY PLACE
❑ INSIGHT IMAGERY (2–20 min)
    THE PATH, THE GUIDE, THE QUESTION

MEDITATION/MINDFULNESS

❐ EIGHT MEDITATIONS (2–20 min
   for one)
   (Name one preferred)
    Body Sense
    Rocking
    Breathing
    Mantra
    Eyes closed image
    Sound
    Eyes open visual stimulus
    Mindfulness
❐ GRADUATED MINDFULNESS
   (25 min)
❐ MINDFUL WALKING (10–15
   min)

Total time of selected exercises: _____

5.   ✎   Add unifying idea. This should be done along with steps 3 and 4, so that the selection and arrangement properly expresses the unifying idea.

         What is your client's unifying idea?

         Now incorporate it into the script, inserting it for every family of techniques.

6.   ✎   Add imagery and meditation details in script. Both should express the unifying idea.

         Imagery theme:

         What is seen:

         What is heard:

         What is felt:

         Fragrances:

7.   ✎   From the list of R-State words and R-Beliefs on the following page, which does the client want to include?

(continued)

TABLE 19.4 *(continued)*

R-STATE WORDS AND AFFIRMATIONS (select no more than 10)

RELAXING WORDS

___ 1. Absorbed	___ 30. Free	___ 59. Pleased
___ 2. Accepted	___ 31. Fun	___ 60. Prayerful
___ 3. Accepting	___ 32. Glorious	___ 61. Refreshed
___ 4. Asleep	___ 33. Glowing	___ 62. Rested
___ 5. Assured	___ 34. Quiet	___ 63. Restored
___ 6. At ease	___ 35. Happy	___ 64. Reverent
___ 7. Awake	___ 36. Harmonious	___ 65. Selfless
___ 8. Aware	___ 37. Healing	___ 66. Sensuous
___ 9. Beautiful	___ 38. Heavy	___ 67. Silent
___ 10. Blessed	___ 39. Hopeful	___ 68. Simple
___ 11. Calm	___ 40. Indifferent	___ 69. Sinking
___ 12. Carefree	___ 41. Infinite	___ 70. Soothed
___ 13. Childlike	___ 42. Inspired	___ 71. Speechless
___ 14. Clear	___ 43. Joyful	___ 72. Spiritual
___ 15. Complete	___ 44. Knowing	___ 73. Spontaneous
___ 16. Confident	___ 45. Laid back	___ 74. Strengthened
___ 17. Contented	___ 46. Light	___ 75. Thankful
___ 18. Creative	___ 47. Limp	___ 76. Timeless
___ 19. Delighted	___ 48. Liquid	___ 77. Tingling
___ 20. Detached	___ 49. Loose	___ 78. Trusting
___ 21. Dissolving	___ 50. Loved	___ 79. Unafraid
___ 22. Distant	___ 51. Loving	___ 80. Untroubled
___ 23. Drowsy	___ 52. Mysterious	___ 81. Warm
___ 24. Energized	___ 53. Mystical	___ 82. Whole
___ 25. Fascinated	___ 54. Optimistic	___ 83. Wonderful
___ 26. Far away	___ 55. Passive	
___ 27. Floating	___ 56. Patient	New Words:
___ 28. Focused	___ 57. Peaceful	
___ 29. Forgetting	___ 58. Playful	

TABLE 19.4 *(continued)*

R-BELIEF AFFIRMATIONS (select no more than three)

Belief #1: View the world with optimism
❏ I can be optimistic about my current hassles
❏ It is important to be optimistic

Belief #2: Accept things the way they are
❏ I can accept things as they are
❏ There's no need to try to change what can't be changed

Belief #3: Be honest with yourself and others
❏ I can accept my thoughts and feelings
❏ I can be honest and open with my feelings

Belief #4: Know when to let go and take it easy
❏ Sometimes it is important to simply take it easy
❏ It is important to know when to stop trying, let go, and relax

Belief #5: Relate to others with love and compassion
❏ The love I give and receive is a source of peace and comfort to me
❏ It is important to treat people with compassion and understanding

Belief #6: Trust the healing wisdom of the body
❏ I trust the body's wisdom and healing powers
❏ There are sources of strength and healing deep within me

Belief #7: Trust God's love and guidance
❏ God guides, loves, and comforts me
❏ I put myself in God's hands

Belief #8: Put your concerns in deeper perspective
❏ Life has a purpose greater than my personal wants and desires
❏ There's more to life than my personal concerns and worries

8.	Add deepening imagery.

	THEME

	BEGINNING FOCUS (COMPLEX, DISCURSIVE, ACTIVE)

	ENDING FOCUS (SINGLE-FOCUSED, EFFORTLESS)

9. ✎ Add concluding segment.

20

Abbreviated Programs

Relaxation scripting takes time, effort, and, above all, substantial trainer commitment and expertise. In this chapter we review strategies that are streamlined and easy, but still enable the client to learn exercises from several families.

RELAXATION PACKAGES

A relaxation package involves presenting complete exercise sequences from three to five families of relaxation. The client practices one sequence a session. After training, the client and trainer determine which sequences were preferred. The trainer presents printed copy or audio instructions for the preferred exercise sequences.

For example, a trainer may select the following sequences for a client: yogaform stretching (abbreviated), autogenic training (verbal), and graduated mindfulness. The trainer and client meet for three sessions, perhaps one week apart. For the first week, the client practices the yogaform stretching (abbreviated) exercises, perhaps using a CD borrowed from the trainer or perhaps relying on a photocopy of instructions. For the second week, the client practices autogenic training (verbal), and in the third week, graduated mindfulness. At the fourth session, client and trainer discuss which exercises worked and which did not. The client may express a dislike for graduated mindfulness, and a preference for the yoga and autogenic exercises. The trainer then (either during the session, or at a subsequent fifth session) would present the client with a printed set of abbreviated (not full) instructions for yoga and autogenic training. This is the client's relaxation package. Because the client has already practiced the exercises, brief printed instructions are usually sufficient.

To elaborate, one begins with initial assessment, a step that is central to making package training work. I recommend the following tools:

- *Relaxation Precautions Fact Sheet.* (Table 16.1)
- *Target Symptoms Fact Sheet.* (Table 17.1) Physical symptoms often respond well to PMR, yogaform stretching, and autogenic training, particularly when these approaches are targeted to the symptom.

In addition, I recommend giving the following:

- *Smith Relaxation Goals Inventory (SRGI).* (Table 17.4) This test directly asks which relaxation goal or set of goals a client prefers.
- *Relaxation Sampler.* The Relaxation Sampler (Appendix) provides five-minute samples of six families of relaxation. Clients can either practice the samples at home or in the office with the trainer. After trying the Sampler, the client indicates on the *Smith Relaxation Preferences Inventory* (Table 17.3) which of the six exercises were definitely preferred and which were definitely disliked. Client and trainer can discuss which exercises seem most appropriate for the goals selected (SRGI).

Once families of exercises have been selected, each should be introduced and practiced in the standard manner, as described in this book.

After each session, give the *Smith Relaxation States Inventory Brief Version or the Smith Relaxation States Inventory Alternate Brief Version (SRSIbv, SrsiABV, Tables 17.7, 17.9)* These inventories (1) train clients to detect and articulate the subtle experiences of relaxation and stress, (2) identify when an exercise is or is not working, and (3) identify any unique effects specific to any specific exercise.

In addition, the trainer observes the client while both practice (using the *Behavioral Signs of Relaxation Rating Scale*, Table 17.2) to detect any signs of tension.

When training is over, the trainer asks which exercises were preferred. Or, a client can make their selections on the *Smith Relaxation Preferences Inventory*. The trainer then presents client with written instructions for preferred exercises.

THE WORLD TOUR

The World Tour format involves first exploring all six families of relaxation, then selecting two to four, and finally practicing the final selections on a rotated basis or in combination. The first step is to present the full instructions for each of six families of techniques. Each approach should be practiced for three sessions, either in individual or group format, before moving on:

Session 1: Full Yogaform Stretching
Session 2: Repeat
Session 3: Repeat
Session 4: Full PMR
Session 5: Repeat
Session 6: Repeat
Session 7: Breathing Exercises
Session 8: Repeat
Session 9: Repeat
Session 10: Verbal Autogenic Training
Session 11: Repeat
Session 12: Repeat
Session 13: Sense Imagery
Session 14: Repeat
Session 15: Repeat
Session 16: Eight Meditations
Session 17: Repeat
Session 18: Repeat

Skipping and Exploring

At any time a client may chose to quit an assigned approach and proceed to the next. For example, after Session 1, a client may decide that she does not like yogaform stretching. Then, Session 2 starts with full PMR.

If a client enjoys a particular family of relaxation, he may chose to take an "extended tour" and devote additional sessions to the variations of that approach. For example, after practicing the assigned three sessions of full PMR, a client may decide that he finds it especially enjoyable and effective. He may then devote Session 4 to abbreviated PMR, and Session 5 to letting go. At Session 6 he would resume the regularly scheduled World Tour and learn Breathing Exercises. At the end of training, all approaches are reviewed, including those explored in the extended tour, and 2–4 are selected.

Rotating and Combining

At the end of the World Tour, the client selects 2–4 exercises to practice. These may be rotated so a different approach is practiced each day. If the selections include one physical exercise (yogaform stretching, PMR, autogenic training, or breathing) and one mental exercise (imagery, meditation), then a combination may be practiced in which one physical approach is practiced in its entirety before one mental approach (for example, full yogaform stretching before imagery). This becomes one's daily practice. If a shorter sequence is requested, some sessions may be devoted exclusively to the mental approach. See Table 19.3 for suggestions on combining and sequencing exercises.

SPOT AND MINI-RELAXATION

Once a relaxation skill has been learned, it should be applied. Our research suggests that one needs to practice at least five days a week in order to have maximum benefit (Smith, 2001). Most relaxation experts suggest at least a month of practice (Smith, 1999b). After introducing a client to several families, two highly streamlined applications are available.

Spot Relaxation

A spot relaxation is a brief (1–3 minute) portable relaxation exercise that can be easily applied in a specific situation. Even without formal training, most people understand the value of taking a good stretch after waking up or breathing deeply a few times after a stressful situation. This strategy of using quick relaxation in specific situations can be substantially enhanced once a client has mastered several families of techniques.

First, explain spot relaxation to the client. Next, give the client a homework assignment in which they are to apply brief exercises or combinations of exercises in different situations over the following week. Emphasize that different situations will call for different exercises. This can be presented as a task of creativity and discovery, one clients usually find to be quite enjoyable. It might be helpful at this point to present Figure 6.1 to illustrate the many possible applications of spot relaxation. To establish the proper frame of mind, you might offer illustrations of what others have tried, for example:

Situation. Babysitting three restless children.
Spot relaxation. Breathing out through the lips. I encourage the children to breathe with me as a sort of game.

Situation. Waiting in the dentist's office for treatment.
Spot relaxation. I shrug and release my shoulders, shake out tension, then fantasize a very distant vacation place.

Situation. Keeping myself from grinding my teeth while I sleep.
Spot relaxation. I do a PMR jaw tense a few times, then a yoga stretch with my jaws, opening them wide.

Situation. In a traffic jam waiting for the cars to move.
Spot relaxation. I see how slowly and smoothly I can breathe while focusing on the car ahead.

Situation. Burnout from homework.
Spot relaxation. After I simply can't think any more, I close my eyes and do a rocking meditation a few minutes. It empties my mind and I can resume refreshed.

Mini-Scripts

Many approaches to stress management, primarily desensitization, incorporate brief periods of relaxation lasting 1–5 minutes. Traditionally, the advice has been to select a cue, such as the word "relax," and consistently think it while engaged in a deep relaxation exercise. Eventually, the cue itself is considered sufficient to evoke relaxation. One simply thinks "relax" when desired (Paul, 1966; Russell & Matthews, 1975).

I prefer creating mini-relaxation scripts tailored to the individual. First, the trainer develops and masters a personalized relaxation sequence using any of the formats described in this book. After the client practices the complete relaxation protocol for a few weeks, both clinician and trainer and client write a mini-relaxation script designed to last from 1–5 minutes. The mini-relaxation should embody the most effective features of the relaxation protocol already developed.

For example, imagine a student has developed a 30-minute relaxation sequence that incorporates the following exercises with the unifying idea of "resting on the warm sand by the beach":

```
PMR Arm and Side (while imagining pushing arms into warm sand)
PMR Back (imagines sinking into sand)
PMR Shoulders (imagines sinking shoulders into sand)
PMR Back of Neck
PMR Front of Neck
AT Warm and Heavy (thinks of body warm and heavy in the sand)
Arm and Side
Stretch(stretches in the sand)
Back Stretch (stretches in the sand)
Legs/Thighs Stretch (moves them through the sand)
Feet Stretch (sinks them in the sand)
Deep Breathing (rests quietly in the sand)
Imagery (entertains entire fantasy of resting on the warm
sand by the beach)
```

The first four exercises are presented with numerous suggestions of the R-States, Physical Relaxation and Disengagement ("Let yourself feel warm and heavy, loose and limp," "Let yourself feel far away"). The imagery segment concludes with phrases suggesting increased R-States, Energized and Rested/Refreshed.

After recording this sequence and practicing it for two weeks, our student decided to make a 3-minute mini-relaxation for use with stress management techniques he was about to learn. In this sequence, he discovered the most powerful components were:

```
PMR Shoulder Squeeze
AT Warm and Heavy
Legs/Thighs Stretch
Imagery
```

All of these are done while fantasizing about resting on a warm beach. This became his mini-relaxation. Here is the entire script:

```
Imagine you are resting on a warm beach in summer. You feel
the comfortable rays of the sun on your skin. Squeeze and shrug
your shoulders really tight. Squeeze out all the tension.
Squeeze further. Then go limp. Let the tension flow out, melted
by the warm sun. Let the tension flow into the sandy beach. Let
```

yourself feel limp and heavy, warm and relaxed. And repeat.
Tighten up your shoulders. Hold the tension. Then go completely
limp, letting the tension flow into the sand. Warm and heavy.
Warm and heavy, feeling far away. Distant and far away from the
world. Relax more and more. As you relax, slowly stretch out your
legs and thighs. Stretch your legs out all the way, pushing them
through the warm sand. As you stretch, feel the tension sink into
the sand brushing against your skin. And slowly, smoothly, and
gently release the stretch. Return your legs to a relaxed and
comfortable position. Enjoy the feelings of warmth and relaxation you have created, far away from the world. In this pleasant
state of mind, let yourself enjoy all that you can sense on this
beautiful beach. The blue sky above, the soft clouds floating
by, the gently waving trees. You can smell the fresh scent of
water, and hear the waves gently lapping against the shore. Enjoy
this setting with all your senses.

When first practicing, our student made an audio recording of the script.
Soon, he realized he did not need the recording and could do the entire
exercise from memory.

I prefer this individualized approach to the traditional cue-controlled approach used in stress management. As you can see, because a client is exposed
to a wide range of exercises (each with different effects), he or she is much
more likely to find exercises that work best. And this individualized process
is completed twice, once for completing a full script, and again two weeks
later when completing a mini-exercise. The trainer has two opportunities to
individualize, vastly increasing the likelihood of selecting a powerful and
effective relaxation.

ACCESS ZONE SCANNING

Access Zone Scanning (Smith, 2004) is a simple exercise sequence based
on the idea of six self-stressing processes (chapter 4) and six corresponding
relaxation access skills. It is a versatile tool that can be used in a variety of
formats—as an introduction to relaxation for clients and groups, and as
a summarizing mini-relaxation for those who have completed training in
several families.

First, the trainer presents the rationale, as described in chapter 16 (Table
16.3). The key points of your introduction should include the following:

We create stress for ourselves in six ways:

1. Stressed Posture
2. Stressed Muscles
3. Stressed Breathing
4. Stressed Body Focus
5. Negative Emotion
6. Stressed Attention

There are six families of relaxation, one for each type of self-stress. So there are six stress-relaxation zones.

1. Relaxed Posture
2. Relaxed Muscles
3. Relaxed Breathing
4. Internal Body Zone Relaxation
5. Relaxed Positive Emotions
6. Calm Focus

Access Zone Scanning targets each of these zones in a simple and enjoyable relaxation sequence.

In Access Zone Scanning, one quietly checks each area of stress, and proceeds with a brief exercise targeted to that zone. If a client discovers that one area of self-stressing is particularly troublesome, then the full exercise sequence may be practiced, using the instructions in the book.

Access Zone Scanning Script

In this exercise are going to relax by scanning for and releasing areas of stress. We will scan our posture. We will scan our muscles. We will scan breathing. We will scan for internal body stress and negative emotion. And we will calmly focus.

Make sure you are sitting in a relaxing place with little distraction. You need a comfortable chair, couch, or bed. Put aside the tasks you have been doing and the tasks you have been completing in your mind. And let yourself sit upright with your feet flat on the floor and your hands in your lap.

Posture

First, let's scan our posture. Notice how you are sitting. Is your posture truly relaxed? Are you slouching? Are your arms or

legs crossed. Let's begin by stretching out any stressed posi-
tions we may have. Slowly, smoothly and gently lift your arms to
your sides. Very gently reach to the sky and stretch all the way.
Feel the stretch in your torso and back. Feel your arms stretch.
Stretch all the way out to your fingertips. And hold the stretch.
   [PAUSE]
And very slowly gently unstretch.
   [PAUSE]
And again, stretch and unstretch, very slowly.
   [PAUSE FOR EXERCISE}
And comfortably sit up straight. Focus on the muscles in the
back of your neck. Slowly, smoothly and gently let your head tilt
back. Feel the gentle stretch in your neck. Do not force your
neck down. Let gravity do the work. Very slowly and easily.
   [PAUSE]
And gently and easily, return your head to an upright
position.
   [PAUSE]
Let's try that once again. Slowly let your head tilt back.
   [PAUSE]
And return your head to an upright position.
   [PAUSE]
Close your eyes.
   [PAUSE]

Breathing

And now we scan our breathing.
Attend to how you are breathing.
Is your breathing slow, easy, and relaxed? Or are you holding
your breath, or breathing in a way that is shallow?
   [PAUSE]
Take in a slow, deep breath, pause, and exhale.
   [PAUSE 3 SECONDS]
Again, this time very slowly, smoothly, and gently, take in
a deep breath. Pause. And exhale.
   [PAUSE 3 SECONDS]
And now breathe naturally easily in and out without effort.
With every outgoing breath, let yourself sink more and more
deeply.

Muscles

And now we scan for muscle tension.
And attend to your hands and fingers.

Gently breathe in.
As you easily breathe out, let go of any tension you feel here.
[PAUSE 5 SECONDS]
Attend to your arms.
Do you notice any tightness or tension there?
Gently breathe in.
As you easily exhale, let go of any tension.
[PAUSE]
Go completely limp
[PAUSE 5 SECONDS]
Attend to your shoulders and neck.
Do you notice any tightness or tension there?
Gently breathe in.
As you easily exhale, let go.
[PAUSE]
Go completely limp
[PAUSE 5 SECONDS]
Attend to the muscles of your face, your jaws, cheeks, eyes, and forehead.
Do you notice any tension?
Gently breathe in.
Easily exhale and let go.
[PAUSE]
Go completely limp.
[PAUSE 5 SECONDS]
Attend to the muscles of your chest and stomach.
Do you notice any tension?
Gently breathe in.
Easily exhale and let go.
[PAUSE]
Go completely limp.
[PAUSE 6 SECONDS]
Attend to the muscles of your thighs, legs, and feet
Do you notice any tension?
Gently breathe in.
Easily exhale and let go.
[PAUSE]
Go completely limp.
[PAUSE 6 SECONDS]
Let yourself become more and more relaxed.
[PAUSE 2 SECONDS]

Internal body zone

And now we scan deep within our bodies.
Attend to your hands and arms.

Let warm blood bring relaxation to your hands and
arms.
[PAUSE]
Warm and heavy.
[PAUSE 5 SECONDS]
Let warm relaxation flow to your hands and arms.
[PAUSE]
Warm and heavy.
[PAUSE 5 SECONDS]
Let warm relaxation flow to you shoulders.
[PAUSE]
Warm and heavy.
[PAUSE 7 SECONDS]
Let relaxation flow to your legs and thighs.
Warm and heavy.
[PAUSE 7 SECONDS]
Let relaxation flow to your feet and toes.
[PAUSE]
Let all the tension of your body flow out through your legs
and feet.
[PAUSE 7 SECONDS]
With every breath, let tension melt, dissolve, and flow out
with your breath.
Let any remaining tension in your body melt, and dissolve into
the air.
[PAUSE]
Let it flow out with your breath.
[PAUSE]
Let yourself settle into relaxation.

Relaxed positive emotion

Let yourself settle into a relaxing fantasy, a safe and peace-
ful faraway place.
A place where the sky is clear and beautiful.
A place filled with lush green trees or grass.
A place with a cooling and refreshing body of water, a lake,
river, or ocean.
A place where you can feel the soothing breeze on your skin.
Where you can hear the quieting sounds in the distance.
Where the relaxing fragrances come and go.
For the next few minutes, enjoy your special relaxing place,
far, far away.
[PAUSE 1 MINUTE]

Positive Focus

And now we are coming to the end of our journey.

What is most relaxing word that comes to you? What word is most relaxing to you?

Or, what relaxing image comes to you? Something very, very simple, like a leaf, a pebble, or drop of water.

Let a special relaxing word, or a special relaxing image come to you now.

[PAUSE]

And gently attend to this word or image. If no word or image comes to you, simply begin to gently rock, very, very gently, back and forth.

And attend to your word or image, or to rocking. That is all. Let all thoughts go. When your mind wanders, simply return, again and again.

[PAUSE 2 MINUTES]

Gently let go of what you are attending to.

We have completed our scanning exercise.

Final scan

Let us do one final scan.

Is your posture relaxed and comfortable? If not, you may shift or adjust yourself.

Do you feel any muscle tension? If so, let go with every outgoing breath.

Are you holding your breath? If so, let go, and breathe slowly and easily.

Let your hands and arms and legs feel warm and heavy, as you sink deep into relaxation.

If any relaxing images or thoughts come to mind, simply note them, as they come and go.

And now take a breath, and stretch.

This completes our relaxation sequence.

21

Workshops and Group Relaxation

The group format is widely used in relaxation training. Groups provide an economical way for educating potential clients, introducing basic principles, and providing actual instruction. Even when introducing or teaching relaxation to more than one individual, it is possible to respect individual differences and tailor training. Here we will consider educational group workshops and instruction groups.

EDUCATIONAL GROUP WORKSHOPS

An important issue to face in constructing a workshop is what information to include. Generally, content and duration is determined by the nature of workshop participants, their reason for attending, and the amount of time available. Clearly health professionals attending a half-day workshop would receive more than potential clients attending a one-hour introduction. This chapter offers a menu of potential workshop topics, termed "modules," and suggests how they might be included.

Module Options

Module 1: The Stress and Relaxation Engines

Explain that relaxation works by triggering a powerful anti-stress relaxation response. Important changes that contribute to a healing, relaxed awareness occur in the brain and body. In addition, the body's "stress alarm" is reset so that one is less sensitive to stressful events (chapter 3).

Module 2: Six Stress Processes and Six Access Skills

This is a natural extension of Module 1 for groups and clients ready for more elaboration. Summarize the points in chapter 4, and briefly explain the six types of self-stressing and the six related relaxation access skills. Then note that each access skill corresponds to a family of widely applied relaxation approaches.

Module 3: Goal-Specific Relaxation Processes

Select a discussion of processes appropriate to the nature of workshop partici- pants. Generally, different groups may have interests various combinations of goals, as summarized in chapter 6:

- Health professionals (goals: stress management and healing)
- Patients (healing)
- Business professionals (health and energy, productivity, and effectiveness)
- Substance abuse groups (calm directed action)
- Weight reduction groups (stress management, calm directed action)
- Artists (creativity and insight)
- Vacationers (spontaneous enjoyment)
- Religious groups (God-based spirituality, meditation and mindfulness)

Identify the goal or goals that apply to the workshop group, and explain specific relaxation processes that contribute to that goal.

Module 4: Six Families of Relaxation

Briefly list and describe the six families of relaxation used by health profes- sionals. Note that recent research has shown that different approaches have different effects. This is a natural extension of Module 2.

Module 5: A Revolution in Relaxation Training:
One Size Doesn't Fit All

For centuries, health professionals and relaxation trainers have used the "one system fits all" philosophy. A stress clinic might teach just muscle relaxation, a yoga retreat only yoga, whereas a psychologist might teach imagery or visualization. This is still practiced in many places and is based on the outdated "generic aspirin" perspective. Specifically, all relaxation families are equally effective at evoking relaxation and, like generic aspirin, it doesn't matter what brand you get. Recent research shows that relaxation is more like a balanced meal, and the six general families are something like basic food groups. Each family is good for a different set of skills. A balanced meal contains something from each food group—vegetables, fruit, protein, etc. A balance relaxation sequence contains something from most families. Just as different people may have different nutritional needs requiring different proportions of various foods (those losing weight eat less fat or carbohydrates, athletes more protein, etc.), people may require different mixes of relaxation.

Module 6: The Relaxation Pyramid—Five Levels of R-States

Begin by showing the Relaxation Pyramid, as described in chapter 5. Include the entire pyramid, with 14 "blocks" with the Aware "circle" to the side. For most explanations, ignore distinctions between columns of states and simply present five levels, with three R-States grouped per level. Alternatively, do not include detailed distinctions between columns and levels (you may even erase the dividing vertical and horizontal lines on your visual presentation. Simply explain that some R-States are more "basic," and more frequently experienced: Sleepiness, Disengagement, Rested/Refreshed, Energized, Physical Relaxation, At Ease/Peace, and Joy. The remaining R-States are somewhat more rare. Emphasize that relaxation can be working very well when R-States near the base are experienced. The fact that one does not experience R-States closer to the peak does not mean that relaxation is not having an effect.

Module 7: Demonstration of Exercises with the Relaxation Sampler or Access Zone Scanning

Present the Relaxation Sampler (see Appendix) or Access Zone Scanning (see chapter 20). Both are 20-minute demonstrations of yoga stretching, PMR, autogenic training, breathing exercises, imagery, and meditation. Give each participant a copy of the Simplified R-State Pyramid Map (Figure 17.1). Participants note on their maps the R-States that were experienced with each technique. Use a simple letter code, in which:

"Y" = Yogaform stretching
"P" = Progressive muscle relaxation

"A" = Autogenic Training
"B" = Breathing
"I" = Imagery
"M" = Meditation/Mindfulness

For the Relaxation Sampler, one pauses after each of the six techniques is demonstrated. During this pause, participants note the effects on their map. For Access Zone Scanning, there are no pauses; instead, the effects are noted at the end of the sequence.

It is important to give participants a chance to discuss their experiences with the Relaxation Sampler or Access Zone Scanning exercise. In groups with more than six participants, I recommend dividing into subgroups of three or four people each. Generally, after practicing relaxation, participants are not inclined to participate in discussion. Dividing into subgroups helps counter this. Depending on the time that is available, one can select one of two processing options.

First, one might ask the entire group if they detected any R-States associated with any exercises. List each of the six families tried. After each one, point to the R-State Pyramid and ask which R-States, if any, were experienced. On the pyramid briefly write the name of each exercise next to its associated R-State.

Alternatively, one might divide a group into subgroups (or use the entire group, if there are six or fewer participants) and have the members complete a group task: "In the next 15 minutes, see if you can decide what each of the different approaches might be good for. When you are finished, each group will present its conclusions to the entire group."

Selecting Modules

All workshops should include some version of Modules 1, 4, 5, and 7. These form the "core relaxation workshop." Additional modules should be incorporated, depending on the time that is available and the interests and natures of workshop participants.

GROUP INSTRUCTION

All formats can be presented to groups. Group training for imagery and scripting can be a challenge. The key alteration of the individual protocol is to have group members vote at each point where a selection has to be made. The voting process involves first asking for nominations, which are then presented for all to see (on a blackboard or flip chart, for example), and second, voting on the nominations. This is relatively easy to apply to imagery.

Group Imagery

Proceed with standard instructions. After the four classes of imagery have been demonstrated (travel, outdoor/nature, water, indoor), the group nominates possible imagery themes. These are then posted for everyone to see. The group then votes on an imagery theme. The trainer asks if any member has any possible disruptive associations or booby traps for the selected image. If any problems are voiced, revisions are entertained. The individual voicing a problem has the option of vetoing the selected theme, in which case the group selects another. If a revised theme is selected and approved, then group members propose details for each sense dimension: what is seen, heard, felt, and smelled. Here, the trainer simply places labels for each dimension on a board and writes down all nominated details for each dimension. Include no more than six and no fewer than three details for any one dimension. There is no vote for sense details. Then the trainer leads the group in an improvised imagery sequence, lasting from 10 to 20 minutes.

In the improvised imagery presentation, the trainer first names the imagery theme, and then proceeds to name each nominated sense suggestion in whatever order makes sense. A skilled trainer will artfully weave suggestions together and embellish upon them in a way consistent with what has been suggested. Once all of the nominated suggestions are presented, the trainer then invites group participants to continue with their imagery for the designated period of time.

In the following example, group members considered several themes and voted on "The Peaceful Forest." They then used brainstorming to generate sense details. The resulting blackboard looked something like Figure 21.1.

The following is a brief illustration of an improvised instruction based on the details generated by group members for their selected theme, "The Peaceful Forest":

> Imagine you are in a peaceful and relaxing forest. You can see the beautiful green trees swaying in the wind. You hear the wind blowing through the leaves and you can feel its gentle touch on your skin. The scent of fresh leaves is clean. You can see the

```
                        GROUP IMAGERY EXERCISE

IMAGERY THEMES                          SENSE DETAILS
 (Vote on these)                        (Do not vote on these)

 Church              Sights        Sounds          Felt Sensations    Fragrances
 Cabin               Green trees   Wind blowing    Wind on skin       Fresh scent
 Ocean Beach         Swaying in wind  Chirping birds  Warm sun on skin  Clean air
✓Forest              Bright blue sky  Rush of brook   Mist on skin
 Submarine trip      Brook
 Hot tub             Clear waters
```

FIGURE 21.1   Example of blackboard summary of group-generated imagery themes and sense details.

bright blue sky above and feel the warm sun against your skin. You
hear the melodic chirping of birds. And the morning air smells
clean. You can see a brook with its clear waters. You hear the
rush of water and feel the delicate mist against your skin. As
you relax, imagine this peaceful and relaxing forest with all
of your senses for the next fifteen minutes. [TRAINER REMAINS
SILENT FOR 15 MINUTES WHILE ALL PRACTICE]

Group Scripting

Group scripting follows a format similar to that of group imagery. First, six
exercises are presented, one per session. Then one session is devoted to
scripting. Generally, standard individual instructions are applied. However,
group nominations and votes are taken at six key decision points:

1. Selecting relaxation goal
2. Identifying R-States consistent with relaxation goal
3. Selecting relaxation exercises
4. Selecting unifying idea
5. Selecting imagery and meditation details
6. Selecting deepening R-State words and affirmations

The trainer adds his or her own deepening imagery. Then, away from the
group, the trainer incorporates group voted details and creates an initial script.

In the following session, the trainer presents his or her proposed group script, while everyone practices. Group members suggest revisions. In the final session, the trainer either presents a script of revised instructions or distributes an audio recording of instructions.

For each script, the Scripting Worksheet can be handed out, discussed, and voted on.

Part V

Special Applications

22

Relaxation for Children

Relaxation training can help children manage the stress of home and school. Allen and Klein (1996) and Forman (1993) offer a set of applications that are perhaps a bit enthusiastic:

- Reducing stress with a planned class activity or instruction
- Recovering from strenuous activity or exercise
- Creating calm after conflict
- Helping enjoy music
- Enhancing school performance
- Staying tense in calm situations
- Dealing with test anxiety
- Enhancing creative writing
- Facilitating listening skills
- Recovering from busy day
- Preparing for sleep
- Facilitating positive thinking
- Enhancing concentration
- Nurturing positive self-concept
- Kindling imagination
- Having fun

For most problems relaxation should be combined with additional active behavioral and cognitive interventions, techniques and strategies targeted to changing specific behaviors and negative thought patterns. For an excellent

293

review of such active approaches, please see Forman (1993) as well as Rapee, Spence, Cobham, and Wignall (2000).

Six Families of Relaxation for Children

This book teaches six general families of relaxation: yogaform stretching, progressive muscle relaxation (PMR), breathing exercises, imagery, autogenic training, and meditation/mindfulness. Our focus is on children older than five years.

When working with children, it is not appropriate to use the formal professional name for each family of techniques. Possible child-friendly names include:

The Squeezies (PMR)
The Warm and Heavies (Autogenic Training)
The Breathies (Breathing Exercises)
The Stretchies (Yogaform Stretching)
Storytelling (Imagery)
Quieting (Meditation/Mindfulness)

I emphasize that each of these six families of relaxation can be successfully taught to children. Our overall objective is to introduce a wide range of approaches, ideally all six. Different approaches to relaxation have different effects, and no single family of techniques works for everyone. In addition, each family has different benefits and can work for different goals. Finally, in my opinion, it is best to integrate and combine the unique strengths of several approaches.

Some important modifications must be made when teaching relaxation to children:

* Because of a child's short attention span, exercises must be shortened and simplified
* Combine families of approaches, especially PMR, breathing, and imagery
* Exercises should not be presented as "fitness regimens" or therapy, but as fun activities
* Incorporate imagery, metaphor, and storytelling whenever possible
* Introduce variety to help maintain attention

- Individualize exercises, incorporating trainee choices
- Incorporate reinforcement and reward for completing an exercise

In addition, the relaxation setting and format should be modified specifi-cally for children:

- Use group training
- Incorporate the entire family with relaxation training, when possible
- Institute a setting that is quiet, free from distraction, and conducive to relaxation. When done in a classroom, change classroom elements to signify it is now relaxation time, not study time
- Incorporate modeling whenever possible; always end the session with words of reinforcement, encouragement, and support
- Ask trainees if they would like music but make sure it is quieting.

Overall Rationale

For children, a minimal exercise rationale is needed. Often accompanying imagery serves as a substitute for a rationale, providing a "story" for what the exercise is doing. Simple versions of arousal reduction and relaxation tuning (chapter 3) can be presented in language appropriate for children. Here is one suggestion:

> Sometimes it is okay to be tense and tight. It is not helpful to be sleepy and dreamy when playing a video game! But there are times when it doesn't feel good to be too tense and tight, like when you have a toothache or itch. These are things you want to get rid of. Your body gets all stirred up inside and this may make you feel ill.
>
> Imagine two cats, Fluffy and Needles. Fluffy is relaxed and peaceful. She calmly walks down the street, very graceful, cool, and calm. She is awake to what is happening. You see, Fluffy is ready to pounce on the first mouse she sees, and zoom away like a bullet when she has to, like when she sees Bluto, the big nasty dog down the street. Now, look at Needles. He is very uptight and tense, like he has a stone stuck in his paw. But he's that way all the time. He's too anxious and wound up for his own good. Needles spends most of his time hunched up like he is ready to attack, or run away, even when everything is safe. He's so wound up that sometimes he even misses a mouse! Sometimes they call him a "fraidy-cat," but the fact is that Needles is just very

nervous, tense, and tight. He hasn't learned how to relax and be cool.

We are going to learn how to be like Fluffy, how to relax when we want, and how to get rid of tightness and tension we don't like. We want to be ready to play and catch that mouse!

R-States for Children

In chapter 5 we considered fifteen R-States, relaxation states of mind associated with the practice of different techniques. R-States most appropriate for children can be presented using the following words and image phrases. Some of the higher R-States are best described with images rather than defining words:

Sleepy: Sleepy, drowsy, dozing off, napping.

Disengagement: Far away. Distant. Dreamy. In a different world. Nice and cozy, like a dog in a doghouse. Like being alone in a cave. Alone in my very own treehouse. My private island world.

Rested/Refreshed: Rested. Refreshed. Clean and new, like after a bath. Like walking through the rain. Like I woke up and am ready for the day.

Energized and Aware (combined R-States Energized and Aware): Energized. Full of pep. Zippy. Ready to go. Awake. Wide-eyed.

Physical Relaxation: Floppy. Loose. Limp. Droopy. Nice and tingly. Like jello. Soft. Squishy.

At Ease/Peace: Safe. Peaceful. Calm. Easy. Calmed down. No worries. No hassles. Not bothered. No hassles.

Joyful: Happy. Fun. Pretty.

Mental Quiet: Very still. Very quiet. Not a sound. Like a simple pond. No one is talking. Very hushed and peaceful. Like a cat in a tree, not moving at all, just aware of it all.

Childlike Innocence: Creative. Playful.

Awe and Wonder: Wonderful! Awesome! Surprising. Wow!

Prayerful: Like being in church, temple, mosque, or synagogue. It is very inspiring. This is very wonderful and holy. God is here.

Deep Mystery: Like a wonderful mystery adventure. A secret chamber of wonders and delights. A magical island far away.

Thankful/Loving: Sharing, thankful, very friendly.

An important part of relaxation is helping trainees learn to identify and differentiate R-States, consider the value and desirability of certain R-States, and discover what relaxation techniques are best for certain R-States. Ask trainees how they feel when they relax. Observe their expressions and tone of voice, and if you think they are experiencing an R-State, ask "Are you feeling happy?" "Are you feeling far away and dreamy?" Reinforce appropriate R-States when they are expressed. Freely introduce appropriate R-States into relaxation instructional scripts.

Progressive Muscle Relaxation (PMR): "The Squeezies"

Progressive muscle relaxation (PMR) may be the most appropriate approach to children who display high levels of stress, including somatic symptoms, worry, and negative emotion such as anxiety, depression, and anger. It is particularly appropriate for children who have difficulties paying attention. PMR is an ideal supplement to therapy.

Special Modifications

- For children eight years of age or younger, focus only on major, easily identified muscle groups.
- Do not do all muscle groups in the first session. Do a few muscle groups in the first session, then add muscle groups in subsequent sessions.
- A mirror can be used to help trainees identify specific target muscle groups.
- Various "squeeze props," pillows, stuffed small animals, toys, and balls can be used with the tense-up phase of each exercise ("Squeeze this ball in your hand . . . let go.")

Specific Rationale

We are going to do an exercise called "the squeezies." You squeeze up a muscle nice and tight (demonstrate with fist) and then let the muscle go completely limp. This is like a bow and arrow. We pull the string of the bow back, making it tense (demonstrate with gesture), then release the string. Twang! The string relaxes, and the arrow goes soaring into the sky. We tense up, and let go, and send our muscles soar like an arrow into calm and relaxation. Or imagine you are holding a rock in your hand over a pond. First squeeze tightly on the rock. All the tension and tightness goes into the rock. Then let go, and the rock goes "plop" into the pond, sinking deeper and deeper, just as you sink into calm and relaxation after letting go.

First, let's try a game. We are going to look for parts of our body that may be tensed up like Needles the cat. Let me demonstrate. Rest your right and left hand in your lap. Which is more tight and tense? [WAIT FOR ANSWER] Now make a fist with your right hand. [DEMONSTRATE] Close your eyes and notice your right hand. Now notice your left hand. Which is more tense? Can you see that the right hand is tense? Now let go of the tension. Make your right hand very loose and limp. Can you feel the difference? In this exercise, we are going to do this to different parts of the body. We will look for hidden tension. Then we will tighten up that part a little, and let it go completely limp so it relaxes.

Then encourage your child to come up with their own words describing tension and relaxation, and use their words when possible. Examples of "tension words" might include:

- Gripping
- Making it tight and hard
- Holding on
- Stiff
- Like a rock
- Wound up
- Clenched
- Screwed up

Encourage Physical Relaxation and Disengagement if the primary goal is to deal with stress, somatic tension, worry, and negative emotion. Focus on Rested/Refreshed and Energized/Aware if the goal is to get ready for school or some vigorous activity. Focus on Happy for creative activities.

Recommended Combinations

Children have shorter attention spans than adults. For this reason, PMR for children is shorter and more condensed than the adult version. We tense up for five seconds, and release tension for ten to fifteen seconds. Body parts are tensed up together. These exercises are best when done in a seated position.

Hands and arms. [DO TWICE ON THE RIGHT SIDE, TWICE ON THE LEFT SIDE]. In this exercise we are going to [OPTIONAL "Take a deep breath and . . . "] make a tight fist with your right hand, like you are squeezing a ball or orange, and bending at the elbow, try to touch your right shoulder with your right hand, like you are pressing the orange against your shoulder, like this. [DEMONSTRATE] And [OPTIONAL "Easily let the air out . . . "] let your arm and hand go completely limp, and flop down onto your lap, like this. Try this right now with me. [DEMONSTRATE] [OPTIONAL "Take a deep breath and . . . "] make a tight fist with your right hand, like you are squeezing a ball or orange, and bending at the elbow, try to touch your right shoulder with your right hand, like you are pressing the orange against your shoulder. Then, let go [OPTIONAL "And easily breathe out."] Let your arm and hand go completely limp, and flop down onto your lap, like this. [DEMONSTRATE] Lets try this again. Together, let's [OPTIONAL "Take a deep breath and . . . "] make a fist and tighten up your arm and fist. Tighten them up right now. Like you are squeezing an orange in your hand and pressing it to your shoulder. Then [OPTIONAL "Let the air out and . . . "] go completely limp and plop onto your lap, like you are letting the orange in your hand fall to the ground. Let your hand and arm relax as I count down: Five . . . loose and relaxed . . . four . . . loose and relaxed . . . three . . . loose and relaxed . . . two . . . loose and relaxed . . . and one . . . loose and relaxed. There, notice how your right hand and arm feel now. Are they more relaxed than they were? Did it hurt? [IF SO, REPEAT, BUT DON'T TIGHTEN UP SO HARD]

Shoulders and back of neck. Now let's do the shoulders and neck. We are going to [OPTIONAL: "Take a deep breath and . . . "] shrug while tilting your head back, like this, [DEMONSTRATE] like you are puppet and strings are pulling your shoulders up to your ears. And [OPTIONAL: "breathe out and . . . "] let go, like the puppet strings are cut. Relax. And now try this with me. [OPTIONAL: "Take a deep breath and . . . "] shrug your shoulders, tilt your head back. Feel a good squeeze, like you are a puppet and strings are pulling your shoulders up to your ears. [DEMONSTRATE WITH CLIENT] Keep the rest of your body relaxed. And [OPTIONAL: "let the air flow out . . . "] let go, like the puppet strings are cut. Your shoulders go flop, and your neck relaxes. You are a floppy relaxed rag doll puppet now. Let your shoulders and neck become more and more relaxed as I count down.

Five . . . loose and relaxed . . . four . . . loose and relaxed . . . three . . . loose and relaxed . . . two . . .
loose and relaxed . . . and one . . . loose and relaxed. Notice how your shoulders and neck feel now. Do they feel more limp
and loose, maybe warm and tingly? Are they more relaxed?

Jaws, nose, and forehead. Now the jaws, nose, and forehead.
Try this with me. We are going to [OPTIONAL: "take a deep breath
and . . . "] screw up your whole face, your jaws, [DEMONSTRATE]
nose, [DEMONSTRATE] and forehead and eyes, [DEMONSTRATE] all
together, like we have eaten a great big piece of very sour lemon.
Scrunch up your whole face, now. And, open your mouth [OPTIONAL:
"and breathe out . . . "] like you are spitting out the lemon.
It feels so good to have that lemon out of your mouth! And let
your face become very smooth and relaxed as I count down:
Five . . . loose and relaxed . . . four . . . loose and relaxed . . . three . . . loose   and   relaxed . . . two
. . . loose   and   relaxed . . . and one . . . loose   and
relaxed.

Stomach, abdomen, and back. Put your right hand on your tummy.
[OPTIONAL: "Take a deep breath and . . . "] Make your tummy really tight, so you can feel how hard it is with your hand. [ALTER-
NATIVE STRATEGY: "Suck your tummy toward your back, so it gets
nice and tight. Make yourself skinny."] Let your entire middle,
from your back to your bellybutton get nice and stiff, like the
trunk of a tree. Let your tummy relax and get nice and loose.
Imagine the hard tree has become soft paper mush. Notice how good
your tummy and back feel as I count down: Five . . . loose
and   relaxed . . . four . . . loose   and   relaxed . . .
three . . . loose and relaxed . . . two . . . loose and relaxed . . . and one . . . loose and relaxed.

Legs and feet. [DO TWICE ON THE RIGHT SIDE, TWICE ON THE LEFT
SIDE] [OPTIONAL: "Take a deep breath and . . . "] push your feet
into the ground. Push with your toes and legs. Push really hard
like you are glued to your chair and can't get up! [DEMONSTRATE]
Make your upper legs, feet, and toes really hard! Then let go
[OPTIONAL "and breathe out . . . "] Let your legs, feet, and
toes, really relax. Imagine the hard glue is melting and is soft
and relaxed. Become more loose and limp as I count down: Five . . . loose and relaxed . . . four . . . loose and relaxed . . . three . . . loose   and   relaxed . . .
two . . . loose and relaxed . . . and one . . . loose and
relaxed.

Review. Let your whole body get loose and relaxed, like a limp,
floppy doll. Your hands and arms. Let them get loose and relaxed,
like a floppy doll. Five . . . loose and relaxed . . . four

. . . loose and relaxed . . . three . . . loose and relaxed
. . . two . . . loose and relaxed . . . and one . . . loose
and relaxed. Your shoulders and neck. Loose and relaxed like a
floppy doll. Five . . . loose and relaxed . . . four . . .
loose and relaxed . . . three . . . loose and relaxed . . .
two . . . loose and relaxed . . . and one . . . loose and relaxed. Your jaws, nose, and forehead. Loose and relaxed like a
floppy doll. Five . . . loose and relaxed . . . four . . .
loose and relaxed . . . three . . . loose and relaxed . . .
two . . . loose and relaxed . . . and one . . . loose and relaxed. Tummy and back. Loose and relaxed like a floppy doll.
Five . . . loose and relaxed . . . four . . . loose and relaxed . . . three . . . loose and relaxed . . . two . . .
loose and relaxed . . . and one . . . loose and relaxed. Legs
and feet. Loose and relaxed like a floppy doll. Five . . . loose
and relaxed . . . four . . . loose and relaxed . . . three
. . . loose and relaxed . . . two . . . loose and relaxed
. . . and one . . . loose and relaxed. Is there any part of your
body that is still tense? Is there any part of the puppet that
is still being pulled by strings?
    [OPTIONAL: "Take a deep breath and . . . "] [OPTIONAL:
"Breathe out and . . . "] Cut the strings, and go completely
floppy with your entire body, completely loose and relaxed.

When tensing up, you may consider the following alternative images:

- Imagine a small bug on your skin. Scrunch up your skin so the bug flies away.
- Tighten and pull in your muscles like a turtle (pulling in its hand and arms, shoulders and neck, face, stomach, legs and feet).
- Imagine your hands and arms (shoulders, face, etc.) are a sponge full of tension. Tighten up and squeeze the sponge.

Alternative "letting go" relaxing images:

- Imagine relaxing fingers gently rubbing your skin, smoothing tension out.
- Imagine a soft gentle kitten brushing against your skin, rushing away tension.
- Imagine a cool (or warm) breeze blowing against your skin, taking tension away.
- Your hands and arms (shoulders, back of neck, etc.) are like a jellyfish, floppy and relaxed.

AUTOGENIC IMAGERY: "THE WARM AND HEAVIES"

Autogenic imagery can be very powerful, used by itself or in combination with PMR. You can target autogenic images to the entire body, or to specific areas of focus in PMR. Most images focus on various ways of experiencing physical relaxation. Here is one sample exercise that uses the image of a floppy doll:

> We are going to do an exercise called "The Warm and Heavies." Let's all imagine we are floppy dolls. First, stand up. Let your hands and arms hang by your sides, like a floppy doll. Shake 'em up a little. Then let them hang, very floppy. Let your shoulders hang very floppy. First, lift them a little, like a little shrug, then let them go floppy and limp. Let your head bow over like the head of a floppy doll. Shake your head a little, then let it go floppy.
>
> Now, let's walk around, like floppy dolls. Very slowly, let your floppy arms and hands hang. Let them flop around a little. Your head stays floppy. Slowly walk, one step at a time, like your legs are very floppy. Very slowly, let's walk and be floppy.
>
> Now let's sit in our chairs, flop down in our chairs. Let your arms hang really limp. Let your head hang. Let your legs get very floppy.
>
> Now imagine the floppy doll is made of candle wax and is beginning to melt. Your arms are warm and heavy, warm and heavy. All the tension flows out of your arms and hands, and out of your fingers. Warm and heavy like melting wax.
>
> Your shoulders are warm and heavy. They are melting like wax. The tension is melting away, down your arms through your fingers, onto the floor. Shoulders are warm and heavy.
>
> Your head and face, are warm and heavy. You can feel the wax melting. It feels so good. Tension is melting. Melting from your head and face.
>
> And now your legs and feet. Your legs and feet are getting warm and heavy. The warm melting wax feels so heavy. It melts down to your toes onto the floor.
>
> Your entire body feels nice and relaxed, warm and heavy, warm and heavy.

Here are some additional images you can use:

• Warm water from a bath touches you and washes away tension and tightness. Your body floats and becomes relaxed.

- A magic wand moves up and down your body. Every part of the body it touches, it carries tension away.
- Sunlight comes in through the window. Slowly it moves up your body. Every part of your body it touches, your body feels nice and warm and toasty as it becomes more relaxed.
- You are by a fireplace with a nice warm fire. The warmth touches each part of your body, melting away tension.
- A warm breeze touches each part of your body, carrying away the tension of the day.
- A soft warm fluffy kitten rolls up on your hand (arms, shoulders, etc.). It feels so good. The kitten begins to purr, and the purring carries away your tension.

BREATHING "THE BREATHIES"

All of the breathing exercises presented in this book can be presented to children. Breathing stretches can be done standing up, either individually or in a group. Breathing exercises can be excellent quick exercises for "cooling off" or reducing the overall level of tension or agitation for individuals or groups of children. They can be used in combination, starting with active stretches, proceeding to diaphragmatic breathing, and ending with passive breathing exercises. Initially, one might apply a sequence including a single exercise from each approach. Eventually, a single exercise preferred by the child can be selected as an abbreviated "cooling off" exercise.

I recommend using the breathing instructions in chapter 11. For all, an initial image might be "breathe out feelings of tension (frustration, anger, etc.), breathe in feelings of calm." Additional supporting images can be tailored to the exercise depending on child preferences:

Group 1: Breathing Stretches

With all the exercises in this group, you may incorporate the following images:

You are a tree bending in the wind. The wind blows away tension, like it blows away dust and leaves.
You are standing under a waterfall or shower (or in the rain). As you breathe out, water runs down your body carrying away tension.

As you bow, tension rolls off with your outgoing breath.
(All are to be done very slowly, smoothly, and gently)

Group 2: Active Diaphragmatic Breathing

The following images are appropriate for active diaphragmatic breathing:

Imagine your stomach is a big beach ball. Put your hands over your stomach and gently squeeze out the air as you breathe out. As you breathe in, let the beach ball fill with air again.
Imagine your middle is a tire filled with air. As you breathe out, the tire leaks, the air goes out, and the tire goes flat. As you breathe in, you are filling the tire with air again.

Group 3: Passive Breathing

Here are some possible passive breathing images:

Imagine sniffing a very delicate flower.
Sniff in the wonderful aroma of what's cooking. Sniff in very slowly, because you can hardly tell what the aroma is.
Imagine blowing on a candle flame, gently so it doesn't go out.
Imagine blowing on the fur of a soft kitten, so gently you don't wake the kitten up.
Imagine blowing on a leaf or feather in your hand, but not so much that it blows away.
Take in a deep breath like you are waking up in the morning.
Take in a deep breath like you have just gone outside and it has just rained. The air is very clean and fresh.
Focus on the flow of breath in and out. Imagine it is a very gentle breeze blowing back and forth.

YOGAFORM STRETCHING: "THE STRETCHIES"

The exercises presented here are simple stretches based on hatha yoga. However, it should be noted that traditional yoga exercises incorporate stretches as well as potentially demanding postures, which may pose a risk to the delicate and growing bones of children. Therefore, I strongly recommend that if traditional hatha yoga is attempted, it should be taught by a qualified health professional experienced with children. The stretches in this book avoid potentially dangerous postures and are relatively safe.

Yogaform stretching exercises are ideal group activities and can be presented as "play." They are appropriate when children need a break from their lessons, or as an energizing warmup for class or sports. They are good for evoking feelings of energy, but less effective for reducing tension, worry, or negative emotions.

As with PMR exercises, we offer abbreviated combinations of stretches. Note that each stretch has a PMR "tense-let go" parallel. Indeed, both exercises can be presented together, with stretching following tensing and letting go. However, unlike PMR, yogaform stretching exercises are done very slowly, smoothly, and gently. Because of this deliberate and graceful quality, supporting imagery can be more extensive. To illustrate, each exercise we present has a name suggestive of the supporting imagery.

Begin in a seated position (or on the floor).

Dancing with the Sun

We are going to do some exercises that are called "stretchies." We will imagine we are outside and the sun is beginning to rise.

Waking and saying "Hello" to the sun (hands and arms). [STAY SEATED] Imagine we have been taking a nap and are ready to wake up. Slowly, smoothly, and gently lift your arms in front of you to say "hello" to the sun. Open them wide! And spread your fingers wide open, like you are greeting and hugging the sunshine. Hold the stretch, letting the sunlight in. Then slowly, smoothly, and gently, close your hands, and let your arms return to your sides.

Now lets try that again while standing.

The Sun greets you with a touch (shoulders and back of neck). [WHILE STANDING] You are waking up, and gently let your head begin to fall forward. Do not force it down, let it slowly pull down on its own, stretching your neck and shoulders. Notice how good it feels. The sun is shining down on your neck and shoulders. The sun touches you with its wonderful, warm, and glowing fingers, dissolving tension, bringing energy.

Laugh with the sun! (jaws, nose, and forehead). Now we are going to do a silly exercise! Imagine the sun is a great big smiling and laughing ball, smiling at you. Open your mouth and eyes really wide, like you are laughing back. Lift your eyebrows! Now stick out your tongue at the sun! Make the sun laugh. And the sunlight touches you and fills you with warmth and happiness. Then slowly, close your eyes and mouth, and relax.

Let the rain roll off! (stomach, abdomen, and back). A rain cloud has come in front of the sun and it is beginning to sprinkle. Slowly, smoothly, and gently bow forward. Do not push yourself down. Just let your back and shoulders bow forward on their own like the earth is pulling them down. And the gentle rain just rolls off your back. Then the rain stops, and you can gently stand up again.

Ready to go! (legs and feet). We are now ready to go. Hold on to something (like a chair or tree) and slowly, smoothly, and gently stretch the right leg out. Let it stretch all the way, stretching out all the kinks so you can move. Then return your right leg. Now let's do that with the left leg.

Now we are awake. The sunlight and the refreshing rain have refreshed us. We have stretched our legs, and are ready to go on with our day.

IMAGERY: "STORYTELLING"

Imagery is best done after a preparatory physical exercise (PMR, autogenic training, breathing, or yogaform stretching). It is not the approach of choice for calming down an overly stimulated class or individual. I recommend imagery as a way of taking a break from activity, or as a preparation for a creativity task (writing, painting, etc.). It can also be a reward for work well done.

My approach to imagery is to tailor both the theme and the details to client preferences. The traditional approach of imposing standard images on everyone risks using images that are not preferred (or even disliked) by clients. Specifically, I first provide generic samples, and then ask the child to select a topic invite him or her to add sense details. It is important to inquire about possible negative associations that could sabotage the imagery sequence. For adults, this book presents four categories of imagery: travel, nature/outdoors, water, and indoors.

I suggest imagery that tells a very simple, quiet, and relaxing story. The story should start with energy and complex detail and gradually evolve so that it is increasingly passive and simple. The "plot" of the story is to find a special relaxing place that is quiet and safe. This imagery strategy is most likely to engage a child's limited attention span and evoke the quiet focus central to relaxation. The following is an abbreviated illustration of the process of introducing sample images, selecting a topic, picking sense details, and then presenting a story.

We are going to have fun with a daydream story. However, unlike some stories, this one is not an exciting adventure or thrilling race. It is a special type of story, one in which you look for and find a very safe and quiet place. In this story you will look for a wonderful, calm, and peaceful place where you can go to completely relax.

First, imagine a magic story person comes to you with four boxes. Each box contains stories, but different types of stories. [YOU MAY BRING FOUR BOXES AS PROPS]

The first box contains stories about traveling. They may involve traveling in a spaceship, far away from the earth into the quiet of space. Or traveling in a train, through the countryside far away. Or maybe in a boat, or airplane or balloon. This box has stories about traveling.

The second box has stories about the outdoors. Perhaps there is a story about a quiet, peaceful forest. Or a wonderful mountaintop. Or a vacation island.

The third box is dripping with water! Why? It has stories about lakes and rivers and oceans. It is a box with a lot of water in it! You might want a story about a peaceful river, or a faraway lake or ocean.

And the fourth box has stories about wonderful, relaxing buildings, like a cabin in the forest or a magical castle.

And now the story person has a question for you. Which box should we open? What kind of story do you want? The travel box? The outdoors box? The lakes and rivers box? Or the box with a house or castle inside. Which do you want?

[THE CHILD SELECTS A STORY BOX. IF IT IS A GROUP, THE GROUP VOTES. WHEN A THEME BOX HAS BEEN SELECTED, OPEN THE BOX AND OFFER SEVERAL STORIES TO SELECT FROM. IN THE FOLLOWING EXAMPLE, THE THEME IS TRAVELING. SEVERAL TRAVEL STORIES ARE THEN SUGGESTED. THE TRAINER WILL HAVE TO INVENT A VARIETY OF STORIES, USING IDEAS SUGGESTED IN CHAPTER 13]

Our magic story person now opens the magic travel box. And inside are three stories. One is about a train that goes through the country, far away from the city. The second is about a big, safe balloon that floats high in the sky. The third is about a bicycle that glides through the park. Which story should we pick? The train? The balloon? The bicycle? Is there a relaxing and peaceful travel story you might want to put in the box?

[THE GROUP OR CHILD THEN SELECTS THE SPECIFIC STORY. NEXT, DISCUSS THE DETAILS WITH THE CHILD OR GROUP. WHAT IS SEEN? WHAT IS HEARD? WHAT IS FELT TOUCHING THE SKIN? WHAT FRAGRANCES DOES ONE SMELL? THE STORYTELLER MAKES NOTE OF THESE DETAILS. IN THE

FOLLOWING EXAMPLE, OUR CHILD OR GROUP HAS PICKED "THE TRAIN" AS
THE PREFERRED THEME.]

What type of train is it? A sleek modern train that slips
through the countryside like a silver river? Maybe it's an old
train, with a chugging steam engine that slowly and smoothly
goes along. [CHILD/GROUP PICKS THE OLD STEAM ENGINE]. What do
you see as the old steam engine chugs through the country. [CHILD
GROUP SUGGESTS "ROLLING HILLS, GREEN GRASS, COWS, CLOUDS, LIT-
TLE HOUSES, A RIVER, SHEEP, LOTS OF BIRDS]. What do you hear
that is relaxing? [THE CHUG CHUG-CHUG OF THE TRAIN. BIRDS. COWS
MOOING. THE WIND RUSHING PAST THE TRAIN.] What do you feel touching your skin? [THE SOOTHING VIBRATION OF THE CHUGGING ENGINE.
THE SOFT LEATHER SEATS THAT ARE SO COZY.] What fragrances do
you smell? [THE WONDERFUL FRAGRANCE OF FRESH GRASS AND TREES.
BURNING WOOD USED TO FIRE THE ENGINE OF THE TRAIN. RAIN.]

THE STORYTELLER THEN HAS THE CHILD OR GROUP CLOSE THEIR EYES
AND BEGINS THE STORY. THE STORY HAS AS ITS GENERAL THEME "FINDING
THE SPECIAL, SAFE, AND QUIET PLACE." INCLUDE THE IMAGES DIS-
CUSSED, MAKING SURE THAT AS THE STORY PROGRESSES, "DEEPENING
IMAGERY" IS DEPLOYED. IMAGES SHOULD BEGIN WITH RELATIVE ENERGY,
ACTIVITY, AND COMPLEX DETAIL, AND THEN BECOME INCREASINGLY CALM
AND FOCUSED UNTIL THE SPECIAL SAFE AND QUIET PLACE IS REACHED OR
IDENTIFIED. UNLIKE ADULT NARRATIVE IMAGERY, THE STORYTELLER
CONTINUES TALKING THROUGHOUT THE EXERCISE. GENERALLY, I DO NOT
RECOMMEND AN EXTENDED QUIET TIME AT THE END OF THE EXERCISE.]

And now, let's close our eyes. We are ready to take a wonderful
journey. It is a special journey where we will discover a special, quiet, and safe place. A place where we can go whenever we
want, far away from the hassles of the day. Imagine you are on a
delightful old train, the kind you might find in a zoo. Only this
train goes way out into the countryside, far away from everything. You are sitting in the best car, near the middle, with
big windows that let you see everything. Your seat is covered
with very soft and comfortable leather. You can feel the relaxing
wiggling and jiggling of the train as it moves along, and the
chugging of the engine. Outside, clouds seem to fly past as the
train gains speed. You see all sorts of wonderful things. It is
wonderfully busy outside. There are lots of things to see. Sheep
and sheepdogs running circles around the flock. Flocks of birds
flying overhead, singing together. Little houses. Grass. You
can smell the wonderful fragrance of the outdoors and the comforting smell of burning wood from the train's engine. Everything is so much fun and alive.

The train moves farther away and deeper into the countryside.
There are fewer things to see. Your ride becomes more and more

quiet. The track becomes smoother, and the train gently glides along. Outside you see rolling fields of grass, with occasional trees. Every once in a while, you see a single deer standing and slowly munching grass. Maybe you see a single bird resting on a treetop, looking at the sky.

Soon the train is completely in the country. It is in its own world. Your ride is completely smooth, as smooth as silk. This is your safe and quiet place. Everything is so peaceful. Rolling fields of grass as far as your eye can see. Everything is calm and simple. And once in a while a little animal peeks up from a clump of grass, winks at you, and dashes away.

If PMR, autogenic training, breathing, or yoga stretching have been explored, selected exercises can be woven into the story to enhance relaxation. Continuing with our example of the train:

Our train is about to leave the station. The conductor is about to start the steam engine. He blows the whistle and, as the train begins, you can hear a "chug" from the engine. The train moves a little. Now, shrug your shoulders really tight and wait for the next chug. "Chug" and the train moves, and you let go of your shoulders. Let them go completely limp. [PMR] And the train smoothly moves on as you relax.

The train is smoothly swaying through the countryside. It turns gently around one big hill. As it turns, reach out your right hand, all the way, as if you were swaying while the train is moving. [YOGAFORM STRETCHING]

The train is very smoothly gliding through the countryside. In your comfortable seat you can feel the soft chugging of the engine. Very gently chugging along. Your body feels very comfortable in its seat. Very comfortable and heavy, and the chugging soothes it. [AUTOGENIC TRAINING]

Slowly breathe out through your lips, as you see the steam from the steam engine float past your window. [BREATHING]

Finally, imagery is an ideal place to select R-State words that are preferred by the child. Presenting a list of words for the child to consider would be too deliberate for most children. Instead, listen for words a child prefers.

MEDITATION/MINDFULNESS: "QUIETING"

For children, one can consider ending any of the preceding approaches to relaxation with one or two minutes of meditation or mindfulness. Try to integrate the meditation or mindfulness exercise selected with what precedes, using breathing meditation with breathing relaxation, rocking meditation with yogaform stretching movement, etc. Ideally, the exercise sequence that comes before meditation should begin with exercises that are relatively energetic and complex, and end (just before meditation) with exercises that are most the simplest and most passive.

The rationale for meditation should explore the notion of meditative Mental Quiet and should incorporate imagery:

> In this exercise you become as quiet and peaceful as possible. Can you think of times that are like this? Maybe you are resting on a very soft sofa and notice that a kitten is sleeping very quietly on your stomach. You want to be very quiet so you do not awaken the kitten. You simply listen to the kitten purring . . . purr . . . purr . . . purr. Or maybe you are on a boat in a pond. You are resting very quietly, and some tiny fish swim up to the boat. You do not want to move at all or the fish will swim away. Can you think of some examples?

To review, this book introduces seven types of concentrative meditation:

- Meditations of the body—body sense meditation, rocking meditation, and breathing meditation
- Meditations of the mind—mantra meditation and image meditation
- Meditations of the senses—meditations on sounds and meditation on a visual image

In addition, we offer a variety of approaches to simply and mindfully attending to the flow of all stimuli. The following examples illustrate how various approaches to relaxation can end with meditation.

> Tense and let go. Let the tension flow. Let yourself sink into relaxation. [PMR] Simply notice how good your muscles feel when they relax. [BODY SENSE MEDITATION]
> Let your hands and arms feel warm and heavy, warm and heavy. You are a tree in the warm sunshine. [AUTOGENIC TRAINING] Let yourself gently rock back and forth, so gently that no one would notice. Let your rocking be very, very quiet. [ROCKING MEDITATION]
> Breathe out through your lips, as if you are breathing on a feather on your hand. [BREATHING] Now simply attend to the air as it moves in and out of your nose. [BREATHING MEDITATION]

Imagine you are in a relaxing train, chugging through the countryside. Your close your eyes, and listen to the gentle and slow chug . . . chug . . . chug. [IMAGERY]. As you sink into relaxation, simply attend to the slow and gentle chug . . . chug . . . chug . . . [MANTRA MEDITATION]

In your relaxing train, you see one very special waterfall far away in the distance. [IMAGERY] Simply attend to the waterfall. Whenever your mind wanders, gently return. [IMAGE MEDITATION]

Slowly bow over as you breathe out, and sit up as you breathe in. [BREATHING] And when you are done, attend to the sound of the wind outside. Just the wind. Whenever you mind wanders, simply return. [SOUND MEDITATION]

And now open your eyes and stretch. [YOGAFORM STRETCHING] Look at the trees outside. Simply attend to how beautiful they are. [MEDITATION ON A VISUAL IMAGE]

Mindfulness meditation can be introduced as a way of creatively attending to something we might ordinarily take for granted, such as a raisin, a painting, or trees.

Taste this raisin. Let the flavors fill your mouth. Notice its texture and flavor. Notice how sweet it is.

Look at this painting. What are all the colors you can see?

Look at the trees outside. What are the different things you see in the tree?

SUMMARY:
MASTERING THE SKILLS OF RELAXATION

Childhood and adolescence are ideal times to teach relaxation. Several very important and basic lessons can be of value throughout life:

1. There are six families of relaxation.
2. Relaxation is good for reducing tension and stress.
3. Relaxation can also do more than reduce tension and stress; it can evoke a variety of positive R-States.
4. Different families of relaxation have different effects, and can be used for different purposes.
5. One can be creative with relaxation, and combine exercises from different families.

THE RELAXATION SAMPLER

For instructors who wish to introduce children to the idea of six families of
relaxation may consider an abbreviated demonstration based on the Relaxation
Sampler (see Appendix). The following script illustrates yogaform stretching,
PMR, autogenic training, breathing exercises, imagery, and meditation.

The Six Magic Stepping Stones in the Cool and Peaceful Park

[START IN STANDING POSITION] We are going to take a vacation
in our minds, a special trip through a wonderful park full of
surprises and delights. It's called The Cool and Peaceful Park.
The park is outdoors, far away from home or school. You are very
safe in this relaxing place.

At the entrance to the park is a huge golden gate, one that
forms a shining half circle, a rainbow-like ring that starts on
the ground, reaches to the sky, and then touches the ground
again. Imagine you are now just under the arch. In front of you
is a beautiful bird standing very quietly. Before you enter, the
bird greets you, and you greet the bird.

The bird slowly lifts its wings into the air. As you watch the
bird, very slowly, smoothly and gently lift both of your arms to
your sides, like the wings of the bird. You are saying hello to
each other. Do this very slowly, so you don't startle the bird
and chase it away. Very easily, higher and higher. Now reach all
the way to the top of the golden door, trying to touch it. Feel
the good stretch all the way. And as the bird slowly returns its
wings, slowly, smoothly, and gently return your arms to your
sides and simply stand comfortably. Now you are ready to move
into the park.

Imagine a park buggy has moved to your side. Sit in the buggy
so you are comfortable. This cart will move you through the park.
[SITTING IN CHAIR] This is a very unusual buggy. In the front is
a conductor who drives. Let's first take a deep breath . . . and
now shrug your shoulders. Create a nice good shrug. And then
go completely limp. Let any tightness go. Let yourself become
relaxed. As you relax, the conductor realizes it is time to begin, and the buggy begins to move.

The buggy moves very slowly into a beam of sunlight. You feel
the sun on your skin. It feels so warm and good. It helps you feel
even more relaxed, like the sunlight is melting tightness and
tension. You feel more comfortable, ready for your journey.

The driver turns to you and smiles. He is ready to start moving
a little faster, still at a very safe speed. You take a deep

breath, and as the buggy begins to move, you gently let the air flow out of your lips, so you can barely hear the hissing. Air gently moves past the buggy as you move smoothly along. Take another deep breath, pause, and let the air flow out through your lips, making a soft hissing sound.

And now the buggy is moving through the park. Let yourself breathe naturally. The buggy travels through different wonderful areas, where you can discover wonderful sounds and sights. What fun and peaceful animals do you see? Maybe a tall giraffe, reaching into the green leaves of a tree. You can hear the leaves crunch as the giraffe munches. You can smell the fresh scent of leaves. You feel the air against your skin. Maybe you see a wonderful pond with golden fish swimming around in circles making little bubbles. You can hear the bubbles as they pop, and the splashing of the fish. You can feel a gentle spray of water on your skin. The water smells so clean and fresh.

And you are now near the end of your trip. The day is coming to a close, and everything around you has become very quiet and still. There is no wind. No sounds. And you see the colorful bird that greeted you at the gateway to the park. The bird lifts its wings one last time. It lifts its wings wide, jumps into the air, and slowly flies higher and higher. It is a wonderful and amazing sight. For a little while, simply look at this very special bird, as it soars higher, above the trees, then above the clouds, and finally becomes a little dot in the sky. Let yourself become very still. Very quiet. Very relaxed. Any little movement, even a thought, and the bird will slip away and you won't see it any more. Very calmly look at the bird and nothing else. See how far you can see the bird as it flies away. And then you say goodbye to the bird, and the park.

[PAUSE 30 SECONDS]

Now, gently let go of what you are attending to. Take a deep breath and stretch. We are finished with our tour through the park. How do you feel? Do you feel relaxed at all? [WAIT FOR ANSWERS. REINFORCE R-STATES DESCRIBED, ENCOURAGING DIVERSE RESPONSES]

There is a special secret about this tour I want to share with you. While we were taking the tour through the park we met many different park creatures. But something else was going on. We did six things that are very good and powerful ways of relaxing. Six ways of moving and thinking that can help us calm down and become cool and peaceful. Here's what we did.

We stretched. [DEMONSTRATE]

We squeezed. [DEMONSTRATE]

We felt warm and heavy. [DEMONSTRATE]

We took a deep breath and breathed out our tension, like this. [DEMONSTRATE]

We enjoyed a little fantasy daydream.

And we ended by putting all our thoughts aside and paying attention to one very simple thing, the bird as it flew away.

Which did you like best? [DISCUSS]

23

Relaxation and Pain Management

Persistent pain is a major reason patients seek professional health care, miss work, display limitations in everyday activities, and suffer from poor physical and psychological health (Gureje, Von Korff, Simon, & Gater, 1998). Perhaps up to 10% of all individuals in the United States suffer from a pain condition on more than 100 days a year (Osterweis, Kleinman, & Mechanic, 1987). Physicians encounter complaints of pain more than any other complaint. Major pain complaints are headache, backache, muscle and joint pain, stomach pain, menstrual cycle pain, and dental pain (Taylor & Curran, 1985). Clearly, pain management is a useful tool for any health professional, and relaxation training is an important part of pain management.

Before continuing, it is important to emphasize that medical evaluation is extremely important for a patient suffering from pain. A qualified physician can help determine the source of pain and recommend appropriate medical treatments, as well as advise which approaches to relaxation should be avoided as potentially dangerous. The medical precautions to relaxation listed in chapter 16 of this book should be studied in detail.

MODELS OF PAIN

First we need to distinguish acute and chronic pain. Acute pain is an immediate symptom typically associated with a specific and identifiable illness or injury and is generally alleviated once the problem is gone. Chronic pain is more enduring, and is often not associated with a specific medical problem. We gain useful insights if we explore the physiological mechanisms of acute and chronic pain.

The Peripheral Nervous System and Pain

Nerves that carry sense impulses (what we see, feel, hear, smell, etc.) to the spine and brain are called peripheral nerves. There are at least two types of peripheral nerve fibers that appear to carry pain messages. A-delta nerve fibers carry impulses at a modest highway speed, perhaps 40 mph. In contrast, C-fibers carry pain impulses at the pace of a stroll, 3 mph. A-fibers quickly inform the brain of pain.

Imagine you are at home with your niece. Suddenly she grabs your hand very tightly, squeezing your fingers together, and you experience a stab of A-fiber pain. This rapid response is highly desirable in order to avoid a serious injury. Slower, chronic pain is more likely to be conveyed by C-fibers, and it is often experienced as discomfort or a dull, cramping, burning, or aching pain. As your niece continues to cling, the quick stab of pain becomes more of an aching, C-fiber pain. Most patients think of their pain as "acute" with a specific cause, even though in fact it may be chronic with ambiguous or indeterminate physical pathology. Many patients may not realize that pain can be real even though there is no tissue damage or injury.

Patients may think of pain as a simple direct result of injury. According to the traditional model, for example, one stubs one's toe, and nerves carry pain messages to the brain. Or using more formal language, the peripheral nervous system (chapter 3) carries pain messages to the brain. Pain continues until the injured body part heals, or the assaulting stimulus goes away. *Although this idea seems to make sense, it is no longer accepted by the experts.* There is more to pain than stubbed toes. Why is it that while talking to your friend during a walk, you may not even notice you have injured yourself? Or that athletes frequently continue playing, not realizing they have been injured? It is not that they have exceptional courage or powers of concentration; they are simply not experiencing the pain of an injury. These are clues that there is more to pain than input from tissue damage.

The Brain/Spinal Cord and Pain

Endorphins and Pain

Pain signals move from A and C fibers to the spinal cord and up to the brain. On their way to the brain, they proceed through the brain stem. Here, the production of special natural morphine-like chemicals can deaden pain. These substances are called endorphins and are chemically very similar to powerful, addictive, narcotic painkillers such as morphine. Narcotics work by blocking the sensitivity to pain of certain nerve cells in the brain. In fact, the word "endorphin" means "endogenous i.e., produced within the body) morphine." Many type of activities can trigger the natural release of endorphins, including stress, strong external stimulation, vigorous exercise, strong emotional excitement, sexual arousal, and deep relaxation. Perhaps the injured basketball player does not experience the pain of her injured ankle because of the excitement, exertion, and stimulation, of the game.

Emotions, the Brain, and Pain

Once they have passed the brain stem, pain signals are further processed by the cerebral cortex and the brain's emotion centers. A-fiber impulses tend to go directly and quickly to the cortex. In the cortex, action decisions are made and executed; one quickly decides what to do (pull one's hand out of the fire, for example). The slower C-fiber impulses go not only to the cortex, but to the brain's stress center, the hypothalamus, and to the emotion centers,the thalamus and the amygdala. As a result, lingering C-fiber pain is more likely to evoke the stress engine, or fight or flight response, discussed in chapter 3, and evoke sustained negative emotion, such as anxiety, depression, or anger.

The moment your niece squeezes your fingers hard, your immediate reaction may be to experience a stab of pain and try to pull your hand away. This is the relatively quick A-fiber-to-cortex pathway we just described. As your niece continues to squeeze, the pain not only shifts to a strong ache (C-fiber pain), but you may feel anger and irritation, and think negative thoughts like "this kid is very rude!" Here, both the brain's thinking and emotion centers are reacting to C-fiber input. If you are experiencing negative emotions, including anxiety, depression, or anger (involving parts of the cortex related to memory as well as parts of the thalamus and amygdala related to emotion), these emotions can sensitize and amplify pain. If you are in a bad mood, perhaps because of a disappointing work evaluation, your niece's hand grab is even more painful.

Attention, the Brain, and Pain

The brain is involved in pain in a different way. Earlier in chapter 3 we noted the importance of the front part of the brain, the prefrontal cortex, in directing and sustaining attention to desired tasks. The spotlight of attention can increase or decrease pain. Put simply, when we focus on pain, pain increases. When we focus on something else, pain decreases. An important part of pain management involves training the brain to sustain attention on a desired task, and thereby not on the pain itself.

The Gate-Control Theory of Pain

There is even more to the story of pain. And we have left the most interesting part for last—what happens to pain between the incoming peripheral A- and C-fiber and the brain. Remember the overall nervous system pathway—nerve impulses travel from peripheral nerves to the spinal cord and up through the brain stem into the brain. We have considered the peripheral A- and C-fiber paths as well as the brain and brain stem. The intermediate part of this journey is the spinal cord. In the spinal cord are special nerve fiber bundles that serve as gateways to the brain. These gates control whether or not a pain stimulus gets to the brain and can alter how pain messages proceed. The relative mix of stimulus input (from pain, sense organs, the brain, emotions, endorphins, etc.) can open or close the pain gates. By altering the mix of stimulus input, you can control much of the experience of pain. This is known as "gate-control theory" (Melzack & Wall, 1965, 1982).

It is easy to see how the pain gates can alter our experience of both acute and chronic pain. Consider our example of your finger-grabbing niece. Just as she grabs your finger, she giggles and distracts you. You do not notice her fingers squeezing yours. The distraction initially closes the pain gates. Imagine she also plants a wonderful, smiling kiss on your cheek. You are filled with love and appreciation, and do not notice the pain. Thoughts and feelings in the brain ("I love that kid! She's so wonderful!") also close the pain gates. While continuing to grab your fingers, she then hugs you with her other arm. Sensations from the hug override the pain sensations from your hand, continue to keep the pain gates closed, and you continue not to feel the pain. She lets go of your hand, and you notice that your fingers are white and there is a thumbprint on your wrist. By now, your brain realizes that the hand grab was completely innocent and you are not injured. What might otherwise be experienced as pain is instead experienced as a strong tingling sensation. The brain, thinking "this is not serious," closes the pain gates once again.

Imagine this same incident, but with one difference that causes the pain gates to open. You are resting on your sofa with your hand and arm dangling over the side, close to the floor. Suddenly you feel something clench on your fingers and wrist. Not knowing what it is, you feel a stab of pain. You think

"Oh no, Fido is biting me!" And the pain grows stronger. You feel a shot of fear over possible infection, and the pain grows even more intense. Your attention is immediately drawn to your hand and the danger it is in, increasing the pain. In this example, thoughts, feelings, and peripheral stimulation open pain gates. (Just to provide a positive ending, let's imagine you turn to look at Fido and discover it is just your niece again. You laugh, and the pain goes away, hastened by a shot of laughter-triggered endorphins. The pain gates close.)

To summarize the useful idea of gate-control theory: Special gates in the spine determine when and how we experience pain. Our thoughts, emotions, endorphins, and directed attention, as well as incoming sensory stimuli from the outside, can open or close the pain gates.

Nonrelaxation Approaches to Pain Management

Many professional options are available for managing pain. A variety of pharmacological agents including narcotics (which operate on the central nervous system) and non-narcotics (which do not). Narcotics include morphine and heroin-like substances and non-narcotics include aspirin and other nonsteroidal anti-inflammatory drugs (NSAIDs), many of which are available over the counter. Unlike narcotics, non-narcotics predominantly operate at the injury site, presumably by inhibiting prostaglandin, a chemical that sensitizes peripheral nerves to pain. Such medications are at times supplemented with agents to reduce anxiety, depression, and muscle tension.

An equally diverse set of non-pharmacological approaches may be used to manage pain. The oldest approach, sensory stimulation, involves stimulating the spinal cord or brain, perhaps by massage, heat packs, cold packs, acupuncture, or superficial electrical stimulation. In terms of gate-control theory, all of these approaches involve increasing peripheral nervous system sensory input to the spinal cord, causing spinal pain gates to close to peripheral pain sensations.

Other non-pharmacological approaches include physical therapy, physical fitness training, hypnosis, biofeedback, cognitive-behavioral approaches, and relaxation. Physical therapy is appropriate for individuals who have a correctable physical impairment that can be improved through specific exercises. A simple example would be a housewife who experiences back pain; a simple physical therapy routine might involve teaching her to walk in a way that reduces back pain.

Simple physical fitness exercises can be effective for some pain problems by reducing some of the physical causes of pain, evoking brain endorphins, and perhaps generating peripheral exercise-related stimulation that may block pain via the spinal pain gates. In general, a healthy body is less prone to painful illness.

Hypnosis involves a trained professional who works with a client in a relaxing setting to enhance the effects of direct suggestion. Once (two centuries ago), hypnosis involved an imposing authoritarian Freud-like hypnotist ordering dramatic, hypnotic commands to a passively compliant client. Today, hypnosis may be authoritarian or non-authoritarian in which client and hypnotist are partners working to explore the possibilities of suggestion. Biofeedback involves external electronic body sensors that can detect signs of change in blood pressure, breathing perspiration, muscle tension, and even brain wave activity. Sensor readings are processed by a computer, and may help clients determine sources of pain and effective approaches to relaxation.

Negative emotions such as anxiety, depression, and anger increase sensitivity to and aggravate pain. Cognitive-behavioral approaches to therapy and stress management are highly effective tools for managing negative emotions. The "four pillars" of such approaches include: relaxation, problem-solving, cognitive restructuring of needless negative thinking, and desensitization/exposure approaches (see Smith, 2002). I strongly recommend this approach as a supplement to relaxation. Cognitive-behavioral approaches can be applied directly to pain. For example, one might:

- Identify specific early warning signs or cues that a potential pain-evoking situation is present or that pain is about to begin. This is the time to take action, by relaxing, coping, or removing the potentially pain-inducing problem.
- Identify hidden rewards for pain, and replace them with rewards for coping. When experiencing pain, we often seek and receive attention and support from others. This may help, but it can serve to reinforce the pain (we unconsciously feel pain again in order to get the good-feeling support). Although social support can be valuable, it can be even more useful when applied to coping. It is preferable to receive praise and support from others for a new strategy you have used to deal with pain, than for simply suffering from pain.
- Identify and change environmental pain-supports. Cold weather, tight-fitting clothes, uncomfortable chairs, and having to stand for long periods of time are just a few of the many environmental conditions that can contribute to pain.

RELAXATION AND PAIN MANAGEMENT

Each of the six families of relaxation offer concrete opportunities for pain management. Relaxation training can affect pain in a variety of ways and involves all of the pain mechanisms we have discussed: generating pain-blocking endorphins, evoking pain-blocking positive emotion, directing attention away from pain, and closing the spinal pain gates with stimulation from the brain and the peripheral nervous system.

The relaxation response, access skills, and psychological R-States can all have an effect on pain. Through trophotropic tuning (chapter 3), one's parasympathetic nervous system (responsible for recovery and rest) becomes more dominant and one is "tuned" more for relaxation, and less for stress and pain. Specific access skills can each contribute to reduced pain: stretching and adjusting posture or position, reducing skeletal muscle tension, relaxing breathing, reducing cognitive autonomic arousal, reducing stressed body focus and sustaining effortless/passive simple focus. As one acquires the access skill of sustained effortless/passive simple focus, the ability to calmly attend to a simple task, one also becomes more resistant to distraction, including pain.

R-States evoked through relaxation techniques may impact pain differently. The R-State, Disengagement (feeling "distant, far away, indifferent"), may enhance detachment from pain. Because of the role of physical tension in pain, Physical Relaxation is clearly desirable in pain reduction. The R-States, Rested/Refreshed and Energized, may enhance the direction of attention to and involvement in activities that can distract one from pain. Joy, Childlike Innocence, Thankfulness and Love, and perhaps most other R-States, can be considered positive states that may block pain impulses. Selfless R-States (Mental Quiet, Childlike Innocence, and Thankful/Loving), as well as spiritual and transcendent states (Deep Mystery, Awe and Wonder, Prayerful, Time-less/Boundless/Infinite) may reduce pain-enhancing self-directed attention and preoccupation. Spiritual and transcendent states also provide a powerful external focus (perhaps one's God or Higher Power) for diverting attention from pain or giving pain a new and more tolerable meaning. Such R-States may also distract one from pain-augmenting catastrophic thinking.

Yogaform Stretching

Traditional hatha yoga should be applied with caution to pain patients because some exercises can augment pain. I recommend consulting a physical thera-pist. Simple stretches may reduce joint symptoms (for example, those associated with arthritis or injury) and skeletal muscle tension. Yoga may be applied in rehabilitation to reduce patterns of posture and movement that contribute to chronic pain. I recommend supplementing stretching with PMR, imagery, and to a lesser extent autogenic training, breathing, and meditation. Research suggests that yogaform stretching enhances the R-State, Energized. When yoga is a preparation for subsequent activity, it may reduce pain by facilitating full engagement in the activity and resistance to distraction. Sustained yoga postures may facilitate diverting attention away from pain.

Progressive Muscle Relaxation

Progressive muscle relaxation (PMR), along with imagery, are the most widely applied approaches to pain management through relaxation. However, PMR must be presented cautiously. Deliberately creating tension in skeletal muscles can aggravate tension associated with pain. Thus, overt PMR exercises should be avoided or taught with caution whenever there is a possibility of present or previous injury or weakness of the skeletal muscles, bones, joints, ligaments, or nerve tissue. Whenever a client complains that an exercise increases pain, the exercise should be terminated. However, one may try minimal PMR or the completely passive version of PMR, a "letting go" exercise in which one releases tension without first tensing up.

There are several good reasons for using PMR for appropriate patients. First, physical tension, or tension of the striated muscles, can aggravate the sensation of pain, opening pain gates and directing attention to an area of pain. Second, patients often unwittingly react to pain by clenching, gripping, bracing, or generating muscle tension. Such self-created tension can become chronic and undetected, thus continuously contributing to sustained pain. One of the primary goals of PMR is to discover such hidden sources of tension before attempting tension release. Third, negative emotional states that aggravate pain are often accompanied by increased tension; and reducing muscle tension can impact negative emotions. In general, patients often experience a self-sustaining cycle of pain–muscle tension–pain, in which pain creates tension, tension aggravates pain, which in turn creates more tension. PMR is perhaps one of the most effective tools for breaking this cycle. Finally, PMR has a demonstrated impact on increasing the R-States, Disengagement and Physical Relaxation, both of which may assist in pain management.

Autogenic Training

Autogenic exercises are similar to PMR in that they are directed to physical sensations. Warmth and heaviness suggestions primarily involve blood flow to skeletal muscles and the skin. However, cardiac and abdominal warmth exercises also target the involuntary internal organs associated with sustained arousal. For some clients, especially those who dislike the overt movement of PMR, autogenic exercises can be highly effective tools for breaking the pain cycle described above. Both verbal ("warm and heavy hands") and visual ("warm hand in the sun or sand") exercises can enhance the effects of visual imagery in directing attention away from and redefining pain. Suggestions of "warmth and heaviness" can redefine a painful experience to one associated with relaxation. I speculate that autogenic training, like PMR, enhances Disengagement and Physical Relaxation.

Breathing Exercises

Breathing exercises combined with yoga stretches are rarely applied in pain management. However, diaphragmatic breathing and passive breathing exercises (breathing through lips, sniffing, blowing, deep breathing, and focused breathing) can be useful portable techniques for reducing tension, diverting attention, and augmenting the effects of PMR and imagery. One can tense up while breathing in, and breathe out while releasing tension. The act of breathing out can be thought of in terms of "breathing out pain." Breathing exercises, like yogaform stretching, can evoke the R-State, Energized.

Imagery

As mentioned above, imagery is deployed widely in pain management. I speculate that it has potential for evoking strong positive R-States and modest levels of Disengagement and Physical Relaxation. The involvement of such R-States can be seen in two general types of imagery application: pain-directed imagery plus self-talk, and traditional sense and insight imagery.

Pain-Directed Imagery Plus Self-Talk

Imagery specifically involving pain can redefine the experience of pain. (McCaul & Malott, 1984). Here the target of attention of is pain; however, a visual image is selected that lessens its impact. This image is enhanced by self-talk repetition of supportive words and phrases.

Numerous imagery techniques are routinely recommended in pain-management texts (Blanchard & Andrasik, 1985; Hansen & Gerber, 1990; Martin, 1993; Philips & Rachman, 1996; Turk & Gatchel, 2002). We review those that are the most frequently deployed.

Learning from pain as teacher. The meaning of pain influences its severity and impact. Knowing your beloved niece is squeezing your hand makes the pain tolerable, more so than the belief that Fido is biting your hand. Often pain patients think of their pain as a terrible and unfair intrusion on life, one with no meaning other than the disruption it causes. Actually, pain can have its positive side. In imagery, one can think of pain as a teacher, a source of insight or options. One might even personify pain in imagery, picturing a "pain teacher" who has a lesson to learn. The lesson may be a concrete coping action ("get more involved with others"), a shift in one's philosophy of life ("accept what is and don't fret about that which cannot be changed"), or perhaps religious insight ("this pain is relatively unimportant in light of God's love and plan for me").

Surviving the pain challenge. Pain can be seen as a survival challenge to "endure without resistance" (Hanson & Gerber, 1990). Key to this image is the notion of facing an unavoidable source of discomfort, and enduring it as best one can. The discomfort must be time-limited. Imagine living in tornado country. The alarm goes off, you go to the underground shelter, and wait for the tornado to pass. While waiting, you take deep breaths, and tell yourself "just hold on, this will be over soon." Then the tornado passes. One might imagine participating in a special sport, or television stunt show where you must put up with a certain degree of pain in order to survive.

Beating the pain enemy. Occasionally, the image of pain as the enemy can help. One might imagine various sources of pain, a dragon or monster for example. And one might rehearse self-statements of encouragement: "Don't let the pain win. Keep calm and cool. Pain will wear itself out and you can go on with your life."

Creating a positive pain situation. One might imagine changing the situational context of pain to a situation where pain has meaning and the situation is interesting or important. One might visualize the pain resulting from:

- Completing a dangerous spy mission: "My arm was hit as I grabbed the spy's notes."
- Engaging in vigorous sports: "While tossing the basketball, I stretched my arm."

- Heroically helping someone: "While saving the child from falling into the lake, I injured my hand."

Imagining a different, modifiable cause. If a patient is preoccupied with thoughts about some diagnosed or undetected medical condition that causes a pain, this imagined cause serves to aggravate and prolong the pain. One is repeating a message that "pain will not change because the cause is unchanging." One might modify pain by visualizing a different plausible cause, and then altering it. For example, someone suffering from arthritic wrist pain may visualize painfully heavy weights on one's wrist, which one visualizes slowly removing. One might imagine rubber bands painfully wrapped around one's wrist, and then visualize slowly cutting the bands, one by one.

Changing one's pain descriptor. Often the words and pictures people use to describe their pain are in themselves aversive, and can thereby magnify pain. Examples of aversive words include:

- Aching
- Stabbing
- Burning
- Pinching
- Binding
- Cutting

Aversive images include:

- Being burned
- Being cut with a knife
- Being poked with a needle
- Being bitten by a dog

Through imagery, one can rehearse replacement words and images that more or less describe the pain, but are not aversive. One might think, for example:

- Pain is cold, like an ice cube pressing my skin.
- Pain is a strong pressure, like a weight
- Pain is dull and numb, like the doctor has injected the pained part with a painkiller

Imagining an object not associated with pain. One might imagine an afflicted body part as an object not associated with pain:

- My hand is like a book, heavy and feeling no pain.
- This arm is not mine, so I do not feel the pain.

Imagining anesthesia. A patient might be instructed to imagine the injection of a powerful painkilling drug, or the application of a painkilling salve.

Self-healing touch. A patient first might be taught to visualize numbness or insensitivity in a hand (providing the hand is not in pain). Once the hand is numb, the patient can then touch an area afflicted with pain and imagine a transfer of imagined pain-reducing properties. For example, a headache patient might first imagine their right hand very cold and numb. They could then touch their head with this hand and imagine the sensations of cold migrating to the head.

Modifying a pain-associated image. A patient can be encouraged to select a visual image that represents pain, for example, a burning red flame or an iceberg. Then the selected image can be gradually modified in a way symbolic of reduced pain. One might image a pain growing smaller, or an iceberg slowly melting.

Imagining a brain pain mechanism. Any of the pain mechanisms we have discussed can be crafted into a visual image for diverting attention from pain. One might imagine:

- The pain gates closing, one by one
- Endorphins secreted by the brain entering the blood stream, closing "pain padlocks"
- The brain's attentional spotlight directed away from pain toward another target stimulus
- The brain's positive-emotion centers secreting comforting and soothing feelings that dissolve pain.

Sense and Insight Imagery

Both sense and insight imagery as described in this book can provide a diversion from pain, possibly evoke pain-blocking positive states, and provide a meaningful context that can reduce pain. Sense imagery involves creating a peaceful setting or situation in which one simply enjoys relaxing sensations. One deliberately includes suggestions of what one sees, feels, hears, and smells. There is no task or objective. One simply enjoys resting on the beach, floating on a raft, sitting on a couch by the fireplace, and so on. Often stimuli can be introduced to soothe or redefine pain sensations ("The warm heat of the fireplace soothes your arm"). The powerful tool of deepening imagery (see chapter 19), in which an image begins relatively discursive and energetic and ends up effortless, singular, and focused, can be used to gently move one away from painful thoughts and increase diverted attention. The range of sense imagery themes is as varied as relaxation in everyday life.

Insight imagery involves a simple relaxing story. One begins by enjoying a relaxing setting in which there is a path. The client travels this path to a special wisdom place, where one finds a guiding person or object (pond, flower, religious symbol, mysterious box, star). One then asks the guide a question about pain: "What is the deeper meaning of pain for me? What is its lesson for me?" Then one meditatively lets answers come and go, as in contemplation (see chapter 24).

Meditation

This book presents a variety of approaches to concentrative and mindfulness mediation. No single approach is best for everyone. All approaches to meditation can divert attention from pain, evoke pain-blocking positive states, and provide a meaning for pain.

In concentrative meditation one focuses on a selected target stimulus, such as an external candle flame or internal mantra. For a pain patient, feelings of pain may well become the primary distraction. Here one treats pain as one would treat any other distraction. With complete indifference, one simply redirects one's attention from the pain back to the target focus of meditation. This may happen hundreds of times in a session. Reassure the trainee that meditative focus comes through practice and is like building a muscle by lifting weights. It is acceptable if pain continues as "background noise" as one sustains attention on one's target focus. Through such a strategy of detachment, one can "decouple" pain sensations from emotional distress, thus reducing suffering even in the presence of painful sensory input.

A variety of images can be used to illustrate this crucial strategy of repeatedly diverting attention away from pain in a calm, nonjudgmental, nonobsessive, noncatastrophizing way:

Treat a pain distraction as any other trivial distraction, for example, a dog may bark in the distance, temporarily disrupting

your attention. When you realize you have been disrupted, simply
return to your meditation without fuss. Pain is like a little
child demanding attention. Just give it a pat on the head, and
continue with your meditation.

Mindfulness meditation offers an unusual strategy for dealing with pain.
Recall that with mindfulness meditation one does not select a target focus,
such as a candle flame or mantra, but calmly and nonjudgmentally attends
to whatever stimulus comes or goes. One is a calm and silent observer of
all sensations that float by. This river of sensations includes pain sensations.

In mindfulness meditation, one calmly and simply attends to a pain sensation whenever it emerges. One attends as along as the sensation attracts
attention, until another stimulus floats by. Most important, one does not think
about or work with any sensation in any way. One does not try to:

- Hold on to a pleasant non-painful sensation
- Figure out pain, or push pain away
- Judge how awful the pain is
- Evaluate whether the pain is less or more intense than before
- Assess if the pain is really serious
- Figure out what the medical cause of the pain might be
- Evaluate how effective meditation is in reducing pain.

One doesn't think at all about the pain. Instead, one quietly attends to
whatever sensation pops into mind. If that sensation is pain, fine. If that
sensation is the smell of coffee, fine. If that sensation is the pressure of your
feet against the floor, fine. If that sensation is the sound of the wind, fine.
If that sensation is the grumbling in your stomach, fine. If that sensation is
a small melody in your mind, fine. Just attend without thought or judgement,
until another sensation moves in on its own. You don't even make a thoughtful
decision to move your attention from pain to another sensation or from
another sensation to pain. You are just a mirror, attending to whatever may
come or go.

Intense pain is often experienced as "solid" or unchanging, a perception
that contributes to further suffering. One can use mindfulness meditation to
counter this perception by attending to the changing sensation of pain, noting
variations in quality, intensity, and duration.

Both concentrative and mindfulness meditation work best after 15 or 20
minutes of physical relaxation, perhaps yogaform stretching, PMR, autogenic

training, or breathing. Through trial and error a client can decide which approach or combination works best.

I also recommend occasionally alternating insight imagery with meditative approaches to pain management. Together, these approaches can be mutually reinforcing and deepening. We will discuss how these two approaches become synergistic in the final chapter, Spirituality, Religion, and Relaxation.

24

Spirituality, Religion, and Relaxation

The role of psychology in religion has inspired much passion and discussion. Generally, there have been three points of view. Some psychologists consider religion to be a pathological obsession with irrational superstitions. Others embrace various versions of the supernatural and paranormal, and seek to understand and possibly enhance the perceived benefits of such beliefs. Third are those who avoid theological and metaphysical questions altogether, and as objective outside observers study the effects of religious belief.

My approach might be considered a fourth way. Let's begin by acknowledging that every major religion has a "great treasure chest" of beliefs and practices. Some, but certainly not all, of these beliefs have supernatural/paranormal aspects.[1] It is useful to begin with a definition:

> The supernatural/paranormal consists of that which is beyond the realm of normal scientific inquiry, has a nonmaterial influence on what we consider desirable or undesirable, and cannot conceivably be disproved through science. This includes notions of (a) an external, intervening god who exists, at least in part, beyond the natural universe and who can violate the laws of physics and change the course of events (through miracles or answered prayers); (b) reincarnation, whereby a nonmaterial entity (the soul) progresses, complete with retained, but sometimes incomplete, memory, from life to life; (c) nonmaterial, miraculous, and magical forces that have a positive or negative influence (on greater strength and health,

331

increased wisdom, higher consciousness, more love, justice, etc.); and (d) karma, that good and bad actions, through nonmaterial means, have positive or negative material consequences in this life and the next.

Most believers have no trouble identifying an interventionist deity, reincarnation, miraculous and magical powers, and karma as "transcending" normal science or as having a potential for good. However, these supernatural/ paranormal ideas are beyond disproof for one simple reason: any challenge can be readily argued away. For example, consider the righteous and devout believer who prays for health, yet succumbs to cancer. Is this evidence against a loving, all-powerful, intervening God? To the believer, this is evidence of nothing, and spiritual counselors can draw from a large number of explanations: "God gives us freedom by not intervening." "God is punishing us for some sin we forgot." "God is teaching us a lesson." "The answer will come in ways you do not expect." "God helps those who help themselves." "God encompasses both good and evil." "God is preparing us, through adversity, for the wonders of the afterlife." "God is simply saying 'no' to our prayer." "We only see this as an unanswered prayer because our minds are so small." "This is all part of God's greater plan." All of these I have heard and read from eminent church leaders. God intervenes physically to answer prayer, and this belief simply cannot be challenged. In the same way, belief in reincarnation, miracles, magic, and karma cannot be challenged.

---

[1]Some may object to linking the concepts "supernatural" and "paranormal." I respect that psychics may not want to appear on the same page as priests and preachers, who in turn may not wish to be bedfellows with psychics. Of course, both groups do have important, unique concerns. In addition, the supernatural does indeed connote a higher power, a larger consciousness, a universal mind; the paranormal connotes events that cannot currently be explained by contemporary science. However, in real life, the distinction between the supernatural and the paranormal is blurred. One can find accounts of the paranormal (miracles, healing, precognitions, resurrections, etc.) in just about every Holy Book (supernatural). Many who believe in the supernatural cite such paranormal feats as supporting evidence. Furthermore, those paranormal phenomena that spark public imagination (and often reported in many contemporary publications and by many churches outside the mainstream traditions) often are tinged with the supernatural. Why is it that some paranormal claims are rarely mentioned today, for example, that bodily essences or fluids are the source of emotional disorders, that the womb can wander in a woman's body? These same claims are resistant to supernatural interpretation. In contrast, other paranormal claims have endured, for example, the notion that one can communicate with the dead, cure illnesses through distant communication, see into the future, read minds, and so on. For each of these, proponents can invoke (at least as an option) a supernatural explanation. Communication with the dead is possible because some individuals never fully reach the afterlife. One can miraculously cure illness by tapping into a great universal healing force. One can see into the future and read minds by tapping into a universal consciousness. Although such supernatural notions are perhaps not as developed as traditional theology, they are still supernatural. Whether we like it or not, religion, as it is practiced today, is both supernatural and paranormal.

Although supernatural/paranormal beliefs may contribute to relaxation by inspiring sustained effortless/passive simple focus, and possibly all fifteen R-States, such beliefs are not a prerequisite for profound relaxation or even spiritual or transcendent experience. Furthermore, I believe it is unwise, and perhaps unethical, for health professionals to claim expertise in realms of the supernatural and paranormal. This role is properly left to priests preachers, and psychics.

However, I do believe we have something of value to say concerning the contents of the great treasure chest of religion that are not intrinsically supernatural/paranormal, for these beliefs and practices can be profoundly valid for both believer and skeptic alike. Also, I will freely use the word "God" and leave it to the reader to fill in the blank, recognizing that in all cases a naturalistic interpretation (God as "inner spirit," "creative unconscious," "flow of being," "higher power," or simply "all sources of life and growth beyond my ego") works just fine.

SPIRITUALITY, RELIGION, AND HEALTH

To begin, there is empirical evidence that personal spirituality, and its manifestation in organized religion, may correlate with physical health and psychological well-being (Hill & Pargament, 2003; Pargament, 1997). How this pattern should be interpreted is ambiguous. Perhaps those who are already healthy and happy are more involved with religion and spirituality, or perhaps religion and spirituality contribute to health and happiness.

Hill and Pargament (2003) propose several mechanisms through which religion and spirituality may enhance health. Some of these mechanisms, such as building support networks and healthy lifestyle habits, are also provided by many secular organizations.

Other mechanisms may be associated with the very nature of religious and spiritual experience. Pargament and Hill conceptualize spirituality as "a search for the sacred," a veneration of that part of life "apart from the ordinary," that is, "God, the divine, Ultimate Reality, and the transcendent" (Pargament, 1997; Hill & Pargament, 2003). Religion and spirituality may enable one to:

- Recognize deeper orienting, motivating, and prompting forces. Such forces enable one to see life in spiritual terms and provide meaning and purpose to oneself and one's activities.
- Feel close to and perhaps experience God. This is sometimes, but not always, associated with feeling a working relationship with an

anthropomorphic God, or simply feeling connected to a greater natural Universe.

Richards and Bergin (1997) suggest a variety of ways of integrating client religious beliefs and practices into treatment, and for our purposes, relaxation. These involve helping clients affirm their spiritual identity, explore how their religion may be a resource, and resolve spiritual concerns related to problems they may have. The activities suggested in this chapter generally address these goals.

However, these are risky waters and one must tread lightly. Those who advocate religion and spirituality need to recognize that fervent promoters have at times promised more than can be delivered. It is tragic when deeply religious parents turn to faithful prayer and deprive their children of medical treatments that can cure deadly diseases. Is it any more ethical for a health professional to direct a client to religion and spirituality for relaxation? Do we risk setting into motion a self-defeating cycle, a "religiosity trap" in which frustration with the fruits of faith contribute to renewed religious zeal, which may be followed by continued frustration, leading to even more zeal, and so on?

This can happen more easily than one might think. Imagine a troubled client who sees a therapist and wants to feel more "inner peace." During the course of therapy, she mentions an interest in various types of prayer and shares that she has been a member of a church for all of her life but quit attending a few years ago. The therapist, believing in the power of relaxation as well as religion and spirituality, gently notes that prayers and church involvement can have a relaxing effect. Taking this as encouragement, the client returns to church, takes a class on prayer, but does not experience her desired "inner peace." Her pastor counsels that "God is all-powerful and answers all prayer," and that as her faith deepens with continued prayer, "God will answer" and she will be at peace. The client continues practicing with increased fervor, again with no effect. She returns to her therapist, who now is in ethical dilemma. He feels responsible for indirectly encouraging her to seek a religious answer, but is utterly unqualified to give religious counsel. What can he say? "God as an all-powerful supernatural entity does not exist." "God is in your mind, something Jungian." "God is telling you to seek answers in yourself and in therapy." "God does not act on our terms." "You belong to the wrong religion." Virtually any answer consistent with his initial subtle religious encouragement requires abandoning the role of objective therapist and taking on the role of pastor, and even making statements about the nature and behavior what is supernatural/paranormal.

Here's a summary of how I introduce religion, spirituality, and relaxation:

Secular psychologists (social workers, counselors, psychiatrists) are not qualified to consider matters of the supernatural and paranormal. However, we recognize that many spiritual activities can be profoundly meaningful and contribute to relaxation, regardless of one's religious orientation. Similarly, music, dance, and poetry are not the exclusive property of any one religion, but can be profoundly meaningful in any religion as well as in the secular world. The techniques we can explore are like music, dance, and poetry. They can work for both faithful and nonfaithful alike. Are you interested in exploring some of these techniques?

SPIRITUALITY AND R-STATES

Thirty years of teaching six families of relaxation to thousands of clients has taught me a lesson. Two levels of R-States, spiritual and transcendent, can emerge spontaneously for any relaxation technique. Spiritual R-States are associated with experiencing a larger, greater "other." Our one transcendent R-State involves just a selfless awareness of this larger, greater other. For purposes of simplicity, we will consider both spiritual and transcendent levels of R-States as "spiritual." They include Deep Mystery, Awe and Wonder, Prayerful, and Timeless/Boundless/Infinite.

Often, relaxation practitioners and trainers alike discount these experiences as interesting, but passing, phenomena. I acknowledge spiritual R-States as having potential meaning and importance. All of the exercises we consider have this as one objective.

When spirituality becomes one's ultimate concern, the remaining R-States can be viewed in terms of preparing the way. To review, I define Level 1 of the R-State Pyramid as Stress Relief. It includes the R-States, Sleepiness, Disengagement, Rested/Refreshed, and Energized. Level 2 is Pleasure and Joy including Physical Relaxation, At Ease/Peace, and Joy (happiness). Levels 1 and 2 provide a foundation for spiritual exploration in that they reflect a release of diverting tensions and openness to new experience. Each R-State prepares us in a different way, by enabling us to recover from fatigue, providing energy and stamina, and beginning the process of exploring worlds of happiness and beauty based on but going beyond simple physical relaxation.

Level 3, Positive Selflessness is closer to spirituality. Here, anything self-centered is a diversion from God-centered or meditative focus. However,

Level 3, Positive Selflessness, is not defined in such negative terms as renouncing compulsive urges, resisting pride, practicing humility or obedient submission, painful renunciation of things the ego may desire, or self-inflicted penance for perceived sins.

Instead, we consider three positive, selfless R-States. Mental Quiet is the simple absence of thought and emotion, both negative and positive. One's mind is completely still, without activity. Even the feelings of "peace" or "rest" are quieted. In a quiet mind, all thought is still, including all self-directed thought. In this sense, quiet is selfless.

Childlike Innocence is the carefree and spontaneous release of burdensome adult-role responsibilities. Such burdens are intrinsically self-centered ("The weight of the world, my family, my future . . . is on MY shoulders.") Of course, no legitimate religion or system of spirituality advocates irresponsible living. However, there is no need to carry the burden of adulthood 24 hours a day, as one's permanent ball and chain. It is often the better part of wisdom to "let go and let God" and become like "the lilies of the field," to trust in forces beyond oneself.

The R-State, Thankful/Loving involves a selfless expression of gratitude, or compassion, towards another. Doing this is a selfless act of directing one's concerns outside of oneself toward the other.

Most systems of spiritual practice recognize the emergence of high levels of R-State as "signs" of spiritual movement or readiness for advanced exercises. At the risk of insulting the growing congregation of guides and gurus, let me propose that the preparatory significance of any specific R-State, or sequence of R-States, is an open, empirical question. For example, we simply do not know if feelings of Thankfulness and Love, or feelings of Deep Mystery, mean one is ready to practice any specific technique.

With this caveat, the R-State Pyramid can be seen in the context of a client's religious beliefs. For example, the R-State, At Ease/Peace, can be the sense of comfort that one is in God's hands. Thankful/Loving can be the expression of deep gratitude for God's forgiveness of sins. Childlike Innocence can be the innocence of Jesus as a child. Awe and Wonder might be the experience of God's power and judgment. Prayfulness can be the experience of confronting an all-powerful anthropomorphic deity. Timeless/Boundless/Infinite and Joy might be the anticipation of a promised afterlife. Again, such interpretations and insights should come from the client, not the health professional.

SPIRITUAL EXPRESSION

Exercises as Metaphors and Prayers

Any family of relaxation exercises can be fashioned into a spiritual metaphor and introduced in prayer. For example, yogaform stretching can be described as follows: "Open your arms and hands as if you were opening to an embracing God." The tense-release cycles of PMR can be expressed as "Hold on to your worries or concerns . . . let go, release them to God." Autogenic training might be expressed thus: "Feel God's loving warmth and comfort supporting you." Breathing could include: "Breathe in the breath of God, the energy of God." Imagery might suggest: "Imagine the story of [insert favorite Holy Book story]." Concentrative meditation might use the phrases: "Let the word 'God' (or Jesus, Buddha, Ghandi, Love, Hillel, etc.) float through your mind." Mindfulness meditation might ask the client to: "Put your judging ego aside and attend to God's world. Do not select anything to attend to; let God do this for you; let God select and draw your attention to parts of the wonders of the universe God wants you to experience."

The Cycle of Renewal

The cycle of renewal is a universal process of healing and growth that involves three stages: withdrawal, recovery, and opening up. One withdraws from the stresses and pressures of the outside world, recuperates and regenerates, and then returns to the world, awakened and energized, open to new challenges and experiences. The simplest prototype of this cycle is the simple nap. Here one withdraws into slumber, experiences the regenerative effects of sleep, and awakens to face the world. This same cycle appears in religious literature from simple activities such as weekly worship services, the spiritual retreat, prayer, and meditation, to encompassing concepts of death and resurrection as well as detachment and enlightenment.

One can select from the six families of relaxation exercises a sequence that expresses the cycle of renewal. For withdrawal, one might select PMR, breathing, and concentrative meditation; for recovery, autogenic training, breathing, and imagery with a recovery theme might be best; and for opening up, imagery with openness to experience as its theme, yogaform stretching, and mindfulness meditation could be effective.

These can be fashioned into a "cycle of renewal" exercise, as follows:

Cycle of Renewal Exercise

In this exercise we will take a journey through the cycle of renewal. Our goal is to put aside the pressures of the day and withdraw into relaxation. We then experience the healing forces of relaxation. We end by returning to and opening up to the world, renewed and energized.

Withdrawal

First, begin by sitting in a comfortable upright position with your feet flat on the floor. You may close your eyes. Let yourself settle into a position that is comfortable.

Progressive Muscle Relaxation and Breathing. Think of all of the pressures and concerns of the day. Think of how we cling to and hold onto them. Focus on your hands, take a deep breath, and make a tight fist with both hands. Let the tension grow, like you are holding on very tightly. And then let go, gently breathe out, and release the tension. Let the concerns of the day begin to dissolve and flow away with your breath. Let yourself sink into your own private world of relaxation. [REPEAT SIMILAR IN- STRUCTIONS FOR ARMS, SHOULDERS, NECK, FACE, LEGS, AND FEET, IN- TEGRATING BREATHING AND USING THE "BRIEF PMR" INSTRUCTIONS IN THE APPENDIX AS A TEMPLATE]

Recovery

Autogenic Training and Breathing. And let yourself sink into relaxation. Notice the healing warmth and heaviness as blood flows to your hands and fingers. There is nothing you have to do. Imagine healing energies touching your body with warmth and heaviness as you sink deeper into relaxation. Let each outgoing breath carry out the negative energies of fatigue and illness. Let each incoming breath bring life and energy. [CONTINUE WITH SIMILAR IMAGERY]

Imagery. Let yourself enjoy a healing fantasy. Imagine a spe- cial healing light touching your body, starting with your fin- gers and hands. Let this warm glowing light touch your arms and your shoulders. Your neck and face. Your abdomen. Your legs and feet. Let it warm your entire body as you sink deeper and deeper.

You are now in a very special place, a garden of life. You can feel the warm sun bathing your skin. You can see the wonderful flowers and trees all around you. You hear the rustling of leaves, and you smell the fresh scent of grass and leaves. A gentle breeze rises and touches your skin, reminding you that it is time to move on. [CONTINUE, PERHAPS INCORPORATING DEEPENING IMAGERY]

Imagery/Mindfulness. Without thought or judgment, simply attend to all the sights, sounds, and sensations in your inner garden of life. Do not attend to any one thing. Simply let stimuli come and go on their own. Simply attend, let go, and attend.

Mindfulness. Take a deep breath, and very slowly open your eyes, as if a window were slowly opening to a new world. And simply attend to what you see. Let sights come and go on their own, without judgment, without thought.

Yogaform Stretching and Breathing. And we finish with a stretch, to embrace the world. Slowly stand. And slowly raise your arms from your sides to the sky. Open your arms and hands all the way, as if you were greeting the sky and the world. Take in a deep breath, taking in the life and energy of the world. As you exhale, slowly return to standing upright with your arms by your sides. You are now ready to enter the world, renewed and refreshed.

Energies

Perhaps one of the most rudimentary supernatural/paranormal ideas is the concept of spiritual energy. Various traditions, new and old, often claim that certain spiritual energies can be accessed and developed through relaxation. Examples of such energy include: auras, bioenergy, chakras, Qi (chi), prana, color energy, crystal powers, enagrams, healing thought fields, healing touch energy, life force, mantra vibrations, magnetic powers, N-rays, orgone energy, pyramid power, quantum healing energy, and so on. As stated at the beginning of this chapter, we will not discuss the supernatural/paranormal subtleties of these ideas. However, I do believe the experience of spiritual energy is very common and is largely a manifestation of the R-State, Physical Relaxation. It is possible to access this experience with metaphors and images that are not supernatural/paranormal. However, the poetic application of spiritually evocative phrases can be an extremely important part of effective technique presentation, as illustrated in the following exercise script.

Spiritual Body Energy

Spiritual Body Energy (SB Energy) is a powerful inner energy we can actually feel. It is an energy related to stress and relaxation.

Spiritual Body Energy is an inner force of healing and renewal, a force we can all tap into. Scientists might call this force a phenomenological manifestation of parasympathetically mediated peripheral subcutaneous vasodilation. However, putting such technical jargon aside, we can say SB Energy is often related to deep relaxation, increased health, and augmented resistance to disease. SB Energy exists within the parameters of the infinite mysteries and wonders of the natural world. It is a very powerful metaphoric realization, amplified by the remarkable powers of imagination, by fantasies that it may have sources in the mystical realm of the metaphysical. Nevertheless, SB Energy can be accessed through a simple series of "SB Energy Flow" exercises.

SE Exercises involve enhancing the experienced movement of SB Energy in a way that maximizes its effects. It is an approach that involves very slowly and gracefully moving and stretching ones arms, legs, and torso in coordination with an imagined relaxing theme, one that is concrete and observable, such as a tree bending in the wind or waves of the sea. Here is a simple example:

First, stand upright in a comfortable position. We will touch and embrace the spiritual energy of the air and draw it into our bodies, minds, and souls.

Breathe in through the nose. Feel the Spiritual Body energy on the inside of your nostrils as air flows in. Feel the air bring in energy and life.

Exhale, and let the barriers and resistance to this energy dissolve and flow out into the air.

And now, slowly push your hands and arms out in front of you. Imagine you are pushing through the spiritual energy of the air. Attend to your hands and fingers. Let go of any resistance to the flow of energy, and let your hands feel warm and heavy . . . warm and heavy. Imagine you are slowly pushing through a fluid that is smooth and thick. You can feel the warmth against your hands as they slowly slide through the spiritual energy in front of you. Feel the warmth and tingling in the palms of your hands as negative energy flows out through your fingers into the air.

And now, with your hands and arms reaching in front of you, open your fingers all the way, and release any tension and resistance you may feel. Let it flow into the air around.

Then slowly and gently cup your hands, turn your palms so they are pointing toward each other, and begin scooping and pulling the spiritual energy of the air in towards you, towards your chest, towards your heart. Feel the warmth of this energy on your hands. They may tingle a bit. Slowly pull the energy, as if you were scooping and pulling energy in towards your heart.

As you pull the energy in, slowly move your cupped hands to your chest and heart. Very gently place them over your chest and heart. You can feel the warmth of energy on your skin. You can feel the energy move from your hands to your heart. And as you breathe in, you breathe in life and energy.

Hold your hands over your chest. Breathe easily. And you breathe out resistance and tension.

Continue with this exercise, reaching out through the spiritual energy of the air, opening your fingers and releasing the negative energy of the body. Slowly scoop in the positive spiritual energy of the air, and very gently pulling it in to your heart and chest. And every time you touch your heart, feel the energy flow from the air to the center of your being.

And remember, you are one with the universe. You embrace the universe, and the universe embraces you.

CONTEMPLATIVE APPROACHES

Contemplation

Contemplation is concentrative meditation with a purpose. In concentrative meditation, one selects a simple focus, often one that has little meaning, such as a candle flame, and calmly restricts attention to it. All associations, both positive and negative, are without consequence, passing distractions. In contemplation one selects a focal stimulus with meaning, such as a painting or religious symbol. One then meditatively attends to the chosen focal object with the passive goal of understanding it more deeply. However, as with meditation, one does not dwell on any arising association; instead, as in meditation, one lets the associations come and go.

Contemplation is a nonanalytic approach to appreciating something. If you were to analytically appreciate a painting, you might study it, try to figure out when it was created, what the participants in the painting are thinking and doing, and so on. Such an analytic approach involves considerable thought. If you were to contemplate a painting, you would put all such analytic thinking aside, and calmly and simply attend to the painting. You would let the painting stir thoughts and feelings, which you would note, let pass, and return to attending. Contemplation is savoring and appreciating something.

Lectio Divina

Lectio divina is an ancient approach to contemplating a written passage— a poem, paragraph, or prayer. First, select the piece of writing you wish to use. For example, you might select a variant of the "serenity prayer" attributed to many sources, including theologian Reinhold Neibuhr (now in the public domain):

> God, grant me
> the serenity to accept the things I cannot change,
> the courage to change the things I can,
> and the wisdom to know the difference.

Select a quiet place and sit. Let yourself settle down. You may apply breathing relaxation, or try concentrative meditation in which your focus is a word or simple phrase with spiritual meaning, for example, the word "serenity" for the serenity prayer. Such a spiritualized form of concentrative meditation is called "centering prayer."

Next, read the passage very slowly, aloud or silently, one word at a time, listening to and contemplatively savoring each word. Let each word resonate in your mind, like the sound of a gentle bell that rings into silence. So, on reading the serenity prayer, you would say:

```
God, grant me . . .
The serenity . . .
to accept . . .
what I cannot change, . . .
the courage . . .
to change what I can, . . .
and the wisdom . . .
to know . . .
the difference.
```

Repeat the passage, slowly and more slowly, two or three times. Let associations, thoughts and pictures, come and go. Do not cling to any association. They are how God speaks to us through the chosen passage, and how we spontaneously reply. Quietly acknowledge each arising association, and give it to God.

Wait for one word or phrase to emerge, usually from the passage that feels special. In our example, the word "acceptance" may emerge as personally very meaningful.

Contemplate this word. That is, gently let the word go over and over in your mind, like a mantra. As before, let go of every distraction, every association, and give it to God. This becomes a sort of very quiet dialog with God.

At the end of this exercise, speak to God. Give God what is new and fresh in your experience, what you have discovered, what new understanding you have of the passage.

For the next few minutes, sit quietly and attend to the world, simply and mindfully, as it is now. You may gently return to reading parts of your passage, to contemplating your special word, to speaking with God, or to savoring Thankfulness and Love (or any of the spiritual or transcendent R-States).

Physical Contemplation

One can practice a variant of lectio divina as a physical sequence of exercises. Here, one selects a sequence of exercises, perhaps from a relaxation script developed from this book. Then, simply treat the sequence as if it were a written passage. First, complete the entire exercise sequence, for example:

```
Tense and release your shoulders.
Tense and release your hands.
Stretch your arms high into the sky and unstretch.
Slowly breathe in and out through your lips.
Gently meditate on the gentle movement of rocking.
```

Then select one piece of the exercise that seems meaningful, say stretching your arms high into the sky and then unstretching. This time you do not actually do the stretch, but think about it. You imagine you are doing it. This is similar to selecting a single special word in lectio divina. Then, proceed with the steps of lectio divina, using your selected imagined movement instead of your selected word.

SPIRITUAL CRISES AND RELAXATION

Richards and Bergin (1997) have suggested that it is appropriate for secular counselors and therapists to help clients with religious crises. However, I believe religious leaders or peers are more appropriate dispensers of strictly religious counsel, such as admonishments to attend church more regularly, give more, pray more, pray for certain things, renounce forbidden activities, engage in fasting, ask for forgiveness, do penance, read the Holy Book more frequently, attend worship groups, and so on. As useful as these options may be, each carries with it an implicit endorsement of a client's religion, and such endorsements are not appropriate for the secular health professional.

However, health professionals can facilitate the process of honest questioning. For the believer, honest questioning is often seen as a great strengthener of faith. For the secular health professional, doubt is a self-affirming act, an act that affirms one's capacity to make authentic choices. Perhaps the honest facing of doubt is where the secular and religious intersect.

Most health professionals are simply not aware of the spiritual doubts of their devout clients. At the most basic level, theistic religion presents three systemic theological challenges. Without offering any answers, let me illustrate each by presenting the thoughts of three inquiring individuals:

> *Gil:* The Holy Book cannot be literally true. If we accept the miracles and fantastic stories of The Holy Book as true, we have established a certain set of criteria for acceptable evidence. If we apply these same criteria elsewhere, we are obligated to accept everything that also meets these criteria, from the annual appearance of Santa Claus to the medieval rationale for burning witches.

> *Ernie:* Why does God create and sustain an ungodly universe? The universe is full of injustice, pain, cruelty, imperfection, error, violence, ugliness, etc. The deserving and righteous can be victims of terrible calamity, whereas true villains can live lives of comfort and luxury. Things that we see as perfect or beautiful, such as a snowflake or a great painting, are often clearly works of natural processes or human genius, or the product of our tendency to perceive order where none exists (seeing angels in clouds or faces on Mars, for example).

> *Lois:* Why are God's answers to prayers so apparently unreliable? It seems the more a prayer is for some change in the physical universe, the less likely we will see an answer. The more a prayer involves evoking some personal psychological change in oneself, the more likely it will be answered, or can be explained. If I pray for miraculous cures for all worthy souls dying of cancer, frankly, I doubt it will happen. If I pray for personal strength in dealing with the fact that many just people suffer unjustly, I feel more confident in some sort of credible response.

I have presented a somewhat emphatic description of these challenges in order to make a point. The three systemic challenges of religion cannot be resolved through deliberate analytic thought or with verbal constructs. Rational inquiry only makes them worse. Two thousand years of theological debate is evidence of this.

We as relaxation trainers are in no position to offer religion-based comfort; to do so would imply that we embrace or reject one or another faith, or that we accept the notion that nonscientific criteria for evaluating claims of the supernatural/paranormal are appropriate in scientific inquiry. We can suggest ways of putting aside the very source of the problem, deliberate and analytic thought, while remaining fully awake and aware of the problem with mental faculties attentive and focused, not compromised by the narrowing pressures of stress and spiritual crisis. This can be a silent act of contemplation, prayer, imagery, or meditation.

Put differently, we can invite clients to learn a different skill of approaching life's deeper issues. This, indeed, is the skill of sustained effortless simple focus. Although, at one level, such focus is a description of a basic relaxation access skill. At a deeper level, it is a type of inquiry. Effortless means putting aside the "effort" of rational, verbal, theological thinking; the "effort" of using mental ideas and constructs to figure things out. "Simple focus" is simply remaining aware, the opposite of discursive thinking, considering one thing after another, dissecting detail, making contrasts and comparisons, exercising judgment and evaluation, and so on. And in order for all of this work to be successful, effortless simple focus must be sustained.

For many of us, the relaxation access skill of sustained effortless simple focus is rarely applied as a tool for probing the mysteries of life. But it can give us access to new ways of viewing old questions. I like to illustrate this with a remarkable contemporary parable, one that heralded the onset of the 21st century. Here is the story of the Hubble Telescope and the Deep Field Survey:

One of the most important astronomical discoveries at the beginning of the 21st century involved an empty spot of space. It is likely that since the beginning of recorded history, humankind has seen absolutely nothing in a certain dark spot of sky, about the size of a pencil eraser, near the handle of the Big Dipper. Even the most powerful telescopes of the 16th, 17th, 18th, 19th, and 20th centuries would have found nothing. Until the Hubble space telescope. This remarkable eye to the universe could do something no Earth-bound telescope could ever do—sustain focus and maintain absolute stillness, unmoved by slight tremors of earthquakes thousands of miles away, and unclouded by the murky flow of atmosphere and pollution and the buzz and glare of civilization. Put simply, the Hubble was above all Earthy distraction, and could truly sustain effortless simple focus.

In an experiment termed the "Deep Field Survey," astronomers decided to train the Hubble on the empty spot for two uninterrupted, undistracted weeks. What the Hubble found changed our view of the universe. Hidden in this dark spot are billions of galaxies, and each galaxy contains billions of stars. The universe is far more immense than we had imagined. And the secret to seeing this is sustained effortless simple focus.

This parable has a postscript. A few years after the Deep Field Survey, the Ultra Deep Field Survey took a longer look at the empty spot and found a few more billion stars and galaxies. But that was not the most startling discovery. The Ultra Deep Field Survey revealed, for the first time, a remarkable glimpse of the very edge of the Big Bang itself, the threshold of the beginning of time. Accessed through sustained effortless simple focus.

Sustained effortless simple focus is a tool that helps us probe the apparently dark and empty regions of life. It is both broadly applicable and nonintrusive. It can comfortably fit within ideological and theological perspectives ranging from fundamentalism to atheism. In sum, we invite a client to put aside needless self-centered rumination, be silent in prayer or meditation, and see what the universe has to reveal.

Let me conclude with a thought. In Zen Buddhism, a "koan" is a paradoxical statement or question offered as a spiritual exercise (e.g., "What is the sound of one hand clapping?"). In spite of urgent pressure to "solve" a koan, it cannot be figured out through ego-driven analytic intellect. Realization of this is a step toward spiritual growth. Perhaps the three systemic challenges to faith are gifts that God has placed in the "great treasure chest." They are, perhaps, the three koans of Western religion.

Appendix

Relaxation Sampler

Required Supplies for Workshop Presentation:

1) The Simplified R-State Pyramid Map (see Figure 17.1)
2) A Candle (for meditation)

Relaxation Sampler

In this exercise we will sample the major approaches to relaxation and meditation used most by health professionals and experts. We will see that different techniques are not like generic anxiety pills, but have different effects. However, to find these differences, we need a special map, the Relaxation States Map.

[DISTRIBUTE THE SIMPLIFIED R-STATE PYRAMID MAP, FIGURE 17.1]

The Relaxation States Map was developed by the Roosevelt University Stress Institute in a ten-year study involving over 10,000 practitioners of dozens of different relaxation techniques. It is a powerful tool that not only helps you determine what approaches work for you, but also tells you what they are good for.

[PUT RELAXATION STATES MAP ON THE BOARD OR DISTRIBUTE]

Here's how we will proceed. First, we will try one exercise, and then pause and reflect on how we felt using the Relaxation States Map.

A Few Good Starting Stretches

Let's start with yoga stretching, a popular oriental approach. Make sure you are seated upright in a comfortable position with your feet flat on the floor. And close your eyes.

Arms and sides.

Now let both your arms fall limply to your sides.

[PAUSE]

Slowly, smoothly and gently circle your arms and hand up and away from your body like the wings of a bird.

[PAUSE]

Let your arms extend straight, and circle higher and higher.
[PAUSE]
Let them circle to the sky.
[PAUSE]
And then circle your arms over your head so your hands points all the way up . . . and arch your body back as you reach and point farther and farther, like a tree arching in the wind.
[PAUSE]
Become aware of the invigorating feelings of stretching.
[PAUSE]
Now gently and easily, sit up straight, and . . .
[PAUSE]
Like the wings of a bird . . .
[PAUSE]
Circle your arms back over your head . . .
to your sides . . .
[PAUSE]
And finally to the resting position.
[PAUSE]
And let your arms hang.
[PAUSE]
[REPEAT]
Back of neck stretch.
Now, while sitting erect, let your head tilt easily toward your chest.
Try not to force it down.
Simply let gravity pull your head down . . .
Farther and farther.
Focus on the stretch in the back of your neck.
The refreshing and renewing energy it releases . . .
As the force of gravity easily and slowly pulls your head down.
When you are ready, gently and easily lift your head.
Lift it until it is again comfortably upright.
[REPEAT]
Front of neck stretch.
Now, like before, let your head tilt, this time backward.
Let gravity pull your head back, but not too far, just enough to feel the stretch.
Do not force it back.
Let gravity do the work for you as it pulls the heavy weight of your head back, farther and farther.
Gently and slightly open your mouth, and let your head relax and fall back.
Focus your mind on the front of the neck stretch as it stretches.

Gently hold the stretch.

Then gently and easily lift your head.

Gradually return it to its upright position.

Take your time. There is no need to hurry.

Now, let go of what you are attending to. How do you feel? Take a look at your relaxation states map. What words fit? Put the letter "Y" for yoga stretching by the words that fit. And then simply sit with your eyes closed.

[PAUSE]

We can now continue.

Progressive Muscle Relaxation

We will now try a different type of exercise, a Western approach called progressive muscle relaxation.

Make sure you are seated upright in a comfortable position with your feet flat on the floor. And close your eyes.

Shoulders.

Begin by focusing on the shoulder muscles.

Squeeze your shoulders, now.

[PAUSE]

Create a nice good shrug.

[PAUSE]

Let the feelings of tightness grow.

[PAUSE]

And let go.

[PAUSE]

Let the tension flow out.

[PAUSE]

Let your tension begin to unwind.

[PAUSE]

Let the muscles begin to smooth out.

[PAUSE]

Let the muscles become more deeply relaxed.

[PAUSE]

[REPEAT]

Both arms.

This time focus on both your arms.

[PAUSE]

Bend your arms at the elbows, trying to touch your shoulder with your hands. Squeeze your lower and upper arm together, now.

[PAUSE]

Press tighter and tighter.

[PAUSE]

Notice the feelings of tension.

[PAUSE]
And let go.
[PAUSE]
Let the tension go.
[PAUSE]
The tension melts away.
[PAUSE]
Let the muscles become more deeply relaxed.
[PAUSE]
[REPEAT]
Back of neck.
Focus on the muscles in the back of the neck.
[PAUSE]
Gently tilt your head back and gently press the back of your head against your neck, now.
[PAUSE]
Tighten up the muscles.
[PAUSE]
Squeeze the muscles more and more.
[PAUSE]
And let go.
[PAUSE]
Let the muscles become more deeply relaxed.
[PAUSE]
Let your entire body become loose and limp.
[PAUSE]
Let yourself sink deeper and deeper into relaxation.
[PAUSE]
Let yourself forget the world.
[PAUSE]
[REPEAT]
Front of neck.
Focus on the muscles of the neck.
[PAUSE]
Bow your head and gently press your chin down to your chest, now.
Tighten up the muscles.
[PAUSE]
Let the tension grow.
[PAUSE]
And let go.
[PAUSE]
Let tension flow away.
[PAUSE]
Let the rest of your body remain relaxed.
[PAUSE]

Let yourself sink deeper and deeper into relaxation.
[PAUSE]
[REPEAT]
And now, how do you feel? On your map, put the letter "P" for Progressive Muscle Relaxation. Then simply sit with your eyes closed.
[PAUSE]

Breathing

Make sure you are seated upright in a comfortable position with your feet flat on the floor. And close your eyes. We are ready to move on breathing exercises, an approach used around the world.
Deep breathing.
Let yourself breathe easily and naturally.
When you are ready, take in a full deep breath, filling your lungs and abdomen with good, refreshing air.
And when you are ready, relax.
And slowly let the air flow out, very smoothly and gently.
And now, just continue breathing normally for a while.
Do not attempt to force yourself to breathe in any particular way.
Just let the air come in and out on its own.
[PAUSE 10 SECONDS]
And, again, when you are ready, take in a full deep breath, filling your lungs with good, energizing air. Feel the calm and strength it brings.
And, when ready, gently and smoothly exhale.
Then resume breathing in a normal way, easily in and out.
[PAUSE 10 SECONDS]
And, again, when you are ready, take in a full deep breath, filling your lung, with good, energizing air. Feel the calm and strength it brings.
And, when ready, gently and smoothly exhale.
[PAUSE]
How do you feel?
[PAUSE]
On your relaxation states map, what words fit? Put the letter "B" for breathing by the words that fit. Then simply sit with your eyes closed.
[PAUSE]

Autogenic Suggestion

And now we are ready to move on to an approach called autogenic suggestion.

Warm and heavy.

With every outgoing breath, let yourself sink into a comfortable state of relaxation.

Simply think the words, "hands and arms, very heavy."

There is no need for you to achieve any effect.

[PAUSE 5 SECONDS]

Hands and arms are very heavy, like gravity is pulling them towards the earth.

[PAUSE 5 SECONDS]

Like a magnet is pulling tension away.

[PAUSE 5 SECONDS]

Arms and legs are getting heavy.

[PAUSE 5 SECONDS]

With every outgoing breath, tension flows away.

[PAUSE 5 SECONDS]

Gravity is pulling your arms down.

[PAUSE 5 SECONDS]

Feel the heavy weight as your arms and legs sink.

[PAUSE 5 SECONDS]

Heavier and heavier.

[PAUSE 5 SECONDS]

Entire body, more and more heavy.

[PAUSE]

Let yourself sink into a distant state of pleasant relaxation with every outgoing breath.

[PAUSE]

There is nothing you have to do.

[PAUSE 5 SECONDS]

Let the words go over and over like an echo.

[PAUSE]

Arms and legs very heavy. Very heavy. Very heavy.

[PAUSE]

There is nothing you have to do.

[PAUSE]

Let tension sink away with every breath.

[PAUSE]

Let gravity pull tension away.

[PAUSE]

As you forget the world . . .

[PAUSE]

You become more calm and relaxed.

[PAUSE]

More quiet.

[PAUSE]

Entire body, very heavy. Very heavy. Very heavy.

[PAUSE 5 SECONDS]
Let yourself sink into a pleasant state of relaxation.
Far, far away from the world.
Very distant and detached, as if nothing seems to matter.
And now let go of what you are attending to. On your relaxation states map, put the letter "A" for autogenic by the words that fit how you feel. Then simply sit with your eyes closed.
[PAUSE]
We can now move on.

Imagery

We are ready to practice imagery and visualization, an approach many people find particularly rewarding.
Make sure you are seated upright in a comfortable position with your feet on the floor. And close your eyes.
This time we are going to enjoy a peaceful fantasy, a relaxing daydream.
In your mind imagine a relaxing outdoor nature setting, one that is very safe and relaxing. This can be a forest, a garden, a mountain, or perhaps the seashore. Imagine a peaceful outdoor setting.
Involve all of your senses. Maybe you see waves of grass or trees extending into the distance. You can hear the wind rushing through grass, trees, or rocks. You can feel a gentle breeze or the warm sun touching your skin. You can smell the peaceful outdoor air.
For the next minute or so let yourself enjoy a daydream about a faraway peaceful outdoor setting of your own. Involve all of your senses.
[PAUSE 1 MINUTE]
And now, how do you feel? On your map, put the letter "I" for imagery by the words that fit. Then simply sit with your eyes closed.
[PAUSE]

Meditation

We are ready to move on to meditation and mindfulness. Make sure you are sitting upright in a comfortable position with your feet flat on the floor. And close your eyes. We will try three types of meditation.
Rocking meditation.
This exercise is called rocking meditation. With your eyes closed, simply attend to your body. As you attend to your body, let go of everything else. Gently begin to rock back and forth.

[PAUSE]

Let each movement become more and more gentle and easy. Let yourself rock effortlessly. Let your body move on its own, in its own way, at its own speed. All you have to do is simply attend.

[PAUSE]

Let each movement become more and more subtle so that someone watching would barely notice you are rocking. All you have to do is quietly attend to the repetitive back and forth movement, like rocking on a boat or a rocking chair. Every time your mind wanders, that's okay. Just gently return to your rocking motion. That is all you need to attend to, rocking back and forth, back and forth, very quietly.

For the next minute or so, let your rocking become barely noticeable. And quietly attend.

[PAUSE 90 SECONDS]

Meditation on a visual image.

We are ready for our next meditation. With your eyes closed, think of the image of a simple spot of light, a candle flame, or a star. Or attend to the word "peace" and let it float through your mind like an echo, over and over.

And calmly attend.

And calmly return after every distraction.

[PAUSE 90 SECONDS]

Gently let go of what you are attending to.

Mindfulness meditation.

We are ready to move on to our last exercise, mindfulness meditation. It is very simple. With your eyes closed, simply attend to the sounds you hear. There is no need to focus on any one sound or try to keep sounds out of mind. Let sounds come to you. All you do is observe. Whenever you notice a sound, simply name it, and continue waiting and observing. Whenever you find yourself thinking about this task or anything else, let go of your thoughts, and resume waiting and observing. Let sounds come to you. Give each sound a name. Continue attending.

[PAUSE 60 SECONDS]

Gently let go of what you are attending to.

How do you feel?

On your map, put the letter "M" for meditation by the words that fit.

Very slowly open your eyes. We have completed our last exercise.

How did this exercise make you feel?

[PAUSE]

Discussion

We have now completed our tour of the most popular approaches to relaxation used by health professionals. Which worked for you? How were they different?

Let's conclude this workshop with another exercise. As a team, I would like you to consider this topic. [IF YOU ARE IN A GROUP WITH MORE THAN SIX PEOPLE, FORM SEPARATE TEAMS OF 3 OR 4 PEOPLE EACH]

Which states on your map seem to go with different approaches to relaxation?

[PAUSE TO COMPLETE EXERCISE]

Let me conclude with a thought about the Relaxation States Map. This map is actually a window of feelings and experiences associated with relaxation and meditation exercises. Different parts of this window are illuminated by different exercises. For those who master complete relaxation, the entire window does not light up; instead, a curtain is pulled back so we can see the light shine through the window in whatever way it happens to shine. This may vary from day to day, technique to technique. Parts of the window may shine during relaxation practice, and parts may shine during the day, adding a new light to what you are doing.

References

Allen, F. (1998). *Health psychology: Theory and practice.* St Leonards NSW, Australia: Allen & Unwin Pty Ltd.

Allen, J. S., & Klein, R. J. (1996). *Ready, set, relax.* Watertown, WI: Inner Coaching.

Benson, H. (1975). *The relaxation response.* New York: Marrow.

Bernstein, D. A., & Borkovec, T. D. (1973). *Progressive relaxation training: A manual for the helping professions.* Champaign, IL: Research Press.

Blanchard, E. B., & Andrasik, F. (1985). *Management of chronic headaches: A psychological approach.* New York: Pergamon.

Brannon, L., & Feist, J. (2000). *Health psychology: An introduction to behavior and health* (4th ed.). Belmont, CA: Wadsworth/Thomson Learning.

Carrington, P. (1978). *Clinical standardized meditation instructor's manual and self-regulating course.* Kendall Park, NJ: Pace Systems.

Conze, E. (1959). *Buddhism: Its essence and development.* New York: Harper & Row.

Coulter, H. D. (2001). *Anatomy of hatha yoga.* Honesdale, PA: Body and Breath.

Davidson, R. J., & Kabat-Zinn, J. (2004). Alterations in brain and immune function produced by mindfulness meditation: Three caveats: Comment response. *Psychosomatic Medicine, 66,* 149–152

DiMatteo, M. R., & Martin, L. R. (2002). *Health psychology.* Needham Heights, MA: Allyn & Bacon.

Dunn, B. R., Hartigan, J. A., & Mikulas, W. L. (1999). Concentration and mindfulness meditation: Unique forms of consciousness? *Applied Psychophysiology and Biofeedback, 24,* 147–165.

Edmonston, W. E. (1986). *The induction of hypnosis.* New York: Wiley.

Eliado, M. (1984). *Patanjali and Yoga.* New York: Funk & Wagnalls.

Everly, G. S. Jr., & Lating, J. M. (2002). *A clinical guide to the treatment of the human stress response, 2nd edition.* New York: Kluwer.

Forman, S. G. (1993). *Coping skills interventions for children and adolescents.* San Francisco: Jossey-Bass.

Fried, R. (1993). The role of respiration in stress and stress control: Toward a theory of stress as a hypoxic phenomenon. In P. M. Lehrer & R. L. Woolfolk (Eds.), *Principles and practice of stress management, 2nd edition.* New York: Guilford.

Friedman, H. S. (2002). *Health psychology* (2nd ed.). Upper Saddle River, NJ: Prentice Hall.

Funderburk, J. (1977). *Science studies yoga.* Glenview, IL: Himalayan Institute.

Gellhorn, E. (1970). The emotions and the ergotropic and trophotropic systems. *Psychologische Forschung, 34,* 48–94.

Gellhorn, E., & Loofbourrow, G. (1963). *Emotions and emotional disorders.* New York: Harper & Row.

Ghonchec, S., & Smith, J. C. (2004). Progressive muscle relaxation, yoga stretching, and AGC relaxation theory. *Journal of Clinical Psychology, 60,* 131–136.

Gureje, O., VonKorff, M., Simon, G. E., & Gater, R. (1998). Persistent pain and well-being: A World Health Organization study in primary care. *Journal of the American Medical Association, 280,* 147–151.

Goodkin, K., & Visser, A. P. (Eds.). (2000). *Psychoneuroimmunology: Stress, mental disorders, and health.* Washington, DC: American Psychiatric Publishing, Inc.

Hansen, R. W., & Gerber, K. E. (1990) *Coping with chronic pain: A guide to patient self-management.* New York: Guilford.

Heide, F. J., & Borkovec, T. D. (1984). Relaxation-induced anxiety: Mechanisms and theoretical implications. *Behaviour Research and Therapy, 22,* 1–12.

Hill, P. C. & Pargament, K. I. (2003). Advances in the conceptualization and measurement of religion and spirituality: Implications for physical and mental health research. *American Psychologist, 58,* 64–74.

Jacobson, E. (1929). *Progressive relaxation.* Chicago: University of Chicago Press.

Jacobson, E. (1938). *Progressive relaxation (2nd ed.).* Chicago: University of Chicago Press.

Jones, F., & Bright, J. (Eds.). (2001). *Stress: Myth, theory and research.* Upper Saddle River, NJ: Prentice Hall.

Kabat-Zinn, J. (1990). *Full catastrophe living.* New York: Dell.

Layman, E. M. (1976). *Buddhism in America.* Chicago: Nelson-Hall.

Lehrer, P. M., Woolfolk, R. L., & Sime, W. E. (Eds.) (2005). *Principles and practice of stress management, 3rd Edition.* New York: Guilford.

Lehrer, P. M., & Woolfolk, R. L., 2nd Edition. (Eds.) (1993). *Principles and practice of stress management.* New York: Guilford.

Lehrer, P. M., & Woolfolk, R. L. (1993). Specific effects of stress management techniques. In P. M. Lehrer & R. L. Woolfolk (Eds.), *Principles and practice of stress management.* New York: Guilford.

Lewis, J. E. (2001). R-States, beliefs, attitudes, and concerns. In J. C. Smith (Ed.), *Advances in ABC Relaxation: Applications and inventories* (pp. 180–182). New York: Springer.

LeShan, L. (1974). *How to meditate.* New York: Batman.

Lichstein, K. (1988). *Clinical relaxation strategies.* New York: Wiley.

Linden, W. (1990). *Autogenic training: A clinical guide.* New York: Guilford.

Linden, W. (1993). The autogenic training method of J. H. Schultz. In P. M. Lehrer & R. L. Woolfolk (Eds.), *Principles and practice of stress management* (pp. 205–279). New York: Guilford.

Luthe, W. (1965). Autogenic training in North America. In W. Luthe (Ed.), *Autogenic training: International edition* (pp. 71–78). New York: Grune & Stratton.

Luthe, W. (Ed.). (1969–1973). *Autogenic therapy* (Vols. 1–8). New York: Grune & Stratton.

McCaul, K. D., & Malott, J. M. (1984). Distraction and coping with pain. *Psychological Bulletin, 95,* 516–533.

Martin, P. R. (1993). *Psychological management of chronic headaches*. New York: Guilford.

Matsumoto, M., & Smith, J. C. (2001). Progressive muscle relaxation, breathing, exercises and ABC relaxation theory. *Journal of Clinical Psychology, 57,* 1551–1557.

Melzack, R., & Wall, P. D. (1965). Pain mechanisms: A new theory. *Science, 150,* 971–979.

Melzack, R., & Wall, P. D. (1982). *The challenge of pain*. New York: Basic Books.

Naranjo, C., & Ornstein, R. (1971). *On the psychology of meditation*. New York: Viking.

Nezu, A. M., Nezu, C. M., Geller, P. A. (2003). *Handbook of psychology: Health psychology. Vol. 4*. New York: Wiley

Osterweis, M., Kleinman, A., & Mechanic, D. (Eds.) (1987). *Pain and disability: Clinical, behavioral, and public policy perspectives*. Washington, DC: National Academy Press.

Pargament, K. I. (1997). *The psychology of religion and coping: Theory, research, and practice*. New York: Guilford.

Patel, C. (1993). Yoga-based therapy. In P. M. Lehrer & R. W. Woolfolk (Eds.), *Principles and practice of stress management* (pp. 89–137). New York: Guilford.

Paul, G. L. (1966, September). The specific control of anxiety: "Hypnosis" and "conditioning". In L. Osease (Chair), Innovations in therapeutic interactions. Symposium presented at the meeting of the American Psychological Association, New York, New York.

Peterson, C. (2000). The future of optimism. *American Psychologist, 55,* 44–55.

Philips, H. C., & Rachman, S. (1996). *The psychological management of chronic pain: A treatment manual (2nd ed.)*. New York: Springer Publishing.

Piiparinin, R. A., & Smith, J. C. (2003). Stress symptoms of two groups before and after the terrorist attacks of 9/11/01. *Perceptual and Motor Skills, 97,* 360–364.

Poppen, R. (1998). *Behavioral relaxation training and assessment, 2nd Edition*. New York: Pergamon.

Prabhavananda, S. (1963). *The spiritual heritage of India*. Garden City, NY: Doubleday.

Rapee, R. M., Spence, S. H., Cobham, V., & Wignall, A. (2000). *Helping your anxious child*. Oakland, CA: New Harbinger.

Richards, P. S., & Bergin, A. E. (1997). *A spiritual strategy for counseling and psychotherapy*. Washington, DC: American Psychological Association.

Russell, R. K., & Matthews, C. O. (1975). Cue-controlled relaxation in *in vivo* desensitization of a snake phobia. *Journal of Behavior Therapy and Experimental Psychiatry, 6,* 49–51.

Salovey, P., Rothman, A. J., Detweiler, J. R., & Steward, W. T. (2000). Emotional states and physical health. *American Psychologist, 55,* 110–121.

Sapolsky, R. M. (1998). *Why zebras don't get ulcers: An updated guide to stress, stress related diseases, and coping* (2nd ed.). New York: W. H. Freeman.

Sarafino, E. P. (1998). *Health psychology: Biopsychosocial interactions* (3rd ed.). New York: John Wiley & Sons, Inc.

Schultz, J. H. (1932). *Das Autogene Training—Konzentrative Selbstentspannung*. Leipzig: Thieme.

Schultz, J. H., & Luthe, W. (1969). *Autogenic therapy, Vol. 1. Autogenic methods*. New York: Grune & Stratton.

Segerstrom, S. C., & Miller, G. E. (2004). Psychological stress and the human immune system: A meta-analytic study of 30 years of inquiry. *Psychological Bulletin, 30,* 601–630.

Seligman, M. E. P., & Csikszentmihalyi, M. (2000). Positive psychology: An introduction. *American Psychologist, 55,* 5–14.

Simonton, O. C., Matthews-Simonton, S., & Craighton, J. (1978). *Getting well again.* Los Angeles: J. P. Tarcher.

Smith, J. C. (1987). *Relaxation dynamics.* Champaign, Il: Research Press.

Smith,.J. C. (1990). *Cognitive-behavioral relaxation training: A new system of strategies for treatment and assessment.* New York: Springer Publishing.

Smith, J. C. (1993b). *Understanding stress and coping.* Englewood Cliffs, NJ: New York.

Smith, J. C. (1999a). *ABC relaxation theory.* New York: Springer Publishing.

Smith, J. C. (1999b). *ABC Relaxation Training.* New York: Springer Publishing.

Smith, J. C. (2001). *Advances in ABC relaxation: Applications and inventories.* New York: Springer Publishing.

Smith, J. C. (2002). *Stress management: A comprehensive handbook of techniques and strategies.* New York: Springer Publishing.

Smith, J. C. (2004). *The Smith Stress Symptoms Inventory.* www.roosevelt-edu/stress

Smith, J. C. (2004a). *The stress management companion.* www.lulu.com/stress.

Smith, J. C., & Sohnle, S. (2001). Stress, relaxation dispositions, and recalled relaxation states for one's preferred relaxation activity. In J. C. Smith (Ed.), *Advances in ABC relaxation training* (pp. 143–148). New York: Springer.

Taylor, H., & Curran, N. (1985). *The Nuprin pain report.* New York: Louis Harris & Associates.

Taylor, S. E. (1999). *Health psychology* (4th ed.). New York: McGraw-Hill.

Turk, D. C., & Gatchel, R. J. (Eds.) (2002). *Psychological approaches to pain management: A practitioner's handbook* (2nd ed.). New York: Guilford.

Vahia, N. S., Doongaji, D. R., Jeste, D. V., Ravindranath, S., Kapoor, S. M., & Ardhapurkar, I. (1973). Psychophysiologic therapy based on the concepts of Patanjacs. *American Journal of Psychotherapy, 27,* 557–565.

Van Dixhoorn, J. (1994). Significance of breathing awareness and exercise training for recovery after myocardial infarction (chapter 9). In J. G. Carlson, A. R. Seifert, & N. Birbaumer (Eds.), *Clinical applied psychophysiology.* New York: Plenum.

Wallace, R. K., & Benson, H. (1972). The physiology of meditation. *Scientific American, 226,* 84–90.

Wallace, R. K., Benson, H., & Wilson, K. (1971). A wakeful hypometabolic physiologic state. *American Journal of Physiology, 221,* 795–799.

Weinstein, M., & Smith, J. C. (1992). Isometric squeeze relaxation (progressive relaxation) versus meditation: Absorption and focusing as predictors of state effects. *Perceptual and Motor Skills, 75,* 1263–1271.

Wolkowitz, O. M., & Rothschild, A. J. (Eds.) (2003). *Psychoneuroendocrinology: The scientific basis of clinical practice.* Washington, DC: American Psychiatric Press.

Wolpe, J. (1958). *Psychotherapy by reciprocal inhibition.* Stanford, CA: Stanford University Press.

Index

ABC Relaxation Theory, 71
ABC₂ Relaxation Theory, 72
Access skills, 29, 44
Access zone scanning, 183, 184, 273, 281
Advanced scripting, 248
Aftereffects of relaxation practice, 77
Allen, F., 27,
Allen, J., 289
Andrasik, F., 320
Assessment, *see* Relaxation, Assessment
    tools
At ease/Peace (R-State), 50
Atheism and spirituality, 53, 327, 342
Autogenic training, suggestion
    Children's version, 298
    Clients, appropriate, 133
    Demonstrating/Warmup, 135
    Duration, 132
    Effects, 37, 131, 132
    Enhancing, 136, 225
    Pain management, 319
    Placement with other approaches, 132
    Portability, 133
    Problems, 136; *see also* Relaxation
        training, troubleshooting
    Rationale for clients, 134

R-States, 132
Script, 137
Training instructions, 134
Voice, 135
Autonomic stress arousal, 22, 24
Awe and Wonder (R-State), 53

Behavioral assessment, 202
Behavioral Signs of Relaxation Rating
    Scale, 202, 203, 268
Beliefs, anti-relaxation, 223
Beliefs, relaxation, 27, 45, 226; *see also*
    Relaxation goals, Outcomes
Benson, H., 10, 28, 71
Bergin, A., 330, 339
Blanchard, E., 320
Breathing exercises (*see also* instructions
    for all other families of
    relaxation)
    Children's version, 299
    Clients, appropriate, 115
    Demonstrating/Warmup, 117
    Duration, 114
    Effects, 34, 113, 114
    Enhancing, 120, 225
    Exercise placement, 114

Breathing exercises *(continued)*
   Pain management, 319
   Placement with other approaches, 114
   Portability, 114
   Problems, 118; *see also* Relaxation
      training, Troubleshooting
   Rationale for clients, 116
   R-States, 114
   Script, 120
   Training instructions, 116
   Voice, 118
Brain, 21, 24
Brannon, L. 27
Brief relaxation training, 185
Bright, J., 27
Buddhism, 27

Calm directed action (Relaxation goal),
   66
Carrington, P., 166, 167
Cascading deepening imagery, 248
Chi, 335
Childlike Innocence (R-State), 52
Children, relaxation and, 289
Clothing and attire in relaxation, 194
Cobham, V., 290
Combination formats, 180
Combining and sequencing exercises, 248
Concentrative meditation, *see* Meditation
Contemplation, 337
Conze, E., 17
Coulter, H., 13
Craighton, J., 12
Creativity and insight (Relaxation goal),
   67
Crises, spiritual, 339
Csikszentmihalyi, M., 45
Curran, N., 311
Cycle of Renewal, 46, 333

Davisdon, R., 41
Deep Mystery (R-State), 53
Deepening countdowns, 252
Deepening cycles, 255
Deepening markers, 253

Deepening metaphors, 251
Deepening techniques, 248
Deepening transitions, 252
Demonstration/Warmup, 77
Detweiler, J. 45
DiMatteo, M., 27
Disengagement (R-State), 47
Doongaji, D., 81
Dunn, B., 41

Eliade, M., 12
Energized (R-State), 47
Enhancing relaxation, *see* Relaxation train-
   ing, enhancing relaxation
Ergotropic tuning, 25; *see also* tropho-
   tropic tuning
Ernie, 3, 64, 340
Evaluating a script, 245
Everly, G., 115

Families of Relaxation, 4, 43, 44
Feist, J., 27
Finger/head-nod signal system, 204
Forman, S., 289, 290
Fried, R., 116
Friedman, H., 27
Funderburk, J., 81

Gatchel, R., 320
Gater, R., 311
Gelhorn, E., 25
Geller, P., 27
General instruction, 77
Gerber, K., 320
Ghonchec, S., 94, 115
Gil, 3, 340
God-based spirituality (Relaxation goal),
   68
Goodkin, K., 27
Group relaxation, 183, 185, 279, 282
Gureje, O., 311

Hansen, R., 320
Happiness, *see* Joy (R-State)
Hartigan, J., 41

Hatha yoga, 13
Healing (Relaxation goal), 61
Health and energy (Relaxation goal), 66
Hill, P., 329
Hinduism, 17
Hubble, story of, 341

Imagery
  Children's version, 302
  Clients, appropriate, 149
  Demonstrating/Warmup, 151
  Duration, 148
  Effects, 38, 147
  Enhancing, 153, 225
  Group training, 283
  Nonrelaxation, 15
  Pain management, 319
  Placement with other approaches, 148
  Portability, 149
  Problems, 152; *see also* Relaxation
        training, Troubleshooting
  Rationale for clients, 150
  R-States, 148
  Script, 154
  Training instructions, 150
  Voice, 152
Insight, *see* Creativity and insight; *also*,
        Imagery

Jacobson, E., 7, 33
Jeste, D., 81
Jones, F., 27
Joy (R-State), 50

Kabat-Zinn, J., 18, 41
Kapoor, S., 81
Klein, R., 289
Kleinman, A., 311
Koan, and Spiritual crises, 342
Kundalini yoga, 11, 15

Lating, J., 115
Layman, E., 17
Lectio Divina, 338
Lehrer, P., 5, 63

LeShan, L., 166
Letting go, 104
Lewis, J., 45
Lichstein, K., 5, 36
Linden, W., 10, 134
Lois, 3, 340
Loofbouroow, G., 25
Luthe, W., 10

Malott, J., 319
Martin, L., 27
Martin, P., 320
Matsumato, M., 94
Matthews, C., 9
Matthews-Simonton, S., 12
McCaul, K., 319
Mechanic, D., 311
Medical model bias, 62
Meditation
  Body, of the, 17
  Children's version, 305
  Clients, appropriate, 163
  Concentrative 16
  Demonstrating/Warmup, 168
  Duration, 162
  Effects, 39, 161
  Enhancing, 169, 225
  Goal of relaxation, 68
  Mind, of the, 17
  Mindfulness, 4, 16, 39, 41, 68, 161
  Pain management, 323
  Placement with other approaches, 162
  Portability, 163
  Problems, 168; *see also* Relaxation
        training, Troubleshooting
  R-States, 162
  Rationale for clients, 164
  Script, 170
  Senses, of the, 17
  Skills of relaxation, 41
  Training instructions, 164
  Voice, 168
Melzack, R., 314
Mental Quiet, 52
Mikulas, W., 41

Miller, G., 26
Mindfulness, 4, 16, 39, 41, 68, 161; *see also* meditation
Mini-scripts, 182, 184, 270
Mystery, *see* Deep Mystery (R-State)

N-States, 271
Naranjo, C., 40
Negative goals of relaxation, 60
Nervous system, components of, 20
Nezu, A., 27

Ornstein, R., 40
Osterweis, M., 311

Package programs, 182, 184, 267
Pain management, 311
Paranormal, 327, 328; *see also* N-States
Pargament, K., 329
Patel, C., 81
Paths of relaxation, 55
Paul, G., 9
Pauses, 228
Positive expressive goals of relaxation, 67
Positive practical goals of relaxation, 66
Positive psychology, 45
Postsession assessment, 78
Peterson, C., 45
Philips, H., 320
Physical relaxation, 49
Physical symptom review, 201
Piiparinen, R., 39
Pleasure and Joy, 47
Prabhavananda, S., 12
Practice, 78
Practice time, 195
Prayer, 327
Prayerful (R-State), 54
Precautions and risks, 187; *see also* Relaxation training, Troubleshooting
Processing technique, 78
Productivity and effectiveness (Relaxation goal), 66
Progressive muscle relaxation
    Children's version, 293

Clients, appropriate, 95
Compared with yoga stretching, 33
Demonstrating/Warmup, 97
Duration, 95
Effects, 33, 93
Enhancing, 104, 225
Letting go, 104
Pain management, 318
Placement with other approaches, 94
Portability, 95
Problems, 103; *see also* Relaxation training, Troubleshooting
Procedural rules, 98
R-States, 94
Rationale for clients, 96, 97
Script, 105
Training instructions, 96
Voice, 103

Qi, 335

R-Beliefs, 226
Rachman, S., 320
Rapee, R., 290
Rationale, presentation of, 77
Ravindranath, S., 81
Recording, making a relaxation; *see* Scripting
Recording a script, 256
Recovery and release, 49
Relaxation engine, 19
    Access skills, 29
    Relaxation response, 28, 62
Relaxation place, 196
Relaxation Precautions Fact Sheet (189)
Relaxation pyramid, 46, 48, 215, 281
Relaxation response, *see* Relaxation engine
Relaxation sampling, 212, 281, 343
Relaxation Scripting Workbook, 237, 238, 257
Relaxation states; R-States, 45
    At ease/Peace, 50
    Awe and Wonder, 53
    Benefits of R-States, 45

Childlike Innocence, 52
Children, terms appropriate for, 292
Deep Mystery, 53
Disengagement, 47
Energized, 47
Joy, 50
Mental Quiet, 52
Mystery, *see* Deep Mystery
Paths of, 55
Physical relaxation, 49
Pleasure and Joy, 47
Prayerful, 54
Pyramid, 46
Recovery and release, 49
Selflessness, 51
Sleepiness, 47
Spirituality, 53
Stress relief, 47
Thankful, loving, 53
Timeless, Boundless, Infinite, At Once,
    35
Transcendence, 54
Value of, 56
Relaxation-induced anxiety, *see* N-States
Relaxation training,
ABC Relaxation Theory, 71
    Comparison of theories, 71
    R-States, 45
    Relaxation pyramid, 46, 48, 215, 281
Assessment tools, 77, 201
    Behavioral assessment, 202
    Behavioral Signs of Relaxation Rat-
        ing Scale, 202, 203, 268
    Finger/head-nod signal system, 204
    Smith Relaxation Inventory Series,
        204, 268
        Smith Relaxation Goals Inventory
            (SRGI), 205, 207, 268
        Smith Relaxation Preferences In-
            ventory (SRPI), 205, 206, 268
        Smith Relaxation States Inventory
            Alternative Brief Version
            (SRSIabv), 205, 213, 235, 268
        Smith Relaxation States Inventory
            Brief Version (SRSIbv), 205,
            210, 235, 268

Smith Relaxation States Inventory
    Revised (SRSIr), 205, 208,
    268
Physical symptom review, 201
Rationale for clients, 198
Relaxation sampling, 212, 281, 343
Target Symptom Fact Sheet, 202
Verbal report, 205
Enhancing relaxation, 217
    Aftereffects, discussion of, 77
    Demonstration/Warmup, 77
    General instruction, 77
    Immediate and gradual enhance-
        ments, 228
    Pauses, 228
    Postsession assessment, 78
    Practice, 78
    Processing technique, 78
    R-Beliefs, 226
    Rationale, 77
    Revising technique, 78
Formats, 179
    Access zone scanning, 183, 184,
        273, 281
    Brief relaxation training, 185
    Combination formats, 180
    Group relaxation, 183, 185, 279, 282
    Mini-scripts, 182, 184, 270
    Package programs, 182, 184, 267
    Revised traditional single-technique
        format, 179, 183
    Scripting, 181, 184, 223; *see also*
        Scripting
    Selection of, 77
    Spot relaxation, 182, 184, 270
    World tour, 182, 1842, 268
    Workshops, 183, 184, 279
Goals, 59
    Calm directed action, 66
    Creativity and insight, 67
    God-based spirituality, 68
    Healing, 61
    Health and energy, 66
    Insight, *see* Creativity and insight
    Meditation and mindfulness, 68

Relaxation training *(continued)*
   Negative goals, 60
   Positive expressive goals, 67
   Positive practical goals, 66
   Productivity and effectiveness, 66
   Rationale for clients, 193
   Sleep and insomnia, 59
   Spontaneous enjoyment, 67
   Stress management, 61
   Transcendent goals, 68
  Orientation, 187
   Clothing and attire, 194
   Explanation of goal-specific relaxation processes, 190
   Explanation of inventories, 198
   Explanation of precautions and risks, 187
   Explanation of selected training formation, 194
   Explanation of stress, relaxation, access skills, 189
   Practice time, 195
   Relaxation place, 196
   Relaxation precautions fact sheet, 189
   Special training requirements, 194
  Troubleshooting
   Autogenic training, 136
   Beliefs, anti-relaxation, 223
   Breathing exercises, 118
   Imagery, 152
   Meditation, 168
   N-States, 271
   Progressive muscle relaxation, 103
   Relaxation-induced anxiety, *see* N-States
   Sleepiness, 220
   Yoga and Yogaform Stretching, 84
  Relaxation voice
   Autogenic training, 135
   Breathing, 118
   Imagery, 152
   Meditation, 168
   Progressive muscle relaxation, 103
   Yogaform stretching, 84

Religion, 327
Revised traditional single-technique format, 179, 183
Revising technique, 78
Richards, P., 330, 339
Rothman, A., 45
Rothschild, A., 27
Russell, R., 9

Salovey, P., 45
Sampling, *see* Relaxation Sampling
Sapolsky, R. 27
Schultz, J., 10
Scripts, verbatim
  Access Zone Scanning, 274
  Autogenic training, for children, 298
  Autogenic training, verbal, 137
  Autogenic training, visual, 141
  Breathing, 120
  Breathing exercises, for children, 299
  Children, overall rationale for relaxation, 291
  Children, rationale for progressive muscle relaxation, 293
  Cycle of renewal exercise, 334
  Goal-specific processes, rationale for clients, 193
  Imagery, for children
  Imagery, sense, 154
  Imagery, insight, 157
  Inventories, explaining, 198
  Letting go, 110
  Meditation, for children, 306
  Meditation, eight meditations, 170
  Mindful walking, 175
  Mindfulness, graduated, 172
  Progressive muscle relaxation, abbreviated, 110
  Progressive muscle relaxation, for children, 295
  Progressive muscle relaxation, full, 105
  Progressive muscle relaxation, letting go, 110
  Religious settings, introducing relaxation in, 331

Sampler, 343
Sampler, relaxation for children, 308
Scripting, client rationale, 235
Spiritual body energy exercise, 335
Yogaform stretching, for children, 301
Yogaform stretching, full, 85
Yogaform stretching, abbreviated, 92
Scripting, 233
    Advanced scripting, 248
    Combining and sequencing exercises, 248
    Deepening techniques, 248
        Cascading deepening imagery, 248
        Deepening countdowns, 252
        Deepening cycles, 255
        Deepening markers, 253
        Deepening metaphors, 251
        Deepening suggestions, 238
        Deepening transitions, 252
        Zoom imagery, 250
    Evaluating a script, 245
    Overview, 234
    Recording a script, 256
    Relaxation Scripting Workbook, 237, 238, 257
Segerstrom, S., 26
Selection of format, 77
Selflessness, 51
Self-stressing, 30
    Attentional processes, 39
    Breathing, 34
    Cognitive affective processes, 38
    Cognitive autonomic processes, 36
    Posture and position, 30
    Skeletal muscles, 33
    Summary, 44
Self-talk, 14, 38, 147
Seligman, M., 45
Simon, G., 311
Simonton, O., 12
Sleep and insomnia (Relaxation goal), 59
Sleep and sleepiness, 59, 220
Sohnle, S., 46
Smith, J., 5, 16, 29, 39, 46, 49, 50, 56, 63, 71, 80, 94, 95, 115, 135, 179, 185, 189, 199, 223, 228, 273, 316
Smith Relaxation Goals Inventory (SRGI), 205, 207, 268
Smith Relaxation Preferences Inventory (SRPI), 205, 206, 268
Smith Relaxation States Inventory—Alternative Brief Version (SRSIabv), 205, 213, 235, 268
Smith Relaxation States Inventory—Brief Version (SRSIbv), 205, 210, 235, 268
Smith Relaxation States Inventory—Revised (SRSIr), 205, 208, 268
Spence, S., 290
Spiritual body energy, 335
Spirituality, 53, 327
Spontaneous enjoyment (Relaxation goal), 67
Spot relaxation, 182, 184, 270
Supernatural, 327, 328
SRGI (Smith Relaxation Goals Inventory), 205, 207, 268
SRPI (Smith Relaxation Preferences Inventory), 205, 206, 268
SRSIabv (Smith Relaxation States Inventory—Alternative Brief Version), 205, 213, 235, 268
SRSIbv (Smith Relaxation States Inventory—Brief Version), 205, 210, 235, 268
SRSIr (Smith Relaxation States Inventory—Revised), 205, 208, 268
Steward, W., 45
Stress, 22
    Ergotrophic tuning, 25
    Illness, link to, 26
    Relaxation, 26, 61
    Self-stressing, 30
    Stress arousal, 22
Stress engine, 19; *see also* access skills
Stress management (Relaxation goal), 61
Stress relief, 47

Target Symptom Fact Sheet, 202
Taylor, S., 27
Taylor, H., 311
Thankful, loving (R-State), 53
Timeless, Boundless, Infinite, At Once
        (R-State), 35
Training requirements, 194
Transcendence, 54
Transcendent goals (Relaxation goal), 68
Trophotropic tuning, 28; *see also* ergo-
        tropic tuning
Troubleshooting, *see* Relaxation,
        Troubleshooting
Turk, D., 320

Vahia, N., 81
Van Dixhoorn, J., 114
Verbal report, assessing relaxation
        through, 205
Vipassana, 17; *see also* Meditation
Visser, A., 27
Voice, *see* Relaxation voice
Von Korff, M., 311
Vogt, O., 10

Wall, P., 314
Wallace, R., 28
Weinstein, M., 95
Wilson, K., 28
Wingall, A., 290
Wolkowitz, O., 27

Wolpe, J., 8
Woolfolk, R., 5, 63
Workbook, Relaxation Scripting, 237,
        238, 257
Workshops, 183, 184, 279
World tour, 182, 184, 268

Yoga, Yogaform stretching
    Children's version, 300
    Clients, appropriate, 81
    Compared with progressive muscle re-
        laxation, 33
    Demonstrating/Warmup, 83
    Duration, 81
    Effects, 31, 32, 79
    Enhancing, 85, 225
    Exercise placement, 80
    Pain management, 317
    Placement with other approaches, 80
    Portability, 81
    Problems, 84; *see also* Relaxation train-
        ing, Troubleshooting
    R-States, 80
    Rationale for clients, 83
    Script, 85
    Training instructions, 83
    Voice, 84

Zazen, 17
Zen meditation, 11
Zoom imagery, 250

Springer Publishing Company

Stress Management

A Comprehensive Handbook of Techniques and Strategies

Jonathan C. Smith, PhD

"...a state-of-the-art book...practical methods of treatment for those who need help managing stress in their lives...ideal as a graduate level text or resource..."
—**Martin Weinstein,** PhD, Associate Professor Roosevelt University, School of Psychology

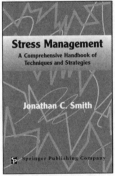

"...an invaluable tool in educating both undergraduate and graduate students, in psychology and across disciplines...clinicians and their clients would be hard-pressed to find a more useful text..."
—**Dena Traylor,** PsyD, Roosevelt University

This clinical manual contains detailed descriptions of tactics for training the user in the methods of relaxation, positive thinking, time management, and more. Features validated self-tests (normed on over 1000 individuals), and first-time-ever stress management motivations and irrational beliefs inventories.

Partial Contents:

Part I. Stress Basics • Stress Competency and the Smith Stress Management Skills Inventory • Stress Concepts, Exercises

Part II. The Four Pillars of Stress Management • Progressive Muscle Relaxation and Autogenic Training • Breathing and Stretching Exercises • Sense Imagery and Meditation • Relaxation, Centering, and Stress Management Exercises • Identifying Clear and Concrete Problem Cues • Stress Inoculation and Relapse Prevention

Part III. Interpersonal Skills: Relationships and Stress Management • Assertiveness, Exercises • Empathy and Assertive Coping • Goals and Priorities • Relaxation Beliefs, Active Coping Beliefs, and Philosophy of Life

2002   280pp   0-8261-4947-2   hardcover

11 West 42nd Street, New York, NY 10036-8002 • **Fax: 212-941-7842**
Order Toll-Free: 877-687-7476 • **Order On-line: www.springerpub.com**

Springer Publishing Company

Advances in the Treatment of Posttraumatic Stress Disorder

Cognitive-Behavioral Perspectives

Steven Taylor, PhD, Editor

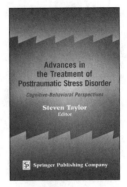

"Steve Taylor...one of the leaders...has brought together an international team of experts to provide us with the very latest in scientifically sound information on the nature and treatment of PTSD. This book is very worthy of the attention of all who work with psychologically traumatized people."

—from the Foreword by **G. Ron Norton,** PhD
Professor Emeritus Department of
Psychology, University of Winnipeg

Are behavioral and cognitive-behavioral therapies sufficiently broad in their effects on trauma-related psychopathology and related factors? This volume considers many of the complexities in treating PTSD, and emphasizes evidence-based approaches to treatment.

A useful resource for clinicians, trainees, as well as investigators doing research into the treatment of PTSD.

Partial Contents:

Part I: Introduction • Current Directions and Challenges in the Treatment of Posttraumatic Stress Disorder, *S. Taylor*

Part II: New Developments • Efficacy and Outcome Predictors for Three PTSD Treatments: Exposure Therapy, EMDR, and Relaxation Training, *S. Taylor*

• PTSD and the Social Support of the Interpersonal Environment: The Development of Social Cognitive Behavior Therapy, *N. Tarrier & A-L Humphreys*

Part III: Treating Special Populations and Problems • Effects of Cognitive-Behavioral Treatments for PTSD on Anger, *S.P. Cahill, S.A. Rauch, E.A. Hembree, & E.B. Foa*

• The Challenge of Treating PTSD in the Context of Chronic Pain, *J. Wald, S. Taylor, & I. C. Federoff*

Part IV: Perspectives on Future Directions • A Glass Half Empty or Half Full? Where We Are and Directions for Future Research in the Treatment of PTSD, *S.P. Cahill & E.B. Foa*

2004   336pp   0-8261-2047-4   Hard

11 West 42nd Street, New York, NY 10036-8002 • Fax: 212-941-7842
Order Toll-Free: 877-687-7476 • Order On-line: www.springerpub.com